Encyclopedia of Colorectal Cancer: Cell and Molecular Biology

Volume II

Encyclopedia of Colorectal Cancer: Cell and Molecular Biology Volume II

Edited by **Teresa Young**

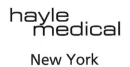

hayle
medical

New York

Published by Hayle Medical,
30 West, 37th Street, Suite 612,
New York, NY 10018, USA
www.haylemedical.com

Encyclopedia of Colorectal Cancer: Cell and Molecular Biology
Volume II
Edited by Teresa Young

International Standard Book Number: 978-1-63241-135-8 (Hardback)

Contents

Preface

Colorectal cancer is a major killer as the cases are increasing worldwide. The researches and studies in this field would be helpful to provide some efficient therapeutic measures for colorectal cancer. This book presents some basic steps being taken in order to understand and diagnose this disease. This book discusses the analysis done by scientists on the data and evidences available related to genes, infections related to colorectal cancer and other factors. A study of cell and molecular biology, examining the tumor microenvironment and the role of intestinal microbes and host-microbial interactions has been described in the book. This text is a valuable account of information for scientists, researchers and medical professionals engaged in this field.

Significant researches are present in this book. Intensive efforts have been employed by authors to make this book an outstanding discourse. This book contains the enlightening chapters which have been written on the basis of significant researches done by the experts.

Finally, I would also like to thank all the members involved in this book for being a team and meeting all the deadlines for the submission of their respective works. I would also like to thank my friends and family for being supportive in my efforts.

Editor

Cell and Molecular Biology

Molecular Traits of the Budding Colorectal Cancer Cells

Boye Schnack Nielsen
Bioneer A/S, Kogle Allé, Hørsholm,
Denmark

1. Introduction

The process of cancer cell metastasis is one of the latest steps in cancer progression that involves escape from the primary tumor through the vascular system to local lymph nodes and distant organs, recently reviewed by Chaffer and Weinberg (Chaffer & Weinberg, 2011). For a cancer cell to metastasize, it must escape the primary tumor by obtaining features that allows detachment from neoplastic epithelial structure, invasion through extracellular matrices, intravasation, survival in the blood circulation, extravasation, establishment or *homing* in a novel organ and local *de novo* proliferation. Colorectal cancers (CRC) comprise different subtypes and vary in the degree of differentiation as well as in the local invasion pattern in the tumor periphery. The invasion pattern is partly related to the metastatic ability of the tumor, and the invasion pattern can be fully discerned by microscopy analysis. Molecular characteristics related to the invasion pattern may help in the histopathological diagnosis to provide a prognostic perspective for the patient and potentially identify which patient would benefit from a certain therapy. For CRC, an invasion pattern related to the ability of cancer cells to form buds and focal single cell invasion into the neighboring stroma has obtained much attention. The invasive cancer cells are known as budding cancer cells and the budding phenomenon describes a morphological event, which is becoming better characterized at the molecular level. In this chapter, I will go through some of the molecular characteristics linked to the budding cancer cells and link the observations to the morphologic and molecular changes related to epithelial-to-mesenchymal transition (EMT) often assigned to locally disseminating cancer cells.

1.1 Identification of budding colorectal cancer cells

Two types of metastatic processes can be considered: active and passive. Passive metastasis occurs when cancer cells enter the vascular system, for example by being captured by disrupted vessels in the tumors, and subsequently being trapped in microvessels for example in the liver or lung, where the cancer cells initially proliferate within the vessel and later on disseminate into the parenchyma of the organ. Active metastasis is considered to involve a certain level of EMT in the primary tumor followed by invasion into the vascular system, extravasation by crossing the vascular wall and invasion into the new organ, and then reverting to an epithelial cancer cell capable of *de novo* proliferation and differentiation to form new tumors.

Budding cancer cells likely belong to the category of active metastasis process because their prevalence is directly linked to metastasis and is independent of the TNM classification (Nakamura et al, 2005; Okuyama et al, 2003; Prall et al, 2005; Ueno et al, 2002). Japanese histopathologists have many years tradition for evaluating growth and invasion patterns in CRC including addressing the clinical implications (Fujimori et al, 2009). A clinical significance of budding cancer cells was first described in colon cancers in 1993 by Hase *et al* (Hase et al, 1993). Hase et al (Hase et al, 1993) defined the budding cancer cells as "small clusters of undifferentiated cancer cells located ahead of the invasive front of the lesion".

Hase et al (Hase et al, 1993) evaluated the degree of budding cancer cells in normal hematoxylin and eosin (H&E) stained sections, an approach being widely used by others (Nakamura et al, 2005; Okuyama et al, 2003; Ueno et al, 2002). Because the budding cancer cells are often present in a dense desmoplastic or highly inflamed stroma and because budding cancer cells can acquire morphologically odd shapes (see below), a precise identification of budding cancer cells in H&E stained sections may not always be straight forward (Turner et al, 2007) at least for non-pathologists. Later studies have employed cytokeratin immunohistochemistry whereby budding cancer cells are much easier identified (Prall, 2007; Prall et al, 2005; Turner et al, 2007; Zlobec et al, 2010). The use of cytokeratin immunohistochemistry to detect cancer cell budding versus evaluation in H&E stained sections may lower the proportion of misclassified cases.

The prevalence of tumor cell budding varies strongly from tumor to tumor and Hase et al (Hase et al, 1993) stratified tumors into BD-1 (none or mild) and BD-2 (moderate or severe) based on the H&E stained sections. Prall et al (Prall et al, 2005) stratified tumors into low and high budding based on sections immunohistochemically stained for cytokeratins and counted all cytokeratin-positive cancer cell clusters with less than 5 nuclei. Hase et al (Hase et al, 1993) classified approximately 25% of all CRC analyzed as BD-2 and Prall et al (Prall et al, 2005) classified approximately 30% as high level budding.

Cancer cell budding as it is observed in colon and rectal adenocarcinomas should not be confused with the diffuse growth pattern, which is common in other gastrointestinal cancers and in contrast to tumors with a solid (or expanding) growth pattern. CRC showing a diffuse growth pattern are low differentiated neoplasms and do not show signs of tubular or glandular formations. Therefore quantitative estimation of cancer cell budding even done using cytokeratin immunohistochemistry should be done with some caution.

The degree of cancer cell budding as stratified into groups with none, mild, moderate and strong budding, or less or more than 5 cells in a cluster, indicate that cancer cell budding is not an "all or none" phenomenon, but reflects gradual differences. Nonetheless, both studies (Hase et al, 1993; Prall et al, 2005) showed that tumors with the highest level of budding significantly more often linked to lymph node metastasis than tumors with a low level of budding. The highest level of budding was, not surprisingly, seen in patients with the poorest survival rate, however, cancer biology reflects individual heterogeneity and in fact, some tumors with low budding also show metastatic events (Hase et al, 1993; Prall et al, 2005; Tanaka et al, 2003; Ueno et al, 2002).

1.2 Histo-morphological characterization

One of the morphological features of the budding cancer cells in CRC is their characteristics of dedifferentiation and acquisition of odd shapes as described at the ultra-structural level by Gabbert et al in 1985 (Gabbert et al, 1985). These authors studied DMH-induced colon cancers in rats and found that poorly differentiated tumors, which showed frequency of lymph vessel invasion, also had isolated cancer cells along the invasive front. Gabbert et al (Gabbert et al, 1985) states about the cancer cells located ahead of the invasive front that "Their nuclei are very large and at their cell surface show no signs of differentiation such as formation of microvilli or formation of a basement membrane are discernible." Thus the cellular characteristics of isolated cancer cells suggested general dedifferentiation compared to the cancer cells placed within the adjacent glandular structures. In addition, the isolated cancer cells at the invasive front showed overt cell shape: "The cell shape of more or less isolated tumor cells at the foremost invasion front is extremely variable ... ranging from a round or oval to a sand glass-like." These observations are consistent with the budding cancer cells in human CRC identified both in H&E stained sections as well as cytokeratin immuno-peroxidase stained sections, see for example the studies by Prall and Turner et al (Prall, 2007; Prall et al, 2005; Turner et al, 2007). According to the histological characteristitcs of the budding CRC cells at the invasive front, the stepwise process of budding-directed growth can be divided into the following steps 1) the budding cancer cells detach from the glandular structures, 2) morphologically change cell shape and 3) invade a short distance, say up to 400μm, through the adjacent tumor-associated stroma and 4) settle and 5) found novel glandular structures. Budding CRC cells are rarely seen in the central areas of the tumors, suggesting that the local environment, the stroma constituting the tumor periphery, is dictating the budding process together with the cancer cells. Interestingly, the morphological characteristics of dedifferentiation and dynamic change in cell shape are consistent with characteristics of cells undergoing EMT as described for cultured cells (Kirkland, 2009; Thuault et al, 2006).

Together with the findings that the prevalence of budding cancer cells is linked to more metastatic cancers, strongly suggests that the budding cancer cells also possess cancer stem cell activity. Thus the budding CRC cells possess all canonical requirements for actively metastasizing cancer cells, including the abilities to undergo EMT and the ability of self-renewal. The stepwise process of the budding cancer cell requires significant molecular changes of the cell: for detachment from neoplastic epithelium, dedifferentiation, EMT, cell migration and invasion, and progenitor activity for *de novo* proliferation. Considering that budding CRC cells undergo such a dramatic transient program, probably within a relatively short time frame, the budding CRC cells as an entire cell population constitute a heterogeneous group of cancer cells that possess a strongly modulating molecular profile. In the following I will go through some of the molecular characteristics reported for the budding CRC cells, first cell surface associated proteins and thereafter intracellular molecules. The molecular characteristics involve proteins that participate in regulating differentiation, transcription, translation, cell migration, cell-cell interactions, and adhesion.

2. Laminin-γ2 (Ln-γ2)

The mRNA encoding the Ln-γ2 chain is the first described molecular marker of the budding CRC cells (Pyke et al, 1994). Pyke et al (Pyke et al, 1994) found Ln-γ2 mRNA positive cancer cells in all of 16 colon cancers varying in the presence of positive cells. In a later report, Pyke et al (Pyke et al, 1995) confirmed that the mRNA expression observed in budding colon cancer cells is followed by protein expression in the same cells using a Ln-γ2 specific antibody. Sordat et al (Sordat et al, 1998) reported similar observations in colon cancers using other Ln-γ2 antibody preparations. Laminins are a group of extracellular glycoproteins being important constituents of basement membrane. They are heterotrimers composed of α, β and γ chains of which there are 5, 4 and 3 isoforms, respectively. The currently used systematic nomenclature defines the composition of a laminin heterotrimers (Aumailley et al, 2005), for example laminin-111 is composed of α1, β1 and γ1 chains and has replaced the earlier used name laminin-1, the most predominant laminin in basement membrane.

The Ln-γ2 chain is only present in the laminin-332 variant, previously known as laminin-5 (Guess & Quaranta, 2009). Laminin-332 links the basement membrane via integrins to hemidesmosomes and thereby stabilizes the polarized positioning of epithelial cell to the basement membrane. Laminins are generally secreted from cells as fully composed heterotrimers, Ln-γ2 being the only exception (Guess & Quaranta, 2009). Ln-γ2 can be secreted as monomer or in complex with the Ln-β3 chain (Guess & Quaranta, 2009) and may have an important significance during budding in CRC (Guess et al, 2009). Pyke et al (Pyke et al, 1995) found Ln-γ2 within the cytoplasm of the budding colon cancer cells and only in rare cases observed basement membrane associated Ln-γ2 immunoreactivity. Sordat et al (Sordat et al, 1998) in contrast found prominent Ln-γ2 immunoreactivity both in the cytoplasm of budding CRC cells and in basement membrane along differentiated tumor cell islands. Today, several monoclonal antibodies against Ln-γ2 are commercially available, some recognize both cytoplasmic and basement membrane associated Ln-γ2, and others are specific for the cytoplasmic precursor form (Hansen et al, 2008; Lindberg et al, 2006). Using Ln-γ2 as marker for budding CRC cells, the antibody employed should therefore be chosen with some consideration.

An interesting finding reported by Sordat et al (Sordat et al, 1998), is that budding cancer cells in addition to express Ln-γ2 also express the Ln-β3 chain, but only at a low level express the Ln-α3 chain. These observations suggest that the secreted Ln-γ2 monomer and Ln-β3-γ2 heterodimer may not function by direct integration into the basement membrane. Other functions have in contrast been found for the secreted Ln-γ2 and Ln-β3 chains. Cell surface directed proteolyic activity performed by matrix metalloproteinase (MMP)-2 (Giannelli et al, 1997) and membrane type-1 (MT1)-MMP (Koshikawa et al, 2000) generates fragments of the Ln-γ2 chain constituting epithelial growth factor (EGF)-like domains that stimulates cell motility. In addition, a cleavage product of Ln-β3 chain generated by MT1-MMP promotes cell migration (Udayakumar et al, 2003). The observations taken together suggest that Ln-γ2 and Ln-β3 chains are contributing to the migratory processes of the budding CRC cells.

In clinical studies, the level of tumor budding in CRC correlated with the level of Ln-γ2 positive budding cells (Shinto et al, 2005). Shinto et al (Shinto et al, 2005) also reported that high-grade Ln-γ2 expression was an independent prognostic indicator, and Aoki et al (Aoki et al, 2002) reported a significant association with synchronous liver metastases. Today, Ln-γ2 expression is considered a strong and potentially clinically applicable prognostic marker that reflects the level of cancer cell budding not only in CRC but also in other cancer types including bladder, esophageal and oral cancer (Guess & Quaranta, 2009).

3. Urokinase Plasminogen Activator Receptor (uPAR)

uPAR (CD87) is a 3-domain highly glycosylated, glycolipid anchored protein. uPAR is a specific high affinity binding receptor for (pro-)uPA, but also binds a number of other proteins in the extracellular matrix, in particular vitronectin (Eden et al, 2011; Gardsvoll & Ploug, 2007). The glycosyl-phosphatidylinositol (GPI) moiety of uPAR attaches the protein to the outer lipid layer of the cell membrane and allows uPAR to move laterally on cell surfaces and hence rapidly concentrate at focal sites where it mediates its uPA-directed activity and its interaction with vitronectin to the extracellular matrix. Active plasmin is generated from circulating plasminogen on the cell surfaces by a cascade mechanism involving plasmin-mediated conversion of pro-uPA to active uPA. uPA directed plasminogen activation is strongly enhanced after binding of uPA to uPAR on the cell surface (Ploug, 2003; Romer et al, 2004).

The active plasmin enzymatically cleaves or degrades fibrin and fibronectin deposited in the extracellular matrix (ECM), laminins, including the Ln-β3 chain (Goldfinger et al, 1998), L1CAM described below (Mechtersheimer et al, 2001), and activates other matrix degrading protease including MMPs. Through activation of pro-MMPs, MMP-3 (stromelysin-1), MMP-9 (gelatinase-B), MMP-13 (collagenase-3) and MMP-2 (Hald et al, 2011; Juncker-Jensen & Lund, 2011; Monea et al, 2002; Suzuki et al, 2007), plasmin may also mediate degradation of other ECM components including fibrillar collagens. In addition, plasmin activates growth factors like TGF-β (Odekon et al, 1994). Active TGF-β can transform fibroblasts into myofibroblasts (Ronnov-Jessen & Petersen, 1993) and initiate the EMT process in mammary epithelial cells (Fuxe et al, 2010; Thuault et al, 2006). Thus acceleration of the plasminogen activation cascade pathway may elevate the pericellular proteolytic activity and cause dramatic changes in cellular phenotypes.

uPAR was described in budding CRC cells first time in 1994 identified both at the mRNA and protein level (Pyke et al, 1995). Direct comparison with Ln-γ2 expression indicated a strong overlap with Ln-γ2 mRNA (Pyke et al, 1995). Later studies have shown co-expression of uPAR and Ln-γ2 in double immunofluorescence analyses in budding CRC cells (Illemann et al, 2009). uPAR is highly expressed at the invasive front of most CRC not only in budding cancer cells, but also in the complex stromal environment constituting inflammatory cells and myofibroblasts. Activated macrophages located at the invasive front of CRC express high levels of uPAR on the cell surface, hampering an easy discrimination between uPAR-positive budding cancer cells and macrophages. Therefore, to unambiguously identify uPAR-positive budding CRC cells, combining antibodies against uPAR and the epithelial marker cytokeratin (or Ln-γ2) in a double immunofluorescence analysis, would be necessary (Illemann et al, 2009; Romer et al, 2004). uPA mRNA is also expressed in the budding CRC cells (Illemann et al, 2009) indicating that uPAR may function directly through mediation of uPA-directed activities.

In normal colon tissue, uPAR is expressed in a group of differentiated epithelial cells located at the luminal edge of the villi. It has been suggested that uPAR on these cells serve to promote detachment of terminally differentiated colonocytes to be shedded into the colon lumen (Pyke et al, 1994). One may speculate that detachment of budding CRC cells from the main neoplastic glandular structures may mimic the shedding of terminally differentiated cells. In the case of cancer invasion the cancer cells are shed into the tumor stroma. However, this hypothesis does not corroborate with the fact that budding CRC cells show characteristics of dedifferentiation. Nevertheless, this is an interesting interpretation and the invasion of budding CRC cells remain an abnormal process.

Tissue extracts from colon cancers contain highly elevated levels of uPAR compared to the normal tissue, and the high uPAR levels are associated with adverse outcome. uPAR levels were found to constitute an independent prognostic parameter, importantly being independent of progression stage (Ganesh et al, 1994). A soluble form of uPAR, generated after enzymatic cleavage by uPA or plasmin (Hoyer-Hansen et al, 1997), can be measured in blood, and studies of plasma samples from colon cancer patients substantiate the prognostic significance of uPAR (Stephens et al, 1999; Thurison et al, 2010). As noted above, several different cell types in colon cancers express uPAR, and therefore the prognostic value of uPAR cannot be ascribed solely to the uPAR-positive budding CRC cells. However, in adenocarcinomas, macrophages are by far the predominant uPAR expressing cell type, and therefore most likely account for the elevated levels of uPAR in tumor tissue extracts and in the blood from the cancer patients (Illemann et al, 2009; Romer et al, 2004). uPAR expressing budding cancer cells may nevertheless also contribute to the malignant stage of CRC. uPAR positive cancer cells likely represent a particular malignant cell population since gastric cancer patients with poor prognosis associated with micro-metastatic disease more frequently had uPAR positive cancer cells identified in the bone marrow (Heiss et al, 2002), and uPAR is indeed expressed on invasive cancer cells in gastric cancer (Alpizar-Alpizar et al, 2010).

4. L1 Cell Adhesion Molecule (L1CAM)

L1CAM (L1, CD171) is one of four single-pass trans-membrane proteins forming the group of L1CAM. L1 was first described in 1984 as a neural cell adhesion molecule distinct from the closely related N-CAM group of proteins (Faissner et al, 1984). The other three members of the L1CAM family are NrCAM, CHL1 and neurofascin. All four genes are thoroughly characterized and highly expressed in the nervous system (Chen & Zhou, 2010). The L1CAMs contain 6 immunoglobulin-like motifs and 4 or 5 fibronectin type III repeats. The Cytoplasmic domain allows binding to cytoskeletal ankyrin and ERM proteins (ezrin-radixin-moesin) that associates with actin filaments (Bretscher et al, 2002). L1 is involved in cell-cell adhesion by homophilic interactions, cell-ECM interactions and cell surface interactions by binding integrins and can directly mediate cytoskeletal changes and signal transduction through its cytoplasmic domain (Chen & Zhou, 2010; Kadmon & Altevogt, 1997; Schmid & Maness, 2008). L1 is highly expressed in normal and diseased brain, and plays a critical role for development and organization of neuronal cell groups (Demyanenko et al, 2001; Sakurai et al, 2001). L1 has functions overlapping with NrCAM identified in double-deficient mice that show postnatal lethality in contrast to the corresponding single deficient mice (Sakurai et al, 2001). L1 has been reported to mediate cell adhesion and transendothelial migration also of dendritic cells (Maddaluno et al, 2009).

Expression of L1 in budding CRC cells has been shown both at the protein (Gavert et al, 2005; Kajiwara et al, 2011) and the mRNA level (Kajiwara et al, 2011). Gavert et al (Gavert et al, 2005) found L1 positive budding cancer cells in 68% of 19 colon cancer cases studied. Kajiwara et al (Kajiwara et al, 2011) studied 275 cases of CRC and also found L1 expression at the invasive front. Furthermore the authors showed that the L1 expression increased according to the grade of tumor budding and that L1 expression was correlated with nodal involvement both at the protein and mRNA level. In normal colon mucosa, L1 is expressed on sporadic intramucosal nerve axons and L1 positive enteric nerve axons were found in the deeper layers of the bowel wall (Gavert et al, 2005). In fact, the authors also noted that L1-positive colon cancer cells invaded along L1 positive nerve axons, and suggested that L1-mediated adhesive interactions between the two cell populations may facilitate the invasion of cancer cells. In this connection, it is curious that also uPAR can be found in enteric nerve bundles (Laerum et al, 2008). It is also interesting to note that L1 has been detected in human and murine myeloid and lymphoid cells (Ebeling et al, 1996; Kowitz et al, 1992) and that no L1 immunoreactivity has been reported in tumor stroma of the CRC. Whether the level of L1 in these cells is below the detection limit, is lost by proteolytic shedding, transcriptional or translational downregulation (Hubbe et al, 1993) remains to be clarified.

Proteolytic shedding of the L1 ectodomain has been reported to be performed by the disintegrin and metalloproteinases (ADAM) ADAM10 (Gutwein et al, 2003; Maretzky et al, 2005; Mechtersheimer et al, 2001), ADAM17 (Maretzky et al, 2005), and plasmin (Mechtersheimer et al, 2001). Shedding of the L1 ectodomain will prevent cell-cell interactions and binding interactions with other cell surface proteins and matrix components affecting the biochemical functions of the protein. Cleavage of L1 by ADAM10 releases an approximately 200kDa L1 fragment that can promote cell migration (Gutwein et al, 2003; Maretzky et al, 2005; Mechtersheimer et al, 2001). Similar activity was reported for the plasmin released L1 fragment (Mechtersheimer et al, 2001). In this connection it is important to note that ADAM10 immunoreactivity has been reported to be co-expressed in budding CRC cells (Gavert et al, 2005), and that cleavage can occur to an extent that a soluble L1 fragment can be measured in serum from cancer patients (Fogel et al, 2003). L1 expression in budding CRC cells may therefore be involved in at least 3 different processes during CRC cell budding: detachment from the differentiated neoplastic glandular structures, cell-cell interactions with L1-positive nerve axons or dendritic cells as well as in the contribution to CRC cell migration upon extracellular enzymatic processing.

5. Matrix Metalloproteinase 7 (MMP-7)

A number of other genes have been found to be focally expressed in the budding colon cancer cells. I have already mentioned some of the MMPs in connection with Ln-γ2 processing and plasmin-activated MMPs. MMP-7 (matrilysin-1) belongs to the group of matrix metalloproteinases (MMPs) (Das et al, 2003; Folgueras et al, 2004), which are zinc dependent endopeptidases known for their ability to cleave several ECM proteins. The activity of MMPs is regulated at the level of pro-MMP conversion and blocking by specific tissue inhibitors of metalloproteinases (TIMP) of which 4 are known (Nagase et al, 2006). MMP-7 can digest several ECM proteins including elastin, collagen IV and vitronectin (Ii et al, 2006). In addition, MMP7 has been shown to play important roles in the regulation of a variety of biochemical processes, such as the activation of MMP-2 and MMP-9 and shedding of Fas-ligand, pro-tumor necrosis factor-α, and E-cadherin (Curino et al, 2004; Ii et al, 2006; Nagase et al, 2006). MMP-7 itself is activated by other endoproteinases including plasmin and trypsin. MMP-7 was recently shown to bind and cleave the Ln-β3 chain. The cleaved Ln-β3 fragments was found to mediate cell migration (Remy et al, 2006). MMP-7 immunoreactivity has been reported in budding CRC cancer cells (Kurokawa et al, 2005; Masaki et al, 2001) and was found to co-localize with laminin-5 and Ln-β3 chain in human xenografted colon tumors (Remy et al, 2006). In the relatively small prognostic study by Masaki et al (Masaki et al, 2001), including 38 patients with early CRC, scoring the MMP-7 immunoreactive budding cancer cells was linked to distant metastasis and adverse outcome. However, MMP-7 immunoreactivity was seen in less than half of the cases with moderate to severe budding as determined on H&E stained sections, indicating that MMP-7 is not consistently expressed in budding CRC. In a study of 494 CRC cases, MMP-7 mRNA was found to be an independent risk factor predicting nodal metastasis (Kurokawa et al, 2005). In the context of budding CRC cells, the ability of MMP-7 to shed E-cadherin and cleave the Ln-β3 chain into a motility stimulating fragment suggest that MMP-7 takes part in the early steps involving detachment from the glandular structures and mobilizing cancer cell migration.

6. Membrane Type-1 Matrix Metalloproteinase (MT1-MMP)

MT1-MMP (MMP-14) immunoreactivity has also been demonstrated in budding CRC cells (Hlubek et al, 2004). MT1-MMP belongs to the group of membrane-bound MMPs and is a trans-membrane protein capable of cleaving fibrillar collagen. This MMP is essential for normal development (Holmbeck et al, 1999). MT1-MMP binds extracellular MMP-2 and TIMP-2 into a ternary complex that is important for the regulation of enzymatic activity on the cell surface (Sato & Takino, 2010; Strongin, 2010). The active enzyme can also cleave a number of other membrane-associated proteins including pro-tumor necrosis factor-α and CD44 (Folgueras et al, 2004). Expression of MT1-MMP mRNA is prominent in colon cancer associated stroma (Okada et al, 1995). As also noted above for evaluation of uPAR expression, strong stromal MT1-MMP expression in the invasive front area will prevent unambiguous identification of the protein in budding cancer cells. Expression of MT1-MMP on the surface of budding CRC cells would allow significant surface associated proteolysis either directly or through activation of MMP-2, which together with TIMP-2 would be provided by adjacent stromal cells (Holten-Andersen et al, 2005; Okada et al, 1995; Poulsom et al, 1992). As already mentioned, MT1-MMP can cleave Ln-γ2 alone or in cooperation with MMP-2, which results in a Ln-γ2 fragment with capacity to stimulate migration (Koshikawa et al, 2005; Koshikawa et al, 2004). More immunohistochemical studies are needed to better clarify the expression patterns of MT1-MMP in budding CRC cells.

The activities of the above mentioned proteins Ln-γ2, uPAR, L1, MMP-7 and MT1-MMP are all taking place on the cell surface and pericellular matrix. The following molecules will be related to intracellular acitivities.

7. β-catenin (Wnt pathway)

β-catenin is an important intracellular protein to consider in the characterization of budding CRC cells. Nuclear β-catenin activates transcription of a number of genes including those encoding Ln-γ2, uPAR and MMP-7 (Brabletz et al, 2004; Crawford et al, 1999; Hlubek et al, 2001; Mann et al, 1999). β-catenin is a protein that binds the cytoplasmic domain of E-cadherin and by concomitantly binding actin filaments contributes to maintain the cytoskeleton and the epithelial integrity. The intracellular localization of β-catenin is linked to the status of Wnt activity directed through the trans-membrane receptor Frizzled. Cellular activation by Wnt cause trans-localization of β-catenin to the nuclei, which through binding to transcription factors, affects transcription. β-catenin is expressed both in the differentiated glandular structures and in the budding CRC cells, but the localization changes from cytoplasmic to nuclear. In the case of budding CRC cells, β-catenin is seen in the nuclei (Brabletz et al, 2001; Brabletz et al, 2004; Gavert et al, 2005; Gavert et al, 2011; Hlubek et al, 2001; Jass et al, 2003). Translocation of β-catenin to the nuclei has been used as a reference marker for CRC cell budding to show co-expression of Ln-γ2 (Hlubek et al, 2001), L1 (Gavert et al, 2011), and disruption of E-cadherin (Brabletz et al, 2001). The EMT process and stem cell characteristics has been associated with the activity of β-catenin in cooperation with TGF-β (Brabletz et al, 2005; Fuxe et al, 2010). For a further discussion on signal transduction in budding CRC cells I suggest to consult the review by Prall (Prall, 2007).

8. Hepatocyte growth factor activator inhibitor type 2-Related Small Peptide (H2RSP)

An interesting novel protein identified to be specifically up-regulated in connection with CRC cell budding is hepatocyte growth factor activator inhibitor type 2-related small peptide (H2RSP) (Uchiyama et al, 2007). The H2RSP gene was first described in 2001 by Itoh et al (Itoh et al, 2001), who observed H2RSP expression in tissues obtained from the gastrointestinal tract. H2RSP protein, which is identical to immortalization-upregulated protein (IMUP-1), is a small protein constituting 106 amino acids. Its interaction partner(s) and function(s) remains to be established. An interaction with single stranded G-rich DNA probably via a lysine-rich domain of the protein was discussed to be involved in nuclear translocation (Uchiyama et al, 2007). Uchiyama et al (Uchiyama et al, 2007) found by immunohistochemistry that H2RSP was located in the cytoplasm of normal un-differentiated epithelial cells in the colon, but found a change in localization to the nuclei in the differentiated epithelial cells. The authors suggested that H2RSP is involved in the transition process from the proliferation phase to terminal differentiation of intestinal epithelium. Looking at colon tumors, they found H2RSP immunoreactivity to be fully lost in the central differentiated tumor areas, but focally upregulated in the invasive front, including in budding CRC cells. In these cells, the H2RSP staining was located in the cytoplasm. The expression of H2RSP coincided with nuclear localization of β-catenin, focal co-expression of p16 and focal loss of proliferation marker Ki67. Thus, H2RSP, as confined to the epithelial cell population, is an interesting marker of budding CRC indicating a stage of dedifferentiation and growth arrest. A potential function in the related hepatocyte growth factor/scatter factor signaling pathway through Met receptor, which is taking place at the cell surface, seems unlikely so far.

9. microRNA-21 (miR-21)

MicroRNAs (miRNA) constitute a group of short, 18-23 base-pair long, non-coding RNAs. MiRNAs are processed from precursor RNA transcripts into mature active forms by a mechanism only partially understood. A generally accepted sequence of steps for the biochemical processing of precursor miRNA to the mature forms is known as the "linear" canonical pathway (Winter et al, 2009). MiRNAs have been found to play particular important roles in cell differentiation by negatively regulating translation (Calin & Croce, 2009; Iorio & Croce, 2009; Lim et al, 2005; Liu & Olson, 2010). miRNAs bind to specific 3'UTR sequences of mRNAs and thereby prevent efficient translation or mediate degradation of target mRNAs. For identification of miRNAs in tissue sections, *in situ* hybridization is an indispensable technique, which different from mRNA *in situ* hybridization cannot be replaced by immunohistochemistry. Specific detection of miRNA *in situ* therefore sets high requirements to the detection probes. Here LNA:DNA chimeric oligo probes have shown to fulfill at least some of the requirement for sufficient specificity and sensitivity (Jorgensen et al, 2010; Kloosterman et al, 2006). In an *in situ* hybridization study of miR-21 expression in stage II CRC, expression of miR-21 was seen in some budding CRC cell located at the invasive front of the tumors (Nielsen et al, 2011). A clear identification and quantitative estimation of the miR-21 positive budding cancer cells was however confounded by high miR-21 signal also in the tumor stroma. Therefore further studies are needed to better address the association of miR-21 to budding CRC cells, including double fluorescence labeling as also discussed above for uPAR. In this case, *in situ* hybridization and immunohistochemistry should be combined as exemplified by Sempere et al (Sempere et al, 2010), who applied this technology in routinely processed clinical paraffin samples.

miR-21 is highly upregulated in CRC compared to normal colon tissue (Nielsen et al, 2011; Schetter et al, 2008) and high expression is linked to adverse outcome in stage II CRC (Nielsen et al, 2011; Schetter et al, 2008). The mechanisms of action of miR-21 in budding cancer cells and in cancer progression in general are unclear. In mice lacking miR-21 (Ma et al, 2011) the number of chemically induced skin tumors was significantly lower than in wild type mice. In keratinocytes from the miR-21 deficient mice, increased expression of SPRY1, PTEN and PDCD4 was found, which is consistent with findings of miR-21 target genes in different human cell lines: *Spry1* in cardiac fibroblasts (Thum et al, 2008), the tumor suppressor *Pten* in hepatocytes and cardiac fibroblasts (Meng et al, 2007; Roy et al, 2009), and the tumor suppressor *Pdcd4* in a variety of cell lines (Asangani et al, 2008; Talotta et al, 2009). In budding CRC cells, miR-21 may suppress the expression level of PTEN and PDCD4 and thereby prevent cell death. miR-21 has also been attributed a central role in TGF-β induced EMT (Zavadil et al, 2007). Whether these regulatory events occur at the invasive front and in budding cancer cells remain to be established.

10. p16, Ki67 and cdx2

In connection with the studies mentioned above a couple of other proteins have been reported to focally change expression pattern in the budding CRC cells. These include p16 (Jass et al, 2003; Uchiyama et al, 2007) and cdx2 (Brabletz et al, 2004). The tumor suppressor p16 plays an important role in regulation of the cell cycle through interaction with p53 and as an inhibitor of cyclin dependent kinase 4 (CDK4). Both Uchiyama et al (Uchiyama et al, 2007) and Jass et al (Jass et al, 2003) noted that p16 was strongly expressed as a cytoplasmic immunoreactivity in the budding CRC cells. The increased expression may block translocation of CDK4 to the nuclei and thereby increase cyclin D1 levels and reduce proliferation (Jass et al, 2003). In fact, the proliferation marker Ki67 is lost in budding CRC cells (Brabletz et al, 2001; Uchiyama et al, 2007). The homeobox *Cdx2* encodes an intestine-specific transcription factor and is considered a tumor suppressor. Cdx2 immunoreactivity was absent in budding CRC cells in contrast to nuclei-related staining in the more differentiated tumor areas (Brabletz et al, 2004). It is intriguing that p16 and Cdx2, as so-called tumor suppressors, present themselves differently with respect to their presence in these highly malignant cells.

Although positive markers of the budding CRC cells provide clues to a mechanistic interpretation, loss of expression or intracellular translocation may provide significant help to characterize the budding process as well. As a final comment, I would like to suggest including the following 3 proteins as reference markers for the dedifferentiated budding CRC cells: Ln-γ2 giving a positive reaction in the cytoplasm, β-catenin giving a positive reaction in the nuclei, and Ki67 being negative (in contrast to the neighboring cancer cells). These markers will complement each other sufficiently as a reference profile and well-characterized antibodies are commercially available and applicable in paraffin embedded specimens.

11. Conclusion

A successful budding CRC cell encounters dramatic challenges during the short local expedition: dedifferentiation and detachment from the established differentiated glandular structure, migration through a foreign stromal tissue rich in inflammatory cells and desmoplastic cells, settlement in the new stromal environment and re-initiation of its own proliferation program. In this chapter I have reviewed current literature in order to compile the molecular traits linked to these cells and put the proteins' function into the budding processes. I propose that budding-initiating factors, such as TGF-β and Wnts, derived from in the stromal environment in the tumor periphery, and that the factors are received by cancer cells with progenitor capacity and which are able to address an activation program involving β-catenin mediated dedifferentiation and migration. From the compiled data, the following sequence of steps could be anticipated: increased levels of ECM degrading proteases, mediated by uPAR/uPA and MT1-MMP/MMP2, and MMP7 taking care of E-cadherin processing. The proliferation program is halted. This could be followed by a discrete EMT program, which transiently changes the morphology of the cells and allows detachment and budding. Upregulation and secretion of Ln-β3 and Ln-γ2 and subsequent extracellular processing will result in strongly motility-inducing fragments that allow migration through the stromal tissue. At the same time L1 is introduced changing the preferred cellular interaction partners to neuronal axons and dendritic cells as well as introducing yet other migration stimulating factors: the ADAM10 and plasmin processed L1 ectodoamins. Budding cancer cells invade as distant as possible into the stroma. One mechanism that could make the invasive cells stop and settle in the stromal environment could be a change in balance between active proteases and protease inhibitors, which may be shifted in favor of the inhibitors. Both PAI-1 and TIMPs are highly expressed in stromal cells at the invasive front (Holten-Andersen et al, 2005; Illemann et al, 2004; Poulsom et al, 1992). Increased protease inhibitor levels would prevent the formation of migration stimulating laminin fragments and also the surface associated proteases needed for invasion through the ECM. After settlement the excess laminins will be deposited and may contribute to form a loose basement membrane for the cancer cell to stick to and polarize, L1 will again be replaced by E-cadherin and proliferation and differentiation programs are reinitiated.

12. References

Alpizar-Alpizar, W., Nielsen, B. S., Sierra, R., Illemann, M., Ramirez, J. A., Arias, A., Duran, S., Skarstein, A., Ovrebo, K., Lund, L. R. & Laerum, O. D. (2010). Urokinase plasminogen activator receptor is expressed in invasive cells in gastric carcinomas from high- and low-risk countries. *Int. J. Cancer*, Vol. 126, No. 2, pp. 405-415.

Aoki, S., Nakanishi, Y., Akimoto, S., Moriya, Y., Yoshimura, K., Kitajima, M., Sakamoto, M. & Hirohashi, S.   (2002). Prognostic significance of laminin-5 gamma2 chain expression in colorectal carcinoma: immunohistochemical analysis of 103 cases. *Dis. Colon Rectum*, Vol. 45, No. 11, pp. 1520-1527.

Asangani, I. A., Rasheed, S. A., Nikolova, D. A., Leupold, J. H., Colburn, N. H., Post, S. & Allgayer, H.   (2008). MicroRNA-21 (miR-21) post-transcriptionally downregulates tumor suppressor Pdcd4 and stimulates invasion, intravasation and metastasis in colorectal cancer. *Oncogene*, Vol. 27, No. 15, pp. 2128-2136.

Aumailley, M., Bruckner-Tuderman, L., Carter, W. G., Deutzmann, R., Edgar, D., Ekblom, P., Engel, J., Engvall, E., Hohenester, E., Jones, J. C., Kleinman, H. K., Marinkovich, M. P., Martin, G. R., Mayer, U., Meneguzzi, G., Miner, J. H., Miyazaki, K., Patarroyo, M., Paulsson, M., Quaranta, V., Sanes, J. R., Sasaki, T., Sekiguchi, K., Sorokin, L. M., Talts, J. F., Tryggvason, K., Uitto, J., Virtanen, I., von der, M. K., Wewer, U. M., Yamada, Y. & Yurchenco, P. D.   (2005). A simplified laminin nomenclature. *Matrix Biol.*, Vol. 24, No. 5, pp. 326-332.

Brabletz, T., Hlubek, F., Spaderna, S., Schmalhofer, O., Hiendlmeyer, E., Jung, A. & Kirchner, T.   (2005). Invasion and metastasis in colorectal cancer: epithelial-mesenchymal transition, mesenchymal-epithelial transition, stem cells and beta-catenin. *Cells Tissues. Organs*, Vol. 179, No. 1-2, pp. 56-65.

Brabletz, T., Jung, A., Reu, S., Porzner, M., Hlubek, F., Kunz-Schughart, L. A., Knuechel, R. & Kirchner, T.   (2001). Variable beta-catenin expression in colorectal cancers indicates tumor progression driven by the tumor environment. *Proc. Natl. Acad. Sci. U. S. A*, Vol. 98, No. 18, pp. 10356-10361.

Brabletz, T., Spaderna, S., Kolb, J., Hlubek, F., Faller, G., Bruns, C. J., Jung, A., Nentwich, J., Duluc, I., Domon-Dell, C., Kirchner, T. & Freund, J. N.   (2004). Down-regulation of the homeodomain factor Cdx2 in colorectal cancer by collagen type I: an active role for the tumor environment in malignant tumor progression. *Cancer Res.*, Vol. 64, No. 19, pp. 6973-6977.

Bretscher, A., Edwards, K. & Fehon, R. G.   (2002). ERM proteins and merlin: integrators at the cell cortex. *Nat. Rev. Mol. Cell Biol.*, Vol. 3, No. 8, pp. 586-599.

Calin, G. A. & Croce, C. M.   (2009). Chronic lymphocytic leukemia: interplay between noncoding RNAs and protein-coding genes. *Blood*, Vol. 114, No. 23, pp. 4761-4770.

Chaffer, C. L. & Weinberg, R. A.   (2011). A perspective on cancer cell metastasis. *Science*, Vol. 331, No. 6024, pp. 1559-1564.

Chen, L. & Zhou, S.   (2010). "CRASH"ing with the worm: insights into L1CAM functions and mechanisms. *Dev. Dyn.*, Vol. 239, No. 5, pp. 1490-1501.

Crawford, H. C., Fingleton, B. M., Rudolph-Owen, L. A., Goss, K. J., Rubinfeld, B., Polakis, P. & Matrisian, L. M.   (1999). The metalloproteinase matrilysin is a target of beta-catenin transactivation in intestinal tumors. *Oncogene*, Vol. 18, No. 18, pp. 2883-2891.

Curino, A., Patel, V., Nielsen, B. S., Iskander, A. J., Ensley, J. F., Yoo, G. H., Holsinger, F. C., Myers, J. N., El-Nagaar, A., Kellman, R. M., Shillitoe, E. J., Molinolo, A. A., Gutkind, J. S. & Bugge, T. H.   (2004). Detection of plasminogen activators in oral cancer by laser capture microdissection combined with zymography. *Oral Oncol.*, Vol. 40, No. 10, pp. 1026-1032.

Das, S., Mandal, M., Chakraborti, T., Mandal, A. & Chakraborti, S. (2003). Structure and evolutionary aspects of matrix metalloproteinases: a brief overview. *Mol. Cell Biochem.*, Vol. 253, No. 1-2, pp. 31-40.

Demyanenko, G. P., Shibata, Y. & Maness, P. F. (2001). Altered distribution of dopaminergic neurons in the brain of L1 null mice. *Brain Res. Dev. Brain Res.*, Vol. 126, No. 1, pp. 21-30.

Ebeling, O., Duczmal, A., Aigner, S., Geiger, C., Schollhammer, S., Kemshead, J. T., Moller, P., Schwartz-Albiez, R. & Altevogt, P. (1996). L1 adhesion molecule on human lymphocytes and monocytes: expression and involvement in binding to alpha v beta 3 integrin. *Eur. J. Immunol.*, Vol. 26, No. 10, pp. 2508-2516.

Eden, G., Archinti, M., Furlan, F., Murphy, R. & Degryse, B. (2011). The Urokinase Receptor Interactome. *Curr. Pharm. Des.* Epub ahead of print.

Faissner, A., Kruse, J., Goridis, C., Bock, E. & Schachner, M. (1984). The neural cell adhesion molecule L1 is distinct from the N-CAM related group of surface antigens BSP-2 and D2. *EMBO J.*, Vol. 3, No. 4, pp. 733-737.

Fogel, M., Gutwein, P., Mechtersheimer, S., Riedle, S., Stoeck, A., Smirnov, A., Edler, L., Ben-Arie, A., Huszar, M. & Altevogt, P. (2003). L1 expression as a predictor of progression and survival in patients with uterine and ovarian carcinomas. *Lancet*, Vol. 362, No. 9387, pp. 869-875.

Folgueras, A. R., Pendas, A. M., Sanchez, L. M. & Lopez-Otin, C. (2004). Matrix metalloproteinases in cancer: from new functions to improved inhibition strategies. *Int. J. Dev. Biol.*, Vol. 48, No. 5-6, pp. 411-424.

Fujimori, T., Fujii, S., Saito, N. & Sugihara, K. (2009). Pathological diagnosis of early colorectal carcinoma and its clinical implications. *Digestion*, Vol. 79 Suppl 1, pp. 40-51.

Fuxe, J., Vincent, T. & Garcia de, H. A. (2010). Transcriptional crosstalk between TGF-beta and stem cell pathways in tumor cell invasion: role of EMT promoting Smad complexes. *Cell Cycle*, Vol. 9, No. 12, pp. 2363-2374.

Gabbert, H., Wagner, R., Moll, R. & Gerharz, C. D. (1985). Tumor dedifferentiation: an important step in tumor invasion. *Clin. Exp. Metastasis*, Vol. 3, No. 4, pp. 257-279.

Ganesh, S., Sier, C. F., Heerding, M. M., Griffioen, G., Lamers, C. B. & Verspaget, H. W. (1994). Urokinase receptor and colorectal cancer survival. *Lancet*, Vol. 344, No. 8919, pp. 401-402.

Gardsvoll, H. & Ploug, M. (2007). Mapping of the vitronectin-binding site on the urokinase receptor: involvement of a coherent receptor interface consisting of residues from both domain I and the flanking interdomain linker region. *J. Biol. Chem.*, Vol. 282, No. 18, pp. 13561-13572.

Gavert, N., Conacci-Sorrell, M., Gast, D., Schneider, A., Altevogt, P., Brabletz, T. & Ben-Ze'ev, A. (2005). L1, a novel target of beta-catenin signaling, transforms cells and is expressed at the invasive front of colon cancers. *J. Cell Biol.*, Vol. 168, No. 4, pp. 633-642.

Gavert, N., Vivanti, A., Hazin, J., Brabletz, T. & Ben-Ze'ev, A. (2011). L1-mediated colon cancer cell metastasis does not require changes in EMT and cancer stem cell markers. *Mol. Cancer Res.*, Vol. 9, No. 1, pp. 14-24.

Giannelli, G., Falk-Marzillier, J., Schiraldi, O., Stetler-Stevenson, W. G. & Quaranta, V. (1997). Induction of cell migration by matrix metalloprotease-2 cleavage of laminin-5. *Science*, Vol. 277, No. 5323, pp. 225-228.

Goldfinger, L. E., Stack, M. S. & Jones, J. C. (1998). Processing of laminin-5 and its functional consequences: role of plasmin and tissue-type plasminogen activator. *J. Cell Biol.*, Vol. 141, No. 1, pp. 255-265.

Guess, C. M., Lafleur, B. J., Weidow, B. L. & Quaranta, V. (2009). A decreased ratio of laminin-332 beta3 to gamma2 subunit mRNA is associated with poor prognosis in colon cancer. *Cancer Epidemiol. Biomarkers Prev.*, Vol. 18, No. 5, pp. 1584-1590.

Guess, C. M. & Quaranta, V. (2009). Defining the role of laminin-332 in carcinoma. *Matrix Biol.*, Vol. 28, No. 8, pp. 445-455.

Gutwein, P., Mechtersheimer, S., Riedle, S., Stoeck, A., Gast, D., Joumaa, S., Zentgraf, H., Fogel, M. & Altevogt, D. P. (2003). ADAM10-mediated cleavage of L1 adhesion molecule at the cell surface and in released membrane vesicles. *FASEB J.*, Vol. 17, No. 2, pp. 292-294.

Hald, A., Rono, B., Melander, M. C., Ding, M., Holck, S. & Lund, L. R. (2011). MMP9 is protective against lethal inflammatory mass lesions in the mouse colon. *Dis. Model. Mech.*, Vol. 4, No. 2, pp. 212-227.

Hansen, L. V., Laerum, O. D., Illemann, M., Nielsen, B. S. & Ploug, M. (2008). Altered expression of the urokinase receptor homologue, C4.4A, in invasive areas of human esophageal squamous cell carcinoma. *Int. J. Cancer*, Vol. 122, No. 4, pp. 734-741.

Hase, K., Shatney, C., Johnson, D., Trollope, M. & Vierra, M. (1993). Prognostic value of tumor "budding" in patients with colorectal cancer. *Dis. Colon Rectum*, Vol. 36, No. 7, pp. 627-635.

Heiss, M. M., Simon, E. H., Beyer, B. C., Gruetzner, K. U., Tarabichi, A., Babic, R., Schildberg, F. W. & Allgayer, H. (2002). Minimal residual disease in gastric cancer: evidence of an independent prognostic relevance of urokinase receptor expression by disseminated tumor cells in the bone marrow. *J. Clin. Oncol.*, Vol. 20, No. 8, pp. 2005-2016.

Hlubek, F., Jung, A., Kotzor, N., Kirchner, T. & Brabletz, T. (2001). Expression of the invasion factor laminin gamma2 in colorectal carcinomas is regulated by beta-catenin. *Cancer Res.*, Vol. 61, No. 22, pp. 8089-8093.

Hlubek, F., Spaderna, S., Jung, A., Kirchner, T. & Brabletz, T. (2004). Beta-catenin activates a coordinated expression of the proinvasive factors laminin-5 gamma2 chain and MT1-MMP in colorectal carcinomas. *Int. J. Cancer*, Vol. 108, No. 2, pp. 321-326.

Holmbeck, K., Bianco, P., Caterina, J., Yamada, S., Kromer, M., Kuznetsov, S. A., Mankani, M., Robey, P. G., Poole, A. R., Pidoux, I., Ward, J. M. & Birkedal-Hansen, H. (1999). MT1-MMP-deficient mice develop dwarfism, osteopenia, arthritis, and connective tissue disease due to inadequate collagen turnover. *Cell*, Vol. 99, No. 1, pp. 81-92.

Holten-Andersen, M. N., Hansen, U., Brunner, N., Nielsen, H. J., Illemann, M. & Nielsen, B. S. (2005). Localization of tissue inhibitor of metalloproteinases 1 (TIMP-1) in human colorectal adenoma and adenocarcinoma. *Int. J. Cancer*, Vol. 113, No. 2, pp. 198-206.

Hoyer-Hansen, G., Ploug, M., Behrendt, N., Ronne, E. & Dano, K. (1997). Cell-surface acceleration of urokinase-catalyzed receptor cleavage. *Eur. J. Biochem.*, Vol. 243, No. 1-2, pp. 21-26.

Hubbe, M., Kowitz, A., Schirrmacher, V., Schachner, M. & Altevogt, P. (1993). L1 adhesion molecule on mouse leukocytes: regulation and involvement in endothelial cell binding. *Eur. J. Immunol.*, Vol. 23, No. 11, pp. 2927-2931.

Ii, M., Yamamoto, H., Adachi, Y., Maruyama, Y. & Shinomura, Y. (2006). Role of matrix metalloproteinase-7 (matrilysin) in human cancer invasion, apoptosis, growth, and angiogenesis. *Exp. Biol. Med. (Maywood.)*, Vol. 231, No. 1, pp. 20-27.

Illemann, M., Bird, N., Majeed, A., Laerum, O. D., Lund, L. R., Dano, K. & Nielsen, B. S. (2009). Two distinct expression patterns of urokinase, urokinase receptor and plasminogen activator inhibitor-1 in colon cancer liver metastases. *Int. J. Cancer*, Vol. 124, No. 8, pp. 1860-1870.

Illemann, M., Hansen, U., Nielsen, H. J., Andreasen, P. A., Hoyer-Hansen, G., Lund, L. R., Dano, K. & Nielsen, B. S. (2004). Leading-edge myofibroblasts in human colon cancer express plasminogen activator inhibitor-1. *Am. J. Clin. Pathol.*, Vol. 122, No. 2, pp. 256-265.

Iorio, M. V. & Croce, C. M. (2009). MicroRNAs in cancer: small molecules with a huge impact. *J. Clin. Oncol.*, Vol. 27, No. 34, pp. 5848-5856.

Itoh, H., Kataoka, H., Yamauchi, M., Naganuma, S., Akiyama, Y., Nuki, Y., Shimomura, T., Miyazawa, K., Kitamura, N. & Koono, M. (2001). Identification of hepatocyte growth factor activator inhibitor type 2 (HAI-2)-related small peptide (H2RSP): its nuclear localization and generation of chimeric mRNA transcribed from both HAI-2 and H2RSP genes. *Biochem. Biophys. Res. Commun.*, Vol. 288, No. 2, pp. 390-399.

Jass, J. R., Barker, M., Fraser, L., Walsh, M. D., Whitehall, V. L., Gabrielli, B., Young, J. & Leggett, B. A. (2003). APC mutation and tumour budding in colorectal cancer. *J. Clin. Pathol.*, Vol. 56, No. 1, pp. 69-73.

Jorgensen, S., Baker, A., Moller, S. & Nielsen, B. S. (2010). Robust one-day in situ hybridization protocol for detection of microRNAs in paraffin samples using LNA probes. *Methods*, Vol. 52, No. 4, pp. 375-381.

Juncker-Jensen, A. & Lund, L. R. (2011). Phenotypic overlap between MMP-13 and the plasminogen activation system during wound healing in mice. *PLoS. One.*, Vol. 6, No. 2, pp. e16954.

Kadmon, G. & Altevogt, P. (1997). The cell adhesion molecule L1: species- and cell-type-dependent multiple binding mechanisms. *Differentiation*, Vol. 61, No. 3, pp. 143-150.

Kajiwara, Y., Ueno, H., Hashiguchi, Y., Shinto, E., Shimazaki, H., Mochizuki, H. & Hase, K. (2011). Expression of l1 cell adhesion molecule and morphologic features at the invasive front of colorectal cancer. *Am. J. Clin. Pathol.*, Vol. 136, No. 1, pp. 138-144.

Kirkland, S. C., (2009). Type I collagen inhibits differentiation and promotes a stem cell-like phenotype in human colorectal carcinoma cells. *Br. J. Cancer*, Vol. 101, No. 2, pp. 320-326.

Kloosterman, W. P., Wienholds, E., de, B. E., Kauppinen, S. & Plasterk, R. H. (2006). In situ detection of miRNAs in animal embryos using LNA-modified oligonucleotide probes. *Nat. Methods*, Vol. 3, No. 1, pp. 27-29.

Koshikawa, N., Giannelli, G., Cirulli, V., Miyazaki, K. & Quaranta, V. (2000). Role of cell surface metalloprotease MT1-MMP in epithelial cell migration over laminin-5. *J. Cell Biol.*, Vol. 148, No. 3, pp. 615-624.

Koshikawa, N., Minegishi, T., Sharabi, A., Quaranta, V. & Seiki, M. (2005). Membrane-type matrix metalloproteinase-1 (MT1-MMP) is a processing enzyme for human laminin gamma 2 chain. *J. Biol. Chem.*, Vol. 280, No. 1, pp. 88-93.

Koshikawa, N., Schenk, S., Moeckel, G., Sharabi, A., Miyazaki, K., Gardner, H., Zent, R. & Quaranta, V. (2004). Proteolytic processing of laminin-5 by MT1-MMP in tissues and its effects on epithelial cell morphology. *FASEB J.*, Vol. 18, No. 2, pp. 364-366.

Kowitz, A., Kadmon, G., Eckert, M., Schirrmacher, V., Schachner, M. & Altevogt, P. (1992). Expression and function of the neural cell adhesion molecule L1 in mouse leukocytes. *Eur. J. Immunol.*, Vol. 22, No. 5, pp. 1199-1205.

Kurokawa, S., Arimura, Y., Yamamoto, H., Adachi, Y., Endo, T., Sato, T., Suga, T., Hosokawa, M., Shinomura, Y. & Imai, K. (2005). Tumour matrilysin expression predicts metastatic potential of stage I (pT1) colon and rectal cancers. *Gut*, Vol. 54, No. 12, pp. 1751-1758.

Laerum, O. D., Illemann, M., Skarstein, A., Helgeland, L., Ovrebo, K., Dano, K. & Nielsen, B. S. (2008). Crohn's disease but not chronic ulcerative colitis induces the expression of PAI-1 in enteric neurons. *Am. J. Gastroenterol.*, Vol. 103, No. 9, pp. 2350-2358.

Lim, L. P., Lau, N. C., Garrett-Engele, P., Grimson, A., Schelter, J. M., Castle, J., Bartel, D. P., Linsley, P. S. & Johnson, J. M. (2005). Microarray analysis shows that some microRNAs downregulate large numbers of target mRNAs. *Nature*, Vol. 433, No. 7027, pp. 769-773.

Lindberg, P., Larsson, A. & Nielsen, B. S. (2006). Expression of plasminogen activator inhibitor-1, urokinase receptor and laminin gamma-2 chain is an early coordinated event in incipient oral squamous cell carcinoma. *Int. J. Cancer*, Vol. 118, No. 12, pp. 2948-2956.

Liu, N. & Olson, E. N. (2010). MicroRNA regulatory networks in cardiovascular development. *Dev. Cell*, Vol. 18, No. 4, pp. 510-525.

Ma, X., Kumar, M., Choudhury, S. N., Becker Buscaglia, L. E., Barker, J. R., Kanakamedala, K., Liu, M. F. & Li, Y. (2011). Loss of the miR-21 allele elevates the expression of its target genes and reduces tumorigenesis. *Proc. Natl. Acad. Sci. U. S. A*, Vol. 108, No. 25, pp. 10144-10149.

Maddaluno, L., Verbrugge, S. E., Martinoli, C., Matteoli, G., Chiavelli, A., Zeng, Y., Williams, E. D., Rescigno, M. & Cavallaro, U. (2009). The adhesion molecule L1 regulates transendothelial migration and trafficking of dendritic cells. *J. Exp. Med.*, Vol. 206, No. 3, pp. 623-635.

Mann, B., Gelos, M., Siedow, A., Hanski, M. L., Gratchev, A., Ilyas, M., Bodmer, W. F., Moyer, M. P., Riecken, E. O., Buhr, H. J. & Hanski, C. (1999). Target genes of beta-catenin-T cell-factor/lymphoid-enhancer-factor signaling in human colorectal carcinomas. *Proc. Natl. Acad. Sci. U. S. A*, Vol. 96, No. 4, pp. 1603-1608.

Maretzky, T., Schulte, M., Ludwig, A., Rose-John, S., Blobel, C., Hartmann, D., Altevogt, P., Saftig, P. & Reiss, K. (2005). L1 is sequentially processed by two differently activated metalloproteases and presenilin/gamma-secretase and regulates neural cell adhesion, cell migration, and neurite outgrowth. *Mol. Cell Biol.*, Vol. 25, No. 20, pp. 9040-9053.

Masaki, T., Matsuoka, H., Sugiyama, M., Abe, N., Goto, A., Sakamoto, A. & Atomi, Y. (2001). Matrilysin (MMP-7) as a significant determinant of malignant potential of early invasive colorectal carcinomas. *Br. J. Cancer*, Vol. 84, No. 10, pp. 1317-1321.

Mechtersheimer, S., Gutwein, P., gmon-Levin, N., Stoeck, A., Oleszewski, M., Riedle, S., Postina, R., Fahrenholz, F., Fogel, M., Lemmon, V. & Altevogt, P. (2001). Ectodomain shedding of L1 adhesion molecule promotes cell migration by autocrine binding to integrins. *J. Cell Biol.*, Vol. 155, No. 4, pp. 661-673.

Meng, F., Henson, R., Wehbe-Janek, H., Ghoshal, K., Jacob, S. T. & Patel, T. (2007). MicroRNA-21 regulates expression of the PTEN tumor suppressor gene in human hepatocellular cancer. *Gastroenterology*, Vol. 133, No. 2, pp. 647-658.

Monea, S., Lehti, K., Keski-Oja, J. & Mignatti, P. (2002). Plasmin activates pro-matrix metalloproteinase-2 with a membrane-type 1 matrix metalloproteinase-dependent mechanism. *J. Cell Physiol*, Vol. 192, No. 2, pp. 160-170.

Nagase, H., Visse, R. & Murphy, G. (2006). Structure and function of matrix metalloproteinases and TIMPs. *Cardiovasc. Res.*, Vol. 69, No. 3, pp. 562-573.

Nakamura, T., Mitomi, H., Kikuchi, S., Ohtani, Y. & Sato, K. (2005). Evaluation of the usefulness of tumor budding on the prediction of metastasis to the lung and liver after curative excision of colorectal cancer. *Hepatogastroenterology*, Vol. 52, No. 65, pp. 1432-1435.

Nielsen, B. S., Jorgensen, S., Fog, J. U., Sokilde, R., Christensen, I. J., Hansen, U., Brunner, N., Baker, A., Moller, S. & Nielsen, H. J. (2011). High levels of microRNA-21 in the stroma of colorectal cancers predict short disease-free survival in stage II colon cancer patients. *Clin. Exp. Metastasis*, Vol. 28, No. 1, pp. 27-38.

Odekon, L. E., Blasi, F. & Rifkin, D. B. (1994). Requirement for receptor-bound urokinase in plasmin-dependent cellular conversion of latent TGF-beta to TGF-beta. *J. Cell Physiol*, Vol. 158, No. 3, pp. 398-407.

Okada, A., Bellocq, J. P., Rouyer, N., Chenard, M. P., Rio, M. C., Chambon, P. & Basset, P. (1995). Membrane-type matrix metalloproteinase (MT-MMP) gene is expressed in stromal cells of human colon, breast, and head and neck carcinomas. *Proc. Natl. Acad. Sci. U. S. A*, Vol. 92, No. 7, pp. 2730-2734.

Okuyama, T., Nakamura, T. & Yamaguchi, M. (2003). Budding is useful to select high-risk patients in stage II well-differentiated or moderately differentiated colon adenocarcinoma. *Dis. Colon Rectum*, Vol. 46, No. 10, pp. 1400-1406.

Ploug, M., (2003). Structure-function relationships in the interaction between the urokinase-type plasminogen activator and its receptor. *Curr. Pharm. Des*, Vol. 9, No. 19, pp. 1499-1528.

Poulsom, R., Pignatelli, M., Stetler-Stevenson, W. G., Liotta, L. A., Wright, P. A., Jeffery, R. E., Longcroft, J. M., Rogers, L. & Stamp, G. W. (1992). Stromal expression of 72 kda type IV collagenase (MMP-2) and TIMP-2 mRNAs in colorectal neoplasia. *Am. J. Pathol.*, Vol. 141, No. 2, pp. 389-396.

Prall, F., (2007). Tumour budding in colorectal carcinoma. *Histopathology*, Vol. 50, No. 1, pp. 151-162.

Prall, F., Nizze, H. & Barten, M. (2005). Tumour budding as prognostic factor in stage I/II colorectal carcinoma. *Histopathology*, Vol. 47, No. 1, pp. 17-24.

Pyke, C., Ralfkiaer, E., Ronne, E., Hoyer-Hansen, G., Kirkeby, L. & Dano, K. (1994). Immunohistochemical detection of the receptor for urokinase plasminogen activator in human colon cancer. *Histopathology*, Vol. 24, No. 2, pp. 131-138.

Pyke, C., Romer, J., Kallunki, P., Lund, L. R., Ralfkiaer, E., Dano, K. & Tryggvason, K. (1994). The gamma 2 chain of kalinin/laminin 5 is preferentially expressed in invading malignant cells in human cancers. *Am. J. Pathol.*, Vol. 145, No. 4, pp. 782-791.

Pyke, C., Salo, S., Ralfkiaer, E., Romer, J., Dano, K. & Tryggvason, K. (1995). Laminin-5 is a marker of invading cancer cells in some human carcinomas and is coexpressed with the receptor for urokinase plasminogen activator in budding cancer cells in colon adenocarcinomas. *Cancer Res.*, Vol. 55, No. 18, pp. 4132-4139.

Remy, L., Trespeuch, C., Bachy, S., Scoazec, J. Y. & Rousselle, P. (2006). Matrilysin 1 influences colon carcinoma cell migration by cleavage of the laminin-5 beta3 chain. *Cancer Res.*, Vol. 66, No. 23, pp. 11228-11237.

Romer, J., Nielsen, B. S. & Ploug, M. (2004). The urokinase receptor as a potential target in cancer therapy. *Curr. Pharm. Des*, Vol. 10, No. 19, pp. 2359-2376.

Ronnov-Jessen, L. & Petersen, O. W. (1993). Induction of alpha-smooth muscle actin by transforming growth factor-beta 1 in quiescent human breast gland fibroblasts. Implications for myofibroblast generation in breast neoplasia. *Lab Invest*, Vol. 68, No. 6, pp. 696-707.

Roy, S., Khanna, S., Hussain, S. R., Biswas, S., Azad, A., Rink, C., Gnyawali, S., Shilo, S., Nuovo, G. J. & Sen, C. K. (2009). MicroRNA expression in response to murine myocardial infarction: miR-21 regulates fibroblast metalloprotease-2 via phosphatase and tensin homologue. *Cardiovasc. Res.*, Vol. 82, No. 1, pp. 21-29.

Sakurai, T., Lustig, M., Babiarz, J., Furley, A. J., Tait, S., Brophy, P. J., Brown, S. A., Brown, L. Y., Mason, C. A. & Grumet, M. (2001). Overlapping functions of the cell adhesion molecules Nr-CAM and L1 in cerebellar granule cell development. *J. Cell Biol.*, Vol. 154, No. 6, pp. 1259-1273.

Sato, H. & Takino, T. (2010). Coordinate action of membrane-type matrix metalloproteinase-1 (MT1-MMP) and MMP-2 enhances pericellular proteolysis and invasion. *Cancer Sci.*, Vol. 101, No. 4, pp. 843-847.

Schetter, A. J., Leung, S. Y., Sohn, J. J., Zanetti, K. A., Bowman, E. D., Yanaihara, N., Yuen, S. T., Chan, T. L., Kwong, D. L., Au, G. K., Liu, C. G., Calin, G. A., Croce, C. M. & Harris, C. C. (2008). MicroRNA expression profiles associated with prognosis and therapeutic outcome in colon adenocarcinoma. *JAMA*, Vol. 299, No. 4, pp. 425-436.

Schmid, R. S. & Maness, P. F. (2008). L1 and NCAM adhesion molecules as signaling coreceptors in neuronal migration and process outgrowth. *Curr. Opin. Neurobiol.*, Vol. 18, No. 3, pp. 245-250.

Sempere, L. F., Preis, M., Yezefski, T., Ouyang, H., Suriawinata, A. A., Silahtaroglu, A., Conejo-Garcia, J. R., Kauppinen, S., Wells, W. & Korc, M. (2010). Fluorescence-based codetection with protein markers reveals distinct cellular compartments for altered MicroRNA expression in solid tumors. *Clin. Cancer Res.*, Vol. 16, No. 16, pp. 4246-4255.

Shinto, E., Tsuda, H., Ueno, H., Hashiguchi, Y., Hase, K., Tamai, S., Mochizuki, H., Inazawa, J. & Matsubara, O. (2005). Prognostic implication of laminin-5 gamma 2 chain expression in the invasive front of colorectal cancers, disclosed by area-specific four-point tissue microarrays. *Lab Invest*, Vol. 85, No. 2, pp. 257-266.

Sordat, I., Bosman, F. T., Dorta, G., Rousselle, P., Aberdam, D., Blum, A. L. & Sordat, B. (1998). Differential expression of laminin-5 subunits and integrin receptors in human colorectal neoplasia. *J. Pathol.*, Vol. 185, No. 1, pp. 44-52.

Stephens, R. W., Nielsen, H. J., Christensen, I. J., Thorlacius-Ussing, O., Sorensen, S., Dano, K. & Brunner, N. (1999). Plasma urokinase receptor levels in patients with colorectal cancer: relationship to prognosis. *J. Natl. Cancer Inst.*, Vol. 91, No. 10, pp. 869-874.

Strongin, A. Y., (2010). Proteolytic and non-proteolytic roles of membrane type-1 matrix metalloproteinase in malignancy. *Biochim. Biophys. Acta*, Vol. 1803, No. 1, pp. 133-141.

Suzuki, Y., Nagai, N., Umemura, K., Collen, D. & Lijnen, H. R. (2007). Stromelysin-1 (MMP-3) is critical for intracranial bleeding after t-PA treatment of stroke in mice. *J. Thromb. Haemost.*, Vol. 5, No. 8, pp. 1732-1739.

Talotta, F., Cimmino, A., Matarazzo, M. R., Casalino, L., De, V. G., D'Esposito, M., Di, L. R. & Verde, P. (2009). An autoregulatory loop mediated by miR-21 and PDCD4 controls the AP-1 activity in RAS transformation. *Oncogene*, Vol. 28, No. 1, pp. 73-84.

Tanaka, M., Hashiguchi, Y., Ueno, H., Hase, K. & Mochizuki, H. (2003). Tumor budding at the invasive margin can predict patients at high risk of recurrence after curative surgery for stage II, T3 colon cancer. *Dis. Colon Rectum*, Vol. 46, No. 8, pp. 1054-1059.

Thuault, S., Valcourt, U., Petersen, M., Manfioletti, G., Heldin, C. H. & Moustakas, A. (2006). Transforming growth factor-beta employs HMGA2 to elicit epithelial-mesenchymal transition. *J. Cell Biol.*, Vol. 174, No. 2, pp. 175-183.

Thum, T., Gross, C., Fiedler, J., Fischer, T., Kissler, S., Bussen, M., Galuppo, P., Just, S., Rottbauer, W., Frantz, S., Castoldi, M., Soutschek, J., Koteliansky, V., Rosenwald, A., Basson, M. A., Licht, J. D., Pena, J. T., Rouhanifard, S. H., Muckenthaler, M. U., Tuschl, T., Martin, G. R., Bauersachs, J. & Engelhardt, S. (2008). MicroRNA-21 contributes to myocardial disease by stimulating MAP kinase signalling in fibroblasts. *Nature*, Vol. 456, No. 7224, pp. 980-984.

Thurison, T., Lomholt, A. F., Rasch, M. G., Lund, I. K., Nielsen, H. J., Christensen, I. J. & Hoyer-Hansen, G. (2010). A new assay for measurement of the liberated domain I of the urokinase receptor in plasma improves the prediction of survival in colorectal cancer. *Clin. Chem.*, Vol. 56, No. 10, pp. 1636-1640.

Turner, R. R., Li, C. & Compton, C. C. (2007). Newer pathologic assessment techniques for colorectal carcinoma. *Clin. Cancer Res.*, Vol. 13, No. 22 Pt 2, pp. 6871s-6876s.

Uchiyama, S., Itoh, H., Naganuma, S., Nagaike, K., Fukushima, T., Tanaka, H., Hamasuna, R., Chijiiwa, K. & Kataoka, H. (2007). Enhanced expression of hepatocyte growth factor activator inhibitor type 2-related small peptide at the invasive front of colon cancers. *Gut*, Vol. 56, No. 2, pp. 215-226.

Udayakumar, T. S., Chen, M. L., Bair, E. L., Von, B., Cress, A. E., Nagle, R. B. & Bowden, G. T. (2003). Membrane type-1-matrix metalloproteinase expressed by prostate carcinoma cells cleaves human laminin-5 beta3 chain and induces cell migration. *Cancer Res.*, Vol. 63, No. 9, pp. 2292-2299.

Ueno, H., Murphy, J., Jass, J. R., Mochizuki, H. & Talbot, I. C. (2002). Tumour 'budding' as an index to estimate the potential of aggressiveness in rectal cancer. *Histopathology*, Vol. 40, No. 2, pp. 127-132.

Winter, J., Jung, S., Keller, S., Gregory, R. I. & Diederichs, S. (2009). Many roads to maturity: microRNA biogenesis pathways and their regulation. *Nat. Cell Biol.*, Vol. 11, No. 3, pp. 228-234.

Zavadil, J., Narasimhan, M., Blumenberg, M. & Schneider, R. J. (2007). Transforming growth factor-beta and microRNA:mRNA regulatory networks in epithelial plasticity. *Cells Tissues. Organs*, Vol. 185, No. 1-3, pp. 157-161.

Zlobec, I., Molinari, F., Martin, V., Mazzucchelli, L., Saletti, P., Trezzi, R., De, D. S., Vlajnic, T., Frattini, M. & Lugli, A. (2010). Tumor budding predicts response to anti-EGFR therapies in metastatic colorectal cancer patients. *World J. Gastroenterol.*, Vol. 16, No. 38, pp. 4823-4831.

Glutathione-S-Transferases in Development, Progression and Therapy of Colorectal Cancer

Tatyana Vlaykova[1], Maya Gulubova[2], Yovcho Yovchev[3],
Dimo Dimov[4], Denitsa Vlaykova[1,6],
Petjo Chilingirov[5] and Nikolai Zhelev[7]
[1]Dept. Chemistry and Biochemistry, Medical Faculty, Trakia University, Stara Zagora,
[2]Dept. General and Clinical Pathology, Medical Faculty, Trakia University, Stara Zagora,
[3]Dept. General Surgery, Medical Faculty, Trakia University, Stara Zagora,
[4]Dept. Internal Medicine, Medical Faculty, Trakia University, Stara Zagora,
[5]Oncology Center, Stara Zagora,
[6]Regional Hospital, Burgass,
[7]University of Abertay Dundee,
[1,2,3,4,5,6]Bulgaria
[7]UK

1. Introduction

Etiologically, sporadic colorectal cancer (CRC) is a complex, multifactorial disease that is linked to both exogenic and endogenic factors. Accumulating evidence indicates that susceptibility to cancer in general, and to CRC in particular, is mediated by genetically determined differences in the effectiveness of detoxification of potential carcinogens and reactive oxygen species. The antioxidant enzymes and phase I and II biotransformation enzymes are important candidates for involvement in susceptibility to sporadic CRC, due to their ability to regulate the metabolism of a wide range of environmental exposures (Perera, 1997; Potter, 1999; McIlwain et al., 2006; Di Pietro et al., 2010). In addition to carcinogens and reactive oxygen species, the majority of anticancer drugs applied in the chemotherapy are also substrates and are biotransformed by xenobiotic-metabolizing enzymes, leading to their activation and/or detoxification (O'Brien &Tew, 1996; Eaton &Bammler, 1999; Townsend &Tew, 2003; Hayes et al., 2005; Michael &Doherty, 2005; Townsend et al., 2005). In this respect, great efforts have been focused to clarify the effects of genetic variations, expression and activity of xenobiotic-metabolizing enzymes in development, progression and therapy of cancers with different histological origin, including CRC (Ranganathan &Tew, 1991; Tew &Ronai, 1999; Welfare et al., 1999; Cotton et al., 2000; de Jong et al., 2002; Dogru-Abbasoglu et al., 2002; Stoehlmacher et al., 2002; Ates et al., 2005; Romero et al., 2006; Liao et al., 2007; Pistorius et al., 2007; Koutros et al., 2009; Di Pietro et al., 2010; Economopoulos & Sergentanis, 2010).

2. Role of GSTs in cell processes

Glutathione-S-transferase (GST, EC. 2.5.1.18) isoemzymes are involved in phase II xenobiotic biotransformation. GSTs belong to a large superfamily of dimeric enzymes, which play an important role in cell defense system. So far, 24 isoenzymes have been described in humans, classified into 11 classes: 7 cytosolic - alpha (α, A), mu (μ, M), pi (π, P), sigma (σ, S), theta (θ, T), zeta (ζ, Z), and omega (ω, O), one mitochondrial - kappa (κ, K), and three microsomal classes, also referred to as membrane-associated proteins in eicosanoid and glutathione metabolism (MAPEG) (Sheehan et al., 2001; Hayes et al., 2005; McIlwain et al., 2006; Laborde, 2010) The most abundant mammalian GST enzymes belong to cytosolic classes alpha, mu, and pi, and their regulation has been studied in details (Hayes &Pulford, 1995). Most of the cytosolic GST classes are coded by several genes, gathered in clusters and thus these enzymes have several subunits, which form a number of homo- and/or heterodimeric isoenzymes (Table 1) (McIlwain et al., 2006; Laborde, 2010).

GST classes	Subunits	Gene (locus) designation	Chromosome location of the genes/gene clusters
Cytosolic			
GST-alpha (GSTα, GSTA)	1,2,3,4,5	GSTA1, GSTA2, GSTA3, GSTA4, GSTA5	6p12
GST-mu (GSTμ, GSTM)	1,2,3,4,5	GSTM1, GSTM2, GSTM3, GSTM4, GSTM5	1p13
GST-omega (GSTω, GSTO)	1,2	GSTO1, GSTO2,	10q25.1
GST-pi (GSTπ, GSTP)	1	GSTP1	11q13
GST-sigma (GSTσ, GSTS)	1	GSTS ([a] HPGDS; PGDS)	4q22.3
GST-theta (GSTθ, GSTT)	1,2	GSTT1, GSTT2	22q11.2
GST-zeta (GSTξ, GSTZ)	1	GSTZ1	14q24.3
Mitochondrial			
GST-kappa (GSTκ, GSTK)	1	GSTK1	7q34
Microsomal			
[b]MAPEG		[c] MGST1, [c] MGST2, [d] ALOX5AP (FLAP) [e] LTC$_4$S [c] MGST3 [f] PGES (PTGES)	12p12.3-p12.1 4q28.3 13q12 5q35 1q23 9q34.3

[a]HPGDS - hematopoietic prostaglandin D synthase (PGDS - prostaglandin D synthase)
[b]MAPEG - membrane-associated proteins in eicosanoid and glutathione metabolism
[c]MGST - microsomal glutathione S-transferase
[d]ALOX5AP (FLAP) - arachidonate 5-lipoxygenase-activating protein
[e]LTC4S - leukotriene C4 synthase
[f]PGES - prostaglandin E synthase

Table 1. Classes, subunits and gene location of human GSTs

GSTs catalyze the conjugation of reduced glutathione with a variety of endogenic and exogenic electrophilic compounds, including several carcinogens and antineoplastics (Hayes &Strange, 1995; Hayes et al., 2005; Michael &Doherty, 2005). This process results in alteration, usually a reduction, of the reactivity of the compounds and makes them more water soluble and favors their elimination.

GSTs can also function as peroxidases and isomerases (Hayes &Pulford, 1995; Cho et al., 2001). Thus GSTA1-1 and GSTA2-2 efficiently catalyze the reduction of fatty acid and phospholipid hydroperoxides (Zhao et al., 1999). Moreover, it has been shown that GSTA3-3 is essential in obligatory double-bond isomerizations of precursors of testosterone and progesterone in steroid hormone biosynthesis (Johansson &Mannervik, 2001). Although the exact physiological function of omega-class GSTs remains undefined (Board et al., 2000; Board, 2011), it has been demonstrated that they can catalyze a range of thiol transferase and reduction reactions that are not catalyzed by members of the other classes: GSTO1 has GSH-dependent reductive activity to dehydroascorbate and to monomethylarsenic acid (V) (Board, 2011). GSTZ1 has isomerase activity and catalyzes the conversion of maleylacetoacetate to fumarylacetoacetate in the catabolic pathway of phenylalanine and tyrosine and also catalyzes the GSH-dependent transformation of α-halogenated acids (McIlwain et al., 2006).

There are six MAPEG (membrane associated proteins in eicosanoid and glutathione metabolism) subfamily members localized to the endoplasmic reticulum and outer mitochondrial membrane. Three of them are involved in the production of leukotrienes and prostaglandin E, whereas the other three have glutathione S-transferase and peroxidase activities, thus implicated in the protection of membranes from oxidative stress (Morgenstern et al., 2011).

In addition to their catalytic functions GSTs have several complementary functions. Some of the GSTs can serve as nonenzymatic binding proteins (known as ligandins) interacting with various lipophilic compounds including steroid and thyroid hormones (Litwack et al., 1971; Ishigaki et al., 1989; Cho et al., 2001; Vasieva, 2011). Moreover, GST isoenzymes can play a regulatory role in cellular signaling by forming protein:protein interactions with key signaling tyrosine kinases, involved in controlling stress response, apoptosis, inflammation, cellular differentiation and proliferation (Adler et al., 1999; Cho et al., 2001; Wang et al., 2001; Townsend &Tew, 2003; Townsend et al., 2005; McIlwain et al., 2006; Laborde, 2010; Vasieva, 2011).

There is strong evidence that GST-pi can bind by protein:protein interaction, sequester and inhibit c-Jun N-terminal kinase (JNK)/stress-activated protein kinases (SAPKs). JNK is a MAP kinase that phosphorylates c-Jun, a component of the activator protein-1 (AP-1) transcriptional factor, resulting in the induction of AP-1-dependent target genes which play role in cell survival and apoptosis. Thus JNK is implicated in pro-apoptotic/survival signaling pathways and may be required for induced cytotoxicity of a variety of antitumor drugs (Adler et al., 1999; Wang et al., 2001; Townsend &Tew, 2003; Townsend et al., 2005; McIlwain et al., 2006; Laborde, 2010; Vasieva, 2011).

Recently, GST-pi was shown to affect the apoptosis pathways also by physical association with TNF receptor associated factor 2 (TRAF2), an adaptor protein which mediates the signal transduction of different receptors and is required for the activation of ASK1 (apoptosis signal-regulating kinase 1) (Wu et al., 2006; Laborde, 2010; Sau et al., 2010;

Vasieva, 2011). ASK1 is a MAP kinase kinase kinase (MAP3 kinase, MAPKKK) that can phosphorylate MKK4/7 and MKK3/6 (MAP kinase kinases, MAP2Ks, MAPKK) which are involved in stress-induced activation of JNK- and p38 signaling pathways, respectively (Dorion et al., 2002; Wu et al., 2006; Sau et al., 2010).

Isoenzymes of the alpha and mu classes have also been shown in vitro to bind to JNK-Jun complexes and inhibit the activation of c-Jun by JNK, however their inhibitory activity was weaker than GST-pi (Villafania et al., 2000; Laborde, 2010). In addition, it has been noted that GST-mu interacts physically with N-terminal portion of ASK1, thus inhibiting its activity and the ASK1-elicited MKK4/7–JNK and MKK3/6–p38 signaling pathways (Dorion et al., 2002).

Another binding partner of GST-pi is the antioxidant enzyme 1-cys peroxiredoxin (1-cysPrx, Prx VI), which is a member of the peroxiredoxin superfamily and is able to protect cells from membrane peroxidation via GSH-dependent peroxidase activity on phospholipid hydroperoxides. The process of heterodimerization of 1-cysPrx with GST-pi leads to activation involving also the S-glutathionylation of 1-cysPrx (Manevich et al., 2004; Vasieva, 2011).

GST-pi has also been found to function in the S-glutathionylation of oxidized cysteine residues of several target proteins following oxidative and nitrosative stress thus playing a direct role in the control of posttranslational S-glutathionylation reactions (McIlwain et al., 2006; Townsend et al., 2006; Townsend et al., 2009; Tew et al., 2011). S-glutathionylation occurs on cysteine moieties located in relatively basic environment in response to oxidative (ROS) or nitrosative stress (RNS) signaling events. Glutathiolylation is reversible process that can occur spontaneously by GSH or catalytically by thioredoxin (Trx), glutaredoxin (Grx) or sylphoredoxin (Srx). Thus besides the phosphorylation/dephosphorylation, the cells are provided with additional dynamic system of controlling the protein activity (Townsend et al., 2009). Proteins sensitive to modification by S-glutathionylation are variety of enzymes with thiols in the active centers, cytoskeleton proteins, signaling proteins – particularly kinases and phosphatases, transcriptional factors, Ras oncogenic proteins, heat shock proteins, ion channels, and calcium pumps (Tew et al., 2011). Since a number of proteins that are S-glutathionylated are involved in growth regulatory pathways, the over-expression of GST-pi in cancers may account for the impaired balance between cell death, proliferation and differentiation and could contribute to tumor development, progression and treatment response (Townsend et al., 2009; Tew et al., 2011).

GST-pi was also shown to bind proteins and compounds containing iron and nitric oxide and thus may influence the NO metabolism and NO signaling (Vasieva, 2011). It has been shown that the natural low molecular mass NO carriers, dinitrosyl-iron complexes (DNIC) and S-nitrosoglutathion (GSNO) bind with high affinity to one active site of the dimeric GST-pi enzyme, while the enzyme maintains its detoxification activity (Lo Bello et al., 2001; Townsend et al., 2006; Vasieva, 2011). Hence, GST-pi (GSTP1-1) may act as a NO carrier, which determines it as a player of a number of processes as formation of nitrothiols, nitrosylation of proteins, NO mediated iron mobilization from cells, and Zn-homeostasis (Vasieva, 2011).

It has also been reported that certain GSTs play novel roles implicated in cell defense: GST-theta was suggested to inhibit the pro-apoptotic action of Bax (Kampranis et al., 2000), and GST-omega (GSTO1-1) was shown to modulate ryanodine receptors (RyR), which are calcium release channels in skeletal and cardiac sarcoplasmic reticulum, suggesting protective functions of GSTO1-1 in mammalian cells from radiation damage and Ca^{2+} induced apoptosis (Dulhunty et al., 2001)

Thereby, these multiple functionalities of the members of GST family, in addition to the well-characterized catalytic activities, could contribute and be of importance in GST-highly expressing tumors for development and progression of cancers and for acquisition of resistance to applied chemotherapeutics.

3. Polymorphic variants of GSTs

Numerous polymorphisms have been described in the genes encoding GSTs as most of them have been associated with a lack or an alteration of enzymatic activity toward several substrates (Ali-Osman et al., 1997; Whyatt et al., 2000; Hayes et al., 2005; McIlwain et al., 2006).

3.1 *GSTP* class

The GST-pi class is encoded by a single gene spanning approximately 3 kb and located on chromosome 11 (11q13). Two *GSTP1* single nucleotide polymorphisms (SNPs) have been identified. They are characterized by transitions at $A^{1578}G$ (exon 5, $A^{313}G$) and $C^{2293}T$ (exon 6, $C^{341}T$), resulting in amino acid substitutions Ile[105]Val and Ala[114]Val, respectively, which appear to be within the active site of the GST-pi protein (Ali-Osman et al., 1997; Watson et al., 1998; Hayes et al., 2005; McIlwain et al., 2006). These two SNPs lead to the following four alleles: *GSTP1*A* (105Ile, 114Ala), *GSTP1*B* (105Val, 114Ala), *GSTP1*C* (105Val, 114Val), and *GSTP1*D* (105Ile, 114Val).

It has been proven that the substitutions due to SNPs in *GSTP1* are functional: the substitution of Ile to Val at position 105 (*GSTP1* Ile[105]Val) results in altered enzyme activity to variety of electrophilic molecules (Hayes et al., 2005; McIlwain et al., 2006). Thus, there is a strong experimental evidence that the two proteins, encoded by the allelic variants, 105Ile and 105Val of the human *GSTP1* gene, differ significantly in their catalytic activities toward a model substrate; the GST-pi 105Val variant has lower activity toward 1-chloro-2,4-dinitrobenzene, a standard substrate, than its 105Ile counterpart (Ali-Osman et al., 1997; Townsend &Tew, 2003, Coles, 2000 #47). On the other hand, the same variant (105Val) displays greater activity toward polycyclic aromatic hydrocarbon (PAH) diol epoxides (Sundberg et al., 1998; Coles et al., 2000; Bostrom et al., 2002). The GST-pi 105Val enzyme variant is found to be more active than 105Ile variant in conjugation reactions with the bulky diol epoxides of PAHs, being up to 3-fold as active toward the *anti-* and *syn*-diol epoxide enantiomers with R-absolute configuration at the benzylic oxiranyl carbon (Sundberg et al., 1998; Coles et al., 2000). The bay-region diol epoxides of PAHs are known to be ultimate mutagenic and carcinogenic metabolites (Sundberg et al., 1998; Bostrom et al., 2002).

The frequency of *GSTP1* 105Ile allele in different Caucasian groups varied from 0.63 to 0.77, whereas the frequency of the variant *GSTP1* 105Val allele ranged between 0.23 and 0.37 (Table 2) (Katoh et al., 2008). In our previous study we determined the frequency of Ile[105]Val *GSTP1* genotypes in 126 ethnic Bulgarian individuals from the region of Stara Zagora (0.54 for Ile/Ile, 0.39 for Ile/Val and 0.07 for Val/Val) (Vlaykova et al., 2007). The obtained figures are consistent with those published for the controls in the case-control study of Bulgarian patients with Balkan endemic nephropathy (Andonova et al., 2004), and for other Caucasian type control cohorts in Finland (Mitrunen et al., 2001), Edinburgh area, Scotland (Harries et al., 1997), Newcastle and North Tyneside, England (Welfare et al., 1999), East Anglia region (Loktionov et al., 2001), etc. (Table 2). Based on these similarities we can conclude that despite the heterogeneous origin ethnic Bulgarians do not differ from other Caucasians in frequency of Ile[105]Val *GSTP1* genotypes and could be included in larger interinstitutional case-control studies for investigation of the effect of this polymorphism on the susceptibility to different diseases, including cancers.

Country/racial origin	Allele frequencies			Genotype frequencies			
	105Ile (%)	105Val (%)	p-value	105 Ile/Ile (%)	105 Ile/Val (%)	105Val/ Val (%)	p-value
Bulgaria/Caucasian (Vlaykova et al., 2007)	73	27		54	39	7	
Bulgaria/Caucasian (Andonova et al., 2004)	66	34	0.284	47	38	15	0.182
Finland/Caucasian (Mitrunen et al., 2001)	74	26	0.873	55	38	7	0.989
Scotland (UK)/Caucasian (Harries et al., 1997)	72.2	27.8	0.899	51	42.5	6.5	0.906
Surrey, UK/Caucasian (Kote-Jarai et al., 2001)	70.4	29.6	0.684	51.2	38.5	10.3	0.702
Newcastle, UK/Caucasian (Welfare et al., 1999)	66.5	33.5	0.318	45	43	12	0.312
East Anglia, UK/Caucasian (Loktionov et al., 2001)	65.5	34.5	0.252	40	49	11	0.128
Germany/ Caucasian (Steinhoff et al., 2000)	73	27	1.00	55	36	9	0.827
Sweden/ Caucasian (Sorensen et al., 2007)	69	31	0.534	49	40	11	0.564
Austria/ Caucasian (Gsur et al., 2001)	63.3	36.7	0.142	39.2	48.2	12.6	0.085
Portugal/ Caucasian (Jeronimo et al., 2002)	67	33	0.356	43.3	47.5	9.2	0.315
American non-Hispanic/ Caucasian (Agalliu et al., 2006)	66	34	0.284	43	46	11	0.258

Table 2. Allele and genotype frequencies of the *GSTP1* Ile[105]Val gene polymorphism in Bulgarians compared to other Caucasian populations.

3.2 *GSTM* class

GSTM1 together with the other four *GSTM* class members (*GSTM2, GSTM3, GSTM4* and *GSTM5*) are mapped to 1p13.3 (Pearson et al., 1993; McIlwain et al., 2006; Laborde, 2010). The close proximity of *GSTM1* and *GSTM2*, as well as the presence of two almost identical 4.2-kb regions flanking the *GSTM1* gene have been suggested to be the reasons for the observed entire *GSTM1* gene deletion resulting in a null *GSTM1* allele (*GSTM1*0*) (Pearson et al., 1993; Bolt &Thier, 2006). Furthermore, a transversion of G with C at position 534 (534G>C, formerly noted as 519G>C) was described leading to a substitution of 172Lys with 172Asn (formerly Lys[173]Asn) (McLellan et al., 1997; Bolt &Thier, 2006; McIlwain et al., 2006; Gao et al., 2010). This SNP results in two new alleles - *GSTM1*A* and *GSTM1*B*, which were reported to be functionally identical (McLellan et al., 1997). In addition, a duplication of *GSTM1* gene has been identified and characterized (*GSTM1*1x2* allele) in people who displayed ultrarapid GSTM1 activity (McLellan et al., 1997).

Thus, four allele loci have been described in the human *GSTM1* - *GSTM1*A, GSTM1*B, GSTM1*0* and *GSTM1*1x2*, which determine several phenotypes. The frequencies of *GSTM1* alleles and genotypes display race and ethnic variations: 42% to 60% of Caucasians, 41% to 63% of Asians and only 16% to 36% of Africans are homozygous for *GSTM1*0* (null *GSTM1* genotype) (O'Brien &Tew, 1996; Cotton et al., 2000; He et al., 2004; Hayes et al., 2005; Bolt &Thier, 2006; McIlwain et al., 2006; Katoh et al., 2008; Gao et al., 2010). Our results showed that the frequency of *GSTM1* genotype in Bulgarian control individuals (36% and 42%) (Figure 1A) (Dimov et al., 2008; Emin et al., 2009; Vlaykova et al., 2009) is commensurable to that reported for some other European populations (Cotton et al., 2000; Ates et al., 2005; Katoh et al., 2008; Gao et al., 2010).

Polymorphic variants have been described for the other GSTM members: *GSTM2, GSTM3, GSTM4* and *GSTM5* (Inskip et al., 1995; Mitrunen et al., 2001; Reszka &Wasowicz, 2001; Hayes et al., 2005; Reszka et al., 2007; Yu et al., 2009; Moyer et al., 2010). The most extensive studies have been performed on *GSTM3* polymorphisms. This gene has an insertion/deletion polymorphism (rs1799735, *GSTM3*A/*B*) with a wild-type *GSTM3*A* allele and a variant one, *GSTM3*B*, which differ in the rate of expression. The variant *GSTM3*B* allele has 3 bp deletion in intron 6, which introduces a recognition site for YY1 transcriptional factor and results in enhanced expression of the enzyme protein. (Inskip et al., 1995; Loktionov et al., 2001; McIlwain et al., 2006; Reszka et al., 2007). Recently, several SNPs in *GSTM3* have been identified and studied for their functional activity and in association with variety of diseases. These are the rare Gln[174]Trp (G[174]W), the more common Val[224]Ile (V[224]I) substitutions, and the transversion of A with C at -63 position in promoter region of *GSTM3* (-62A>C) (Liu et al., 2005; McIlwain et al., 2006). The variant 174Trp allele, as well as the wild-type 224Val allele, were reported to exhibit decreased catalytic activity, whereas the variant -63C allele was associated with increased expression of the gene (Liu et al., 2005; McIlwain et al., 2006).

3.3 *GSTT* class

A null polymorphism has also been described in *T1* locus of *GSTT* cluster at 22q11.2. Analogously to *GSTM1*, *GSTT1* consisting of 5 exons, is flanked by two highly homologous 18 kb regions (HA3 and HA5). The null *GSTT1*0* allele is possibly caused by a homologous recombination resulting in 54 kb deletion containing the entire *GSTT1* gene (Sprenger et al.,

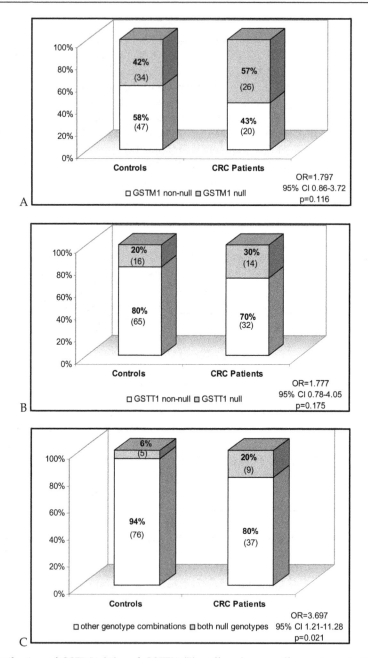

Fig. 1. Distribution of GSTM1 (A) and GSTT1 (B) null and non-null genotypes in Bulgarian patients with CRC and control individuals. Frequency of carriers of GSTM1 and GSTT1 double null genotype among the patients and controls (C). Data are presented in percentages and in real numbers (in brackets); the ORs and the 95% CI are also given.

2000; Bolt &Thier, 2006). A SNP (310A>C) in exon 3 of *GSTT1* is the reason for substitution of Tre104 with Pro104 (Tre[104]Pro) in GST-theta protein, which was associated with a decrease in the catalytic activity possibly due to a conformational changes of the protein molecule (Alexandrie et al., 2002). The frequency of the null *GSTT1* genotype has also been found to vary significantly between different races and ethnic groups: between 13% and 31% (with some exceptions) in Caucasians in Europe and USA and between 35% and 48% in Asians (O'Brien &Tew, 1996; Cotton et al., 2000; He et al., 2004; Hayes et al., 2005; Bolt &Thier, 2006; McIlwain et al., 2006; Katoh et al., 2008). Our preliminary results concerning a small Bulgarian control group showed homozygosity for *GSTT1*0* (*GSTT1* null genotype) in a rate of only 7% (Dimov et al., 2008; Vlaykova et al., 2009). However, when the control group was extended the frequency of *GSTT1* null genotype turned out to be 20% (Figure 1B) (Emin et al., 2009) which is comparable to other Caucasian populations (Bolt &Thier, 2006; Katoh et al., 2008).

Polymorphic variants have been described also in the second theta-class GST gene, *GSTT2*. Coggan et al. reported a pseudogene (*GSTT2P*), which rises from G to T transition at nt 841 (841G>T) in intron 2 of *GSTT2* and C to T transition at nt 3255 (3255C>T) in exon 5 of *GSTT2P* changing 196Arg to a stop codon. In addition a G to A transition at nt 2732 (2732G>A) in exon 4 of *GSTT2* was defined that results in substitution of 139Met to 139Ile (Met[139]Ile) (Coggan et al., 1998). However, there is still no clear evidence that the latter SNP may have influence on the enzyme function. In the meantime, the defined promoter polymorphisms in *GSTT2* (-537G>A, -277T>C, -158G>A, and -129T>C) were shown to affect the gene expression (Guy et al., 2004; Jang et al., 2007).

3.4 *GSTA* class

Although, variety of polymorphisms of alpha-class GST genes has been defined, their functional activity has not yet been comprehensively investigated. Nevertheless, it is already proven that the SNPs in the promoter (5'-regulatory) region of *GSTA1* (-567, -69, and -52) and specifically the substitution at -69C>T (determining a variant *GSTA1*B* allele), result in enhanced promoter activity and increased expression (Coles et al., 2001; Sweeney et al., 2002; McIlwain et al., 2006). However, for 10 SNPs in the coding regions (exons) of *GSTA1* and *GSTA2* was shown to have no significant functional effects (Tetlow et al., 2001). In a later study, the new Pro[110]Ser polymorphism in *GSTA2* was found to affect the catalysis with several substrates, as the Ser containing isoform has significantly diminished enzyme activity (Tetlow &Board, 2004). Similar decrease in the glutathione-conjugating activity was also shown for the Leu containing isoform of Ile[71]Leu (I[71]L) polymorphism of *GSTA3* (Tetlow et al., 2004).

3.5 *GSTO* class

The omega-class GSTs are coded by 2 genes (*GSTO1* and *GSTO2*) both composed of six exons and spread by 7.5 kb on chromosome 10q25.1 (Whitbread et al., 2003; Whitbread et al., 2005). A total of 26 putative variants have been identified in the coding region of *GSTO1* in different databases. Among them only 10 have been confirmed candidates and only one GSTO1*A140D (A[140]D, Ala[140]Asp, 419C>T) has been found in the ethnic group studies (Whitbread et al., 2003). In addition a 3-bp deletion polymorphism (AGg from the final GAG codone [155E, 155Glu]) has been identified in the boundary of *GSTO1* exon4 and intron 4.

This deletion has the potential to alter the existing splice site, may reform a new splice donor site and causes the deletion of 155Glu (*GSTO1*E155del*) resulting in a loss of heat stability and increased enzyme activity toward 2-hydroxyethyl disulphide (HEDS) and CDNB (Whitbread et al., 2003). Only one variant in GSTO2 has been confirmed and identified in the population studies: this variation results from an A>G transition at nt 424 (424A>G) and causes a substitution of 142Asn to 142Asp (Asn142Asp, N142D) (Whitbread et al., 2003).

3.6 *GSTZ* class

A number of genetic polymorphisms in the gene encoding glutathione S-transferase-zeta (*GSTZ1*) have been defined: G-1002A, Glu32Lys, Gly42Arg, Thr82Met. The latter three SNPs are functional and determine four *GSTZ1* alleles referred to as *GSTZ1*A* (32Lys, 42Arg, 82Thr), *GSTZ1*B* (32Lys, 42Gly, 82Thr), *GSTZ1*C* (32Glu, 42Gly, 82Thr), and *GSTZ1*D* (32Glu, 42Gly, 82Met) (Blackburn et al., 2001). The *B*, *C* and *D* alleles have been associated with a lower activity to dichloroacetic acid compared to *GSTZ1A* (Blackburn et al., 2001), but non of these SNPs affect significantly the risk of bladder cancer in Spain (Cantor et al., 2010) and breast cancer in Germany (Andonova et al., 2009).

4. Role of GSTs polymorphisms as risk factors for development, progression and therapeutic response of CRC

4.1 *GSTP1*

Epidemiological studies of *GSTP1* (*GSTP1 Ile105Val*) and colorectal cancer risk have suggested a deleterious effect of the low activity genotypes, but findings have been inconsistent (Harries et al., 1997; Welfare et al., 1999; Kiyohara, 2000; Ates et al., 2005; Gao et al., 2009; Economopoulos &Sergentanis, 2010).

The results of our case-control study (Vlaykova et al., 2007) based on 80 patients with primary sporadic CRC and 98 unaffected control individuals showed that the genotype distribution is consistent with those published for other Caucasian type control cohorts. We also found a statistically significant prevalence of heterozygous *GSTP1* genotype by itself (*105Ile/Val* – co-dominant model) and the prevalence of variant allele-containing *GSTP1* genotypes (*105Ile/Val* or *105Val/Val* – dominant model) in control group compared to the CRC cases. This suggests a protective effect of the variant 105*Val* allele lowering the risk for developing of CRC. Based on our observations and on the experimental evidence reported by other research groups for greater activity of the enzyme encoded by the valiant *105Val* allele toward polycyclic aromatic hydrocarbon (PAH) diol epoxides (Sundberg et al., 1998; Coles et al., 2000; Bostrom et al., 2002), we suggest that the heterozygous *GSTP1* genotype may determine a better protection toward GST-pi-metabolized chemical toxins and reactive oxygen species (Vlaykova et al., 2007). This genotype may provide enzyme with an adequate detoxification of some and relatively weak activation of other carcinogens, depending on their characteristics.

Two recent large meta-analyses summarized the results focused on the role of *GSTP1* *Ile105Val* from 16 published case-control studies involving a total of 4386 colorectal cancer patients and 7127 controls (Gao et al., 2009) and 19 studies with altogether 5421 cases and 7671 controls (Economopoulos &Sergentanis, 2010) .The results of the meta-analysis performed by Gao et al. (Gao et al., 2009) sowed no strong evidence that the *105Val* allele conferred increased susceptibility to colorectal cancer compared to *105Ile* allele either in the whole pooled case-controls groups or in the stratified one: by race - Caucasian and Asian descent; by the type of controls - in healthy and hospital controls. They also did not find evidence for an association with colorectal cancer in dominant (OR= 1.02, 95% CI:0.94, 1.10) and co-dominant (OR= 0.88 , 95% CI: 0.77, 1.01) models for the effect of Val. Only a slight, but significant, protective effect of Val allele was observed in the recessive model 0.86 (95% CI: 0.76–0.98). The final conclusion of this large meta-analysis was that *GSTP1 Ile[105]Val* polymorphism is unlikely to increase considerably the risk of sporadic colorectal cancer (Gao et al., 2009).

Similar are the results and final conclusion of the recent meta-analysis performed by Economopoulos et al. (Economopoulos &Sergentanis, 2010): there were no significant effects of *105Val* allele on the risk of colorectal cancer either in dominant model (OR=1.025, 95% CI: 0.922–1.138), co-dominant model (OR=1.050, 95% CI: 0.945–1.166), or in the recessive model (OR=0.936, 95% CI: 0.823–1.065). Hence, the conclusions confirmed that the *GSTP1 Ile[105]Val* status did not seem to confer additional risk for colorectal cancer (Economopoulos &Sergentanis, 2010).

4.2 *GSTM1* and *GSTT1*

Because GST-mu and GST-theta are important in the detoxification of carcinogens implicated in colorectal cancer, the absence of these enzymes is assumed to increase the risk of this common malignancy. In this regard a number of epidemiological studies have investigated the association of *GSTM1* and *GSTT1* genetic polymorphisms with colorectal cancer risk, however the results from these studies have also been with quite controversial conclusions (Cotton et al., 2000; Economopoulos &Sergentanis, 2010; Gao et al., 2010). The preliminary results from our study including very limited number of patients and controls (45 and 42), showed a statistically significant case-control difference in the presence of *GSTT1* null genotype (0.30 vs. 0.07, p=0.006), and only a tendency for prevalence of *GSTM1* null genotype in CRC patient (0.57 vs. 0.36, p=0.052) (Vlaykova et al., 2009). The combined null genotypes were determined only in patients (0.20), whereas none of the control individual was with such genotype (p<0.0001). We found a 5.69-fold (95% CI, 1.59-20.00) and 2.34-fold (95% CI, 0.99-5.49) increased risk associated with *GSTT1* and *GSTM1* null genotypes, respectively and 21.533-fold (95% CI, 3.56-128.71) increased risk associated with the combined null genotypes. The colorectal cancer was diagnosed earlier in patients with *GSTM1* null genotype and those patients had tumors in more advanced stage (III or IV) (p=0.033) and were with more aggressive phenotype, such as presence of lymph vessel invasion (p=0.042) than the patients with non-null genotype.

A slight difference was obtained when the control group was extended to 81 persons (Figure 1A, 1B and 1C): the null *GSTT1* and *GSTM1* genotypes turned out only to tend to associate with an increased risk of colorectal cancer (OR=1.797, 95% CI 0.86-3.72, p=0.116 for *GSTM1*, and OR=1.777, 95% CI 0.78-4.05, p=0.175 for *GSTT1*), however the carriers of *GSTM1* and *GSTT1* double null genotype had significantly higher risk of development of the disease (OR=3.697, 95% CI 1.21-11.28, p=0.021) (Figure 1C). As a conclusion, we suggested that the inherited simultaneous lack of GST-theta and GST-mu detoxifying enzymes due to the presence of homozygous null genotypes may be associated with development of sporadic colorectal cancer (Vlaykova et al., 2009).

Our findings are analogous to the one of meta-analyses performed on a large number of published case-control studies. The results of these meta-analyses support the suggestion that GSTM1 and GSTT1 null polymorphisms are associated with increased risk of CRC, especially in the Caucasian population (Economopoulos &Sergentanis, 2010; Gao et al., 2010). Economopoulos et al. have summarized the results from 44 studies for GSTM1 and 34 for GSTT1 null polymorphisms and concluded that GSTM1 null genotype carriers exhibited increased colorectal cancer risk in Caucasian population (OR=1.15, 95% CI: 1.06-1.25), but not in Chinese subjects (OR=1.03, 95% CI: 0.90-1.16). They reported similar results for GSTT1 null polymorphism: OR=1.31, 95% CI:1.12-1.54 for Caucasian population and OR=1.07, 95% CI:0.79-1.45 for Chinese subjects (Economopoulos &Sergentanis, 2010). Gao at al., carried out a meta-analysis of GSTM1 genotype data from 36 studied including 9149 patients with CRC and 13 916 control individuals (Gao et al., 2010). The results indicated that GSTM1 null genotype was associated with CRC (OR=1.13, 95% CI: 1.03-1.23) in the pooled cases and controls from a number of different ethnics groups. However, the significance of this association remained for Caucasians, but not for Asians (Gao et al., 2010).

4.3 *GSTA1, GSTM3, GSTO2*

According to our knowledge there are only a limited number of studies aiming to evaluate the possible role of polymorphisms in the genes encoding other GST isoforms as predisposing factors for colorectal cancer. The polymorphisms in GSTA1 have been explored in colorectal cancer only by four research teams (Sweeney et al., 2002; van der Logt et al., 2004; Martinez et al., 2006; Kury et al., 2008) . The Sweeney at al. have found that the GSTA1*B/*B (promoter polymorphisms) genotype is associated with an increased risk of colorectal cancer, particularly among consumers of well-done meat and have suggested that GSTA1 genotype, in addition to the CYP2A6 phenotype should be evaluated as markers for susceptibility to dietary carcinogens (Sweeney et al., 2002). However, other studies did not find any associations between the GSTA1 polymorphisms and the risk of CRC (van der Logt et al., 2004; Martinez et al., 2006; Kury et al., 2008).

Kury et al., and Martinez at al, have also attempted to elucidate the influence of GSTM3 genetic variants on colorectal cancer risk, however no correlation between these polymorphisms and CRC susceptibility was found (Martinez et al., 2006; Kury et al., 2008). Similarly, no effect of GSTM3 polymorphism was found in a large study investigating the role of single SNPs within 11 genes of phase I and 15 genes of phase II of xenobiotic metabolism (Landi et al., 2005). Opposite results have been reported for GSTM3*A/GSTM3*B alleles (the latter arising from a 3 bp deletion in intron 6): patients who were carriers of genotypes with at least one GSTM3*B allele (GSTM3 AB and GSTM3 BB combined) had advanced tumour T-stage, increasing Dukes' stage, higher frequency of distant metastases and shorter survival (Holley et al., 2006) Thus, the GSTM3 AA genotype was suggested to be associated with improved prognosis of CRC especially in patients with GSTM1 null genotype (Holley et al., 2006). Analogous results have been reported by Loktionov et al. who found associations between GSTM3*B frequency in patients with distal colorectal cancers particularly when combined with the GSTM1 null genotype (Loktionov et al., 2001).

A very recent study investigated the association between *GSTO2 N142D (Asn142Asp)* genetic polymorphism and susceptibility to colorectal cancer and reported that ND and DD genotypes were not associated with CRC risk, in comparison with the NN genotype. However subjects with NN genotype and positive family history were at high risk to develop colorectal cancer in comparison with subjects with DD or ND genotypes and negative family history. Thus, GSTO2 NN genotype was suggested to increase the risk of colorectal cancer in persons with positive family history for cancer in the first degree relatives (Masoudi et al., 2010).

The common characteristic of the theta-class GSTs is their high affinity for the organic hydroperoxide species and particularly toward cumene hydroperoxide (GSTT2), underling the importance of GSTT2 activity in protection of cells against toxic ROS and lipid peroxidation products (Tan &Board, 1996), which are a major source of endogenous DNA damage and thus contribute significantly to cancer genesis and progression. In this respect efforts have been done to determine whether *GSTT2* promoter SNPs (-537G>A, -277T>C and -158G>A) are associated with colorectal cancer risk (Jang et al., 2007). Jang at al., reported that -537A allele was associated with colorectal cancer risk, while the -158A allele was protective against colorectal cancer, finally suggesting that SNPs and haplotypes of the *GSTT2* promoter region are associated with colorectal cancer risk in the Korean population (Jang et al., 2007). However, in a Caucasian population there was no such association of GSTT2 polymorphisms with the risk of CRC (Landi et al., 2005)

5. Role of GST-pi in cancer progression

The isoenzyme of class pi, GST-pi, acidic cytosolic protein, possesses unique enzymatic properties: broad substrate specificity (e.g. alkylating antitumor agents such as cisplatin derivatives), glutathione peroxidase activity towards lipid hydroperoxides, and high sensitivity to reactive oxygen species (ROS) (Tsuchida &Sato, 1992; de Bruin et al., 2000; Hoensch et al., 2002). As it was discussed above, GST-pi acts also non-catalytically as intracellular binding protein for a large number of non-substrate molecules of either endogeneous or exogenous origin, thus contributing to their intracellular transport, sequestration and disposition (Laisney et al., 1984; de Bruin et al., 2000; Hayes et al., 2005). Besides that, GST-pi plays a regulatory role in the MAP kinase pathway that participates in cellular survival and death signals via direct protein:protein interaction with c-Jun-N-terminal Kinase 1 (JNK1) and Apoptosis Signal-regulating Kinase (Ask1) (Adler et al., 1999; Tew &Ronai, 1999; Townsend &Tew, 2003; Hayes et al., 2005; Michael &Doherty, 2005).

Therefore, the increased protein levels and activity of GST-pi found in a variety of neoplastic cancers with different histological origins, including colorectal carcinoma (Moorghen et al., 1991; Ranganathan &Tew, 1991; de Bruin et al., 2000; Dogru-Abbasoglu et al., 2002; Murtagh et al., 2005), are debated as factors responsible, at least partly, for the progression and chemotherapy resistance, observed in many cancers (O'Brien &Tew, 1996; Tew &Ronai, 1999; Townsend &Tew, 2003; Michael &Doherty, 2005).

Earlier we reported our preliminary results concerning the survival of 76 patients with primary CRC according to the level of expression of GST-pi determined by immunohistochemistry (Vlaykova et al., 2005). Further we extended the patient population to 132 and found that the tumors varied according to their GST-pi immune staining: there were tumors negative for GST-pi, others had weak staining and finally tumors exhibiting strong and very strong immune reaction for GST-pi (Figure 2).

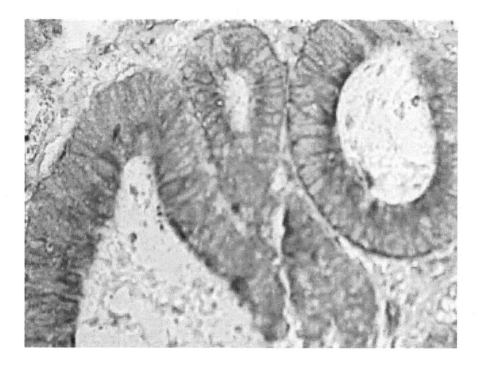

Fig. 2. Intensive cytoplasmic immune reaction for GST-pi in the cells of the tumor glands of a well-differentiated primary colorectal cancer (x 400).

The results concerning survival of the patients with CRC with different level of expression of GST-pi, showed that the higher expression of GST-pi was significantly associated with shorter survival period after surgical therapy (median of 19 months) compared to those negative or with weak GST-pi staining (median of 58 months, p=0.004, Log-rang test) (Figure 3A). This statistically significant association persisted also after stratification for pTNM staging (stage I/II vs. Stage III/IV, p=0.005, Log-rank test) (Figure 3B).

Interestingly, the strong expression of GST-pi retained its impact as unfavorable prognostic factor both for the patients who received an adjuvant chemotherapy (n=63, p=0.008, Log-rank test) (Figure 4A) and for the once without such treatment (n=66, p=0.019, Log-rank test) (Figure 4B). Hence, we suggested that the strong expression of GST-pi may lead to lower effectiveness of the administered anticancer drugs or to inhibiting the apoptosis, thus influencing the survival of the patients.

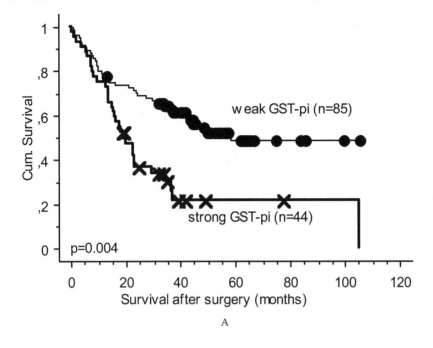

A

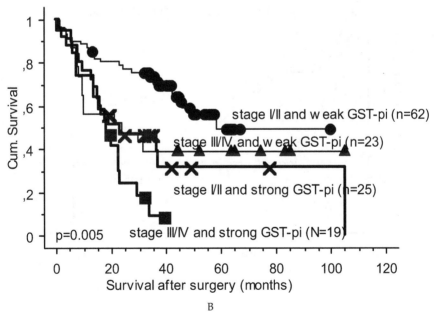

B

Fig. 3. Survival of the whole studied patient population with colorectal carcinoma after surgical treatment according to the level of expression of GST-pi in tumor cells (**A**) and after stratification to pTNM staging (**B**).

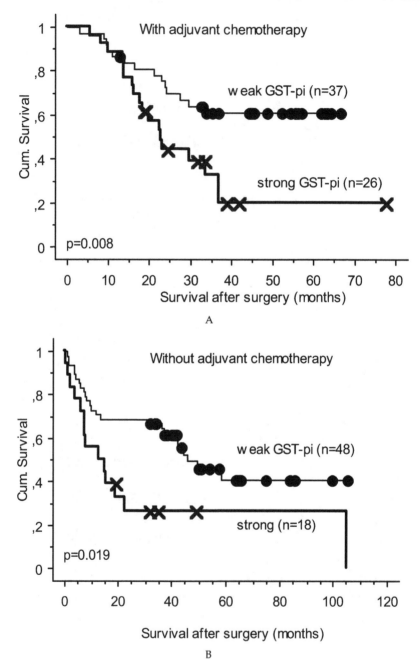

Fig. 4. Survival according to the GST-pi expression of patients with CRC subjected to adjuvant chemotherapy (A), Association between the level of expression of GST-pi and survival of patients, who did not receive adjuvant chemotherapy (B).

Previously, we also described expression of GST-pi in chromogranin A-positive endocrine cells in colorectal cancers, which also expressed some other antioxidant enzymes, such as SOD1 and SOD2 (Gulubova &Vlaykova, 2010). Moreover, we found that patients having tumors with GST-pi-positive endocrine cells have an unfavorable prognosis. We suggest that not the neuroendocrine differentiation in general, but the presence of endocrine cells with activated antioxidant defense and probably higher metabolic activity might determine a more aggressive type of cancer leading to worse prognosis for patients (Gulubova &Vlaykova, 2010).

The observed heterogeneous expression of GST-pi in tumor glands could be due to different genetic or epigenetic factors. We suppose that the reactive oxygen species, which are generated in high amount during the metabolism of tumor cells could be such factors resulting in overproduction of GST-pi . These ROS are found to induce the expression of the genes of GST-pi and other phase II xenobiotic-biotransformating enzymes (O'Brien &Tew, 1996; Tew &Ronai, 1999; Hoensch et al., 2002). There is a growing evidence that these genes have regulatory sequences recognized by Nrf2 transcription factor, which in turn is regulated by the antioxidant response element (ARE) (O'Brien &Tew, 1996; Tew &Ronai, 1999; Hoensch et al., 2002). Another Zn-dependent mechanism for ROS-induced expression of genes coding GST-pi and other antioxidant enzymes has been proposed (Chung et al., 2005).

Another factor, resulting in overproduction of GST-pi, could be its gene amplification. Such genetic change has been proven for squamous cell carcinoma of head and neck. *GSTP1* amplification has been shown to be a common event and proposed to be associated with cisplatin resistance and poor clinical outcome in head and neck cancer patients treated with cisplatin-based therapy (Wang et al., 1997; Cullen et al., 2003).

On the other hand, the lack of or the low expression of GST-pi could be due to the somatic inactivation by hypermethylation of promoter sequences of GST-pi gene (Yang et al., 2003; Lasabova et al., 2010). Such hypermethylation is the most common event (about 90%) described in prostate adenocarcinoma (Jeronimo et al., 2002).

The results of our studies demonstrated the association between high expression level of GST-pi and unfavorable prognosis for the patients with colorectal carcinoma. This association was valid both for patients who had received adjuvant chemotherapy and for those without such treatment. We suppose that the shorter survival of patients with higher GST-pi could be due to lowering of the effectiveness of administered antineoplastic agents. The high protein level of GST-pi could contribute to this process either via its direct detoxifying effect towards some of the drugs (oxaliplatin) (O'Brien &Tew, 1996; Michael &Doherty, 2005), or via the inhibitory effect of GST-pi on MAP kinase signal pathways of apoptosis, triggered by 5-FU, mitomicin C, camtothecin or other antitumor drugs included in mono- or polychemotherapeutic regiments (Adler et al., 1999; Townsend &Tew, 2003; Hayes et al., 2005; Michael &Doherty, 2005).

The observed association of high GST-pi level with worse prognosis of the patients, who did not received chemotherapy, could also be explained with the ability of this enzyme protein directly to interact with and inhibit proteins involved in regulation of apoptosis (JNK1 and Ask1) (Adler et al., 1999; Townsend &Tew, 2003; Hayes et al., 2005; Michael &Doherty, 2005). In tumors, the high levels of free radicals, which in general are triggering factors and mediators of apoptosis, probably stimulate the expression of GST-pi that can lead to suppression of apoptosis. As a result, the decreased apoptosis can lead to increased tumor burden, which negatively affects patients survival.

6. Conclusions

Colorectal cancer (CRC) is a neoplasm that occurs at high frequency worldwide, including Bulgaria. CRC is a complex and multifactorial disease, since several environmental and endogenous factors, including personal genetic characteristics, are implicated in its etiology, pathogenesis, progression and outcome. The members of the glutathione-S-tranferase (GST) family are important candidates for involvement in susceptibility to carcinogen-associated CRC and for developing of tumor chemotherapy resistance. In this work we presented a short overview of the main cellular functions of some of the GST isoenzymes, their polymorphic nature, and their role as risk factors for development of CRC and of resistance to chemotherapy. We also presented the results of our studies focused on the role of the null *GSTM1* and *GSTT1* polymorphisms, the *Ile*[105]*Val* SNP in *GSTP1* and GST-pi expression as risk and prognostic factors in primary CRC. In conclusion, we suggest that the expression level of GST-pi in primary tumors could be a valuable prognostic factor for patients with colorectal carcinoma both treated with adjuvant chemotherapy and those not subjected to such therapy.

7. References

Adler, V., Yin, Z., Fuchs, S.Y., Benezra, M., Rosario, L., Tew, K.D., Pincus, M.R., Sardana, M., Henderson, C.J., Wolf, C.R., Davis, R.J. & Ronai, Z. (1999). Regulation of JNK signaling by GSTp. *Embo J*, 18, 1321-34.

Agalliu, I., Lin, D.W., Salinas, C.A., Feng, Z. & Stanford, J.L. (2006). Polymorphisms in the glutathione S-transferase M1, T1, and P1 genes and prostate cancer prognosis. *Prostate*, 66, 1535-41.

Alexandrie, A.K., Rannug, A., Juronen, E., Tasa, G. & Warholm, M. (2002). Detection and characterization of a novel functional polymorphism in the GSTT1 gene. *Pharmacogenetics*, 12, 613-9.

Ali-Osman, F., Akande, O., Antoun, G., Mao, J.X. & Buolamwini, J. (1997). Molecular cloning, characterization, and expression in Escherichia coli of full-length cDNAs of three human glutathione S-transferase Pi gene variants. Evidence for differential catalytic activity of the encoded proteins. *J Biol Chem*, 272, 10004-12.

Andonova, I.E., Justenhoven, C., Winter, S., Hamann, U., Baisch, C., Rabstein, S., Spickenheuer, A., Harth, V., Pesch, B., Bruning, T., Ko, Y.D., Ganev, V. & Brauch, H. (2009). No evidence for glutathione S-transferases GSTA2, GSTM2, GSTO1, GSTO2, and GSTZ1 in breast cancer risk. *Breast Cancer Res Treat*, 121, 497-502.

Andonova, I.E., Sarueva, R.B., Horvath, A.D., Simeonov, V.A., Dimitrov, P.S., Petropoulos, E.A. & Ganev, V.S. (2004). Balkan endemic nephropathy and genetic variants of glutathione S-transferases. *J Nephrol*, 17, 390-8.

Ates, N.A., Tamer, L., Ates, C., Ercan, B., Elipek, T., Ocal, K. & Camdeviren, H. (2005). Glutathione S-transferase M1, T1, P1 genotypes and risk for development of colorectal cancer. *Biochem Genet*, 43, 149-63.

Blackburn, A.C., Coggan, M., Tzeng, H.F., Lantum, H., Polekhina, G., Parker, M.W., Anders, M.W. & Board, P.G. (2001). GSTZ1d: a new allele of glutathione transferase zeta and maleylacetoacetate isomerase. *Pharmacogenetics*, 11, 671-8.

Board, P.G. (2011). The omega-class glutathione transferases: structure, function, and genetics. *Drug Metab Rev*, 43, 226-35.

Board, P.G., Coggan, M., Chelvanayagam, G., Easteal, S., Jermiin, L.S., Schulte, G.K., Danley, D.E., Hoth, L.R., Griffor, M.C., Kamath, A.V., Rosner, M.H., Chrunyk, B.A., Perregaux, D.E., Gabel, C.A., Geoghegan, K.F. & Pandit, J. (2000). Identification, characterization, and crystal structure of the Omega class glutathione transferases. *J Biol Chem*, 275, 24798-806.

Bolt, H.M. & Thier, R. (2006). Relevance of the deletion polymorphisms of the glutathione S-transferases GSTT1 and GSTM1 in pharmacology and toxicology. *Curr Drug Metab*, 7, 613-28.

Bostrom, C.E., Gerde, P., Hanberg, A., Jernstrom, B., Johansson, C., Kyrklund, T., Rannug, A., Tornqvist, M., Victorin, K. & Westerholm, R. (2002). Cancer risk assessment, indicators, and guidelines for polycyclic aromatic hydrocarbons in the ambient air. *Environ Health Perspect*, 3, 451-88.

Cantor, K.P., Villanueva, C.M., Silverman, D.T., Figueroa, J.D., Real, F.X., Garcia-Closas, M., Malats, N., Chanock, S., Yeager, M., Tardon, A., Garcia-Closas, R., Serra, C., Carrato, A., Castano-Vinyals, G., Samanic, C., Rothman, N. & Kogevinas, M. (2010). Polymorphisms in GSTT1, GSTZ1, and CYP2E1, disinfection by-products, and risk of bladder cancer in Spain. *Environ Health Perspect*, 118, 1545-50.

Cho, S.G., Lee, Y.H., Park, H.S., Ryoo, K., Kang, K.W., Park, J., Eom, S.J., Kim, M.J., Chang, T.S., Choi, S.Y., Shim, J., Kim, Y., Dong, M.S., Lee, M.J., Kim, S.G., Ichijo, H. & Choi, E.J. (2001). Glutathione S-transferase mu modulates the stress-activated signals by suppressing apoptosis signal-regulating kinase 1. *J Biol Chem*, 276, 12749-55.

Chung, M.J., Walker, P.A., Brown, R.W. & Hogstrand, C. (2005). ZINC-mediated gene expression offers protection against H2O2-induced cytotoxicity. *Toxicol Appl Pharmacol*, 205, 225-36.

Coggan, M., Whitbread, L., Whittington, A. & Board, P. (1998). Structure and organization of the human theta-class glutathione S-transferase and D-dopachrome tautomerase gene complex. *Biochem J*, 334, 617-23.

Coles, B., Nowell, S.A., MacLeod, S.L., Sweeney, C., Lang, N.P. & Kadlubar, F.F. (2001). The role of human glutathione S-transferases (hGSTs) in the detoxification of the food-derived carcinogen metabolite N-acetoxy-PhIP, and the effect of a polymorphism in hGSTA1 on colorectal cancer risk. *Mutat Res*, 482, 3-10.

Coles, B., Yang, M., Lang, N.P. & Kadlubar, F.F. (2000). Expression of hGSTP1 alleles in human lung and catalytic activity of the native protein variants towards 1-chloro-2,4-dinitrobenzene, 4-vinylpyridine and (+)-anti benzo[a]pyrene-7,8-diol-9,10-oxide. *Cancer Lett*, 156, 167-75.

Cotton, S.C., Sharp, L., Little, J. & Brockton, N. (2000). Glutathione S-transferase polymorphisms and colorectal cancer: a HuGE review. *Am J Epidemiol*, 151, 7-32.

Cullen, K.J., Newkirk, K.A., Schumaker, L.M., Aldosari, N., Rone, J.D. & Haddad, B.R. (2003). Glutathione S-transferase pi amplification is associated with cisplatin resistance in head and neck squamous cell carcinoma cell lines and primary tumors. *Cancer Res*, 63, 8097-102.

de Bruin, W.C., Wagenmans, M.J. & Peters, W.H. (2000). Expression of glutathione S-transferase alpha, P1-1 and T1-1 in the human gastrointestinal tract. *Jpn J Cancer Res*, 91, 310-6.

de Jong, M.M., Nolte, I.M., te Meerman, G.J., van der Graaf, W.T., de Vries, E.G., Sijmons, R.H., Hofstra, R.M. & Kleibeuker, J.H. (2002). Low-penetrance genes and their involvement in colorectal cancer susceptibility. *Cancer Epidemiol Biomarkers Prev*, 11, 1332-52.

Di Pietro, G., Magno, L.A. & Rios-Santos, F. (2010). Glutathione S-transferases: an overview in cancer research. *Expert Opin Drug Metab Toxicol*, 6, 153-70.

Dimov, D., Vlaykova, T., Shazie, S. & Ilieva, V. (2008). Investigation of GSTP1, GSTM1 and GSTT1 gene polymorphisms and susceptibility to COPD. . *Trakia J Sci*, 6(4), , 1-8.

Dogru-Abbasoglu, S., Mutlu-Turkoglu, U., Turkoglu, S., Erbil, Y., Barbaros, U., Uysal, M. & Aykac-Toker, G. (2002). Glutathione S-transferase-pi in malignant tissues and plasma of human colorectal and gastric cancers. *J Cancer Res Clin Oncol*, 128, 91-5.

Dorion, S., Lambert, H. & Landry, J. (2002). Activation of the p38 signaling pathway by heat shock involves the dissociation of glutathione S-transferase Mu from Ask1. *J Biol Chem*, 277, 30792-7.

Dulhunty, A., Gage, P., Curtis, S., Chelvanayagam, G. & Board, P. (2001). The glutathione transferase structural family includes a nuclear chloride channel and a ryanodine receptor calcium release channel modulator. *J Biol Chem*, 276, 3319-23.

Eaton, D.L. & Bammler, T.K. (1999). Concise review of the glutathione S-transferases and their significance to toxicology. *Toxicol Sci*, 49, 156-64.

Economopoulos, K.P. & Sergentanis, T.N. (2010). GSTM1, GSTT1, GSTP1, GSTA1 and colorectal cancer risk: a comprehensive meta-analysis. *Eur J Cancer*, 46, 1617-31.

Emin, S., Yordanova, K., Dimov, D., Ilieva, V., Koychev, A., Prakova, G. & Vlaykova, T. (2009). Investigation of the role of null polymorphisms of glutathione-S-transferase genes (GST) for development of COPD and Bronchial asthma. *Eur J Med Res* 14 (Supplement II), 173.

Gao, Y., Cao, Y., Tan, A., Liao, C., Mo, Z. & Gao, F. (2010). Glutathione S-Transferase M1 Polymorphism and Sporadic Colorectal Cancer Risk: An Updating Meta-Analysis and HuGE Review of 36 Case-Control Studies. *Annals of Epidemiology*, 20, 108-121.

Gao, Y., Pan, X., Su, T., Mo, Z., Cao, Y. & Gao, F. (2009). Glutathione S-transferase P1 Ile105Val polymorphism and colorectal cancer risk: A meta-analysis and HuGE review. *European Journal of Cancer*, 45, 3303-3314.

Gsur, A., Haidinger, G., Hinteregger, S., Bernhofer, G., Schatzl, G., Madersbacher, S., Marberger, M., Vutuc, C. & Micksche, M. (2001). Polymorphisms of glutathione-S-transferase genes (GSTP1, GSTM1 and GSTT1) and prostate-cancer risk. *Int J Cancer*, 95, 152-5.

Gulubova, M. & Vlaykova, T. (2010). Expression of the xenobiotic- and reactive oxygen species-detoxifying enzymes, GST-pi, Cu/Zn-SOD, and Mn-SOD in the endocrine cells of colorectal cancer. *Int J Colorectal Dis*, 25, 1397-405.

Guy, C.A., Hoogendoorn, B., Smith, S.K., Coleman, S., O'Donovan, M.C. & Buckland, P.R. (2004). Promoter polymorphisms in glutathione-S-transferase genes affect transcription. *Pharmacogenetics*, 14, 45-51.

Harries, L.W., Stubbins, M.J., Forman, D., Howard, G.C. & Wolf, C.R. (1997). Identification of genetic polymorphisms at the glutathione S-transferase Pi locus and association with susceptibility to bladder, testicular and prostate cancer. *Carcinogenesis*, 18, 641-4.

Hayes, J.D., Flanagan, J.U. & Jowsey, I.R. (2005). Glutathione transferases. *Annu Rev Pharmacol Toxicol*, 45, 51-88.

Hayes, J.D. & Pulford, D.J. (1995). The glutathione S-transferase supergene family: regulation of GST and the contribution of the isoenzymes to cancer chemoprotection and drug resistance. *Crit Rev Biochem Mol Biol,* 30, 445-600.

Hayes, J.D. & Strange, R.C. (1995). Potential contribution of the glutathione S-transferase supergene family to resistance to oxidative stress. *Free Radic Res,* 22, 193-207.

He, J.Q., Connett, J.E., Anthonisen, N.R., Pare, P.D. & Sandford, A.J. (2004). Glutathione S-transferase variants and their interaction with smoking on lung function. *Am J Respir Crit Care Med,* 170, 388-94.

Hoensch, H., Morgenstern, I., Petereit, G., Siepmann, M., Peters, W.H., Roelofs, H.M. & Kirch, W. (2002). Influence of clinical factors, diet, and drugs on the human upper gastrointestinal glutathione system. *Gut,* 50, 235-40.

Holley, S.L., Rajagopal, R., Hoban, P.R., Deakin, M., Fawole, A.S., Elder, J.B., Elder, J., Smith, V., Strange, R.C. & Fryer, A.A. (2006). Polymorphisms in the glutathione S-transferase mu cluster are associated with tumour progression and patient outcome in colorectal cancer. *Int J Oncol,* 28, 231-6.

Inskip, A., Elexperu-Camiruaga, J., Buxton, N., Dias, P.S., MacIntosh, J., Campbell, D., Jones, P.W., Yengi, L., Talbot, J.A., Strange, R.C. & et al. (1995). Identification of polymorphism at the glutathione S-transferase, GSTM3 locus: evidence for linkage with GSTM1*A. *Biochem J,* 312, 713-6.

Ishigaki, S., Abramovitz, M. & Listowsky, I. (1989). Glutathione-S-transferases are major cytosolic thyroid hormone binding proteins. *Arch Biochem Biophys,* 273, 265-72.

Jang, S.G., Kim, I.J., Kang, H.C., Park, H.W., Ahn, S.A., Yoon, H.J., Kim, K., Shin, H.R., Lee, J.S. & Park, J.G. (2007). GSTT2 promoter polymorphisms and colorectal cancer risk. *BMC Cancer,* 7, 16.

Jeronimo, C., Varzim, G., Henrique, R., Oliveira, J., Bento, M.J., Silva, C., Lopes, C. & Sidransky, D. (2002). I105V polymorphism and promoter methylation of the GSTP1 gene in prostate adenocarcinoma. *Cancer Epidemiol Biomarkers Prev,* 11, 445-50.

Johansson, A.S. & Mannervik, B. (2001). Human glutathione transferase A3-3, a highly efficient catalyst of double-bond isomerization in the biosynthetic pathway of steroid hormones. *J Biol Chem,* 276, 33061-5.

Kampranis, S.C., Damianova, R., Atallah, M., Toby, G., Kondi, G., Tsichlis, P.N. & Makris, A.M. (2000). A novel plant glutathione S-transferase/peroxidase suppresses Bax lethality in yeast. *J Biol Chem,* 275, 29207-16.

Katoh, T., Yamano, Y., Tsuji, M. & Watanabe, M. (2008). Genetic polymorphisms of human cytosol glutathione S-transferases and prostate cancer. *Pharmacogenomics,* 9, 93-104.

Kiyohara, C. (2000). Genetic polymorphism of enzymes involved in xenobiotic metabolism and the risk of colorectal cancer. *J Epidemiol,* 10, 349-60.

Kote-Jarai, Z., Easton, D., Edwards, S.M., Jefferies, S., Durocher, F., Jackson, R.A., Singh, R., Ardern-Jones, A., Murkin, A., Dearnaley, D.P., Shearer, R., Kirby, R., Houlston, R. & Eeles, R. (2001). Relationship between glutathione S-transferase M1, P1 and T1 polymorphisms and early onset prostate cancer. *Pharmacogenetics,* 11, 325-30.

Koutros, S., Berndt, S.I., Sinha, R., Ma, X., Chatterjee, N., Alavanja, M.C., Zheng, T., Huang, W.Y., Hayes, R.B. & Cross, A.J. (2009). Xenobiotic metabolizing gene variants, dietary heterocyclic amine intake, and risk of prostate cancer. *Cancer Res,* 69, 1877-84.

Kury, S., Buecher, B., Robiou-du-Pont, S., Scoul, C., Colman, H., Le Neel, T., Le Houerou, C., Faroux, R., Ollivry, J., Lafraise, B., Chupin, L.D., Sebille, V. & Bezieau, S. (2008). Low-penetrance alleles predisposing to sporadic colorectal cancers: a French case-controlled genetic association study. *BMC Cancer, 8*, 326.

Laborde, E. (2010). Glutathione transferases as mediators of signaling pathways involved in cell proliferation and cell death. *Cell Death Differ, 17*, 1373-80.

Laisney, V., Nguyen Van, C., Gross, M.S. & Frezal, J. (1984). Human genes for glutathione S-transferases. *Hum Genet, 68*, 221-7.

Landi, S., Gemignani, F., Moreno, V., Gioia-Patricola, L., Chabrier, A., Guino, E., Navarro, M., de Oca, J., Capella, G. & Canzian, F. (2005). A comprehensive analysis of phase I and phase II metabolism gene polymorphisms and risk of colorectal cancer. *Pharmacogenet Genomics, 15*, 535-46.

Lasabova, Z., Tilandyova, P., Kajo, K., Zubor, P., Burjanivova, T., Danko, J. & Plank, L. (2010). Hypermethylation of the GSTP1 promoter region in breast cancer is associated with prognostic clinicopathological parameters. *Neoplasma, 57*, 35-40.

Liao, L.H., Zhang, H., Lai, M.P., Lau, K.W., Lai, A.K., Zhang, J.H., Wang, Q., Wei, W., Chai, J.H., Lung, M.L., Tai, S.S. & Wu, M. (2007). The association of CYP2C9 gene polymorphisms with colorectal carcinoma in Han Chinese. *Clin Chim Acta, 380*, 191-6.

Litwack, G., Ketterer, B. & Arias, I.M. (1971). Ligandin: a hepatic protein which binds steroids, bilirubin, carcinogens and a number of exogenous organic anions. *Nature, 234*, 466-7.

Liu, X., Campbell, M.R., Pittman, G.S., Faulkner, E.C., Watson, M.A. & Bell, D.A. (2005). Expression-based discovery of variation in the human glutathione S-transferase M3 promoter and functional analysis in a glioma cell line using allele-specific chromatin immunoprecipitation. *Cancer Res, 65*, 99-104.

Lo Bello, M., Nuccetelli, M., Caccuri, A.M., Stella, L., Parker, M.W., Rossjohn, J., McKinstry, W.J., Mozzi, A.F., Federici, G., Polizio, F., Pedersen, J.Z. & Ricci, G. (2001). Human glutathione transferase P1-1 and nitric oxide carriers; a new role for an old enzyme. *J Biol Chem, 276*, 42138-45.

Loktionov, A., Watson, M.A., Gunter, M., Stebbings, W.S., Speakman, C.T. & Bingham, S.A. (2001). Glutathione-S-transferase gene polymorphisms in colorectal cancer patients: interaction between GSTM1 and GSTM3 allele variants as a risk-modulating factor. *Carcinogenesis, 22*, 1053-60.

Manevich, Y., Feinstein, S.I. & Fisher, A.B. (2004). Activation of the antioxidant enzyme 1-CYS peroxiredoxin requires glutathionylation mediated by heterodimerization with pi GST. *Proc Natl Acad Sci U S A, 101*, 3780-5.

Martinez, C., Martin, F., Fernandez, J.M., Garcia-Martin, E., Sastre, J., Diaz-Rubio, M., Agundez, J.A. & Ladero, J.M. (2006). Glutathione S-transferases mu 1, theta 1, pi 1, alpha 1 and mu 3 genetic polymorphisms and the risk of colorectal and gastric cancers in humans. *Pharmacogenomics, 7*, 711-8.

Masoudi, M., Saadat, I., Omidvari, S. & Saadat, M. (2010). Association between N142D genetic polymorphism of GSTO2 and susceptibility to colorectal cancer. *Mol Biol Rep, 27*.

McIlwain, C.C., Townsend, D.M. & Tew, K.D. (2006). Glutathione S-transferase polymorphisms: cancer incidence and therapy. *Oncogene, 25*, 1639-48.

McLellan, R.A., Oscarson, M., Alexandrie, A.K., Seidegard, J., Evans, D.A., Rannug, A. & Ingelman-Sundberg, M. (1997). Characterization of a human glutathione S-transferase mu cluster containing a duplicated GSTM1 gene that causes ultrarapid enzyme activity. *Mol Pharmacol*, 52, 958-65.

Michael, M. & Doherty, M.M. (2005). Tumoral drug metabolism: overview and its implications for cancer therapy. *J Clin Oncol*, 23, 205-29.

Mitrunen, K., Jourenkova, N., Kataja, V., Eskelinen, M., Kosma, V.M., Benhamou, S., Vainio, H., Uusitupa, M. & Hirvonen, A. (2001). Glutathione S-transferase M1, M3, P1, and T1 genetic polymorphisms and susceptibility to breast cancer. *Cancer Epidemiol Biomarkers Prev*, 10, 229-36.

Moorghen, M., Cairns, J., Forrester, L.M., Hayes, J.D., Hall, A., Cattan, A.R., Wolf, C.R. & Harris, A.L. (1991). Enhanced expression of glutathione S-transferases in colorectal carcinoma compared to non-neoplastic mucosa. *Carcinogenesis*, 12, 13-7.

Morgenstern, R., Zhang, J. & Johansson, K. (2011). Microsomal glutathione transferase 1: mechanism and functional roles. *Drug Metab Rev*, 43, 300-6.

Moyer, A.M., Sun, Z., Batzler, A.J., Li, L., Schaid, D.J., Yang, P. & Weinshilboum, R.M. (2010). Glutathione pathway genetic polymorphisms and lung cancer survival after platinum-based chemotherapy. *Cancer Epidemiol Biomarkers Prev*, 19, 811-21.

Murtagh, E., Heaney, L., Gingles, J., Shepherd, R., Kee, F., Patterson, C. & MacMahon, J. (2005). Prevalence of obstructive lung disease in a general population sample: the NICECOPD study. *Eur J Epidemiol*, 20, 443-53.

O'Brien, M.L. & Tew, K.D. (1996). Glutathione and related enzymes in multidrug resistance. *Eur J Cancer*, 6, 967-78.

Pearson, W.R., Vorachek, W.R., Xu, S.J., Berger, R., Hart, I., Vannais, D. & Patterson, D. (1993). Identification of class-mu glutathione transferase genes GSTM1-GSTM5 on human chromosome 1p13. *Am J Hum Genet*, 53, 220-33.

Perera, F.P. (1997). Environment and cancer: who are susceptible? *Science*, 278, 1068-73.

Pistorius, S., Goergens, H., Engel, C., Plaschke, J., Krueger, S., Hoehl, R., Saeger, H.D. & Schackert, H.K. (2007). N-Acetyltransferase (NAT) 2 acetylator status and age of tumour onset in patients with sporadic and familial, microsatellite stable (MSS) colorectal cancer. *Int J Colorectal Dis*, 22, 137-43.

Potter, J.D. (1999). Colorectal cancer: molecules and populations. *J Natl Cancer Inst*, 91, 916-32.

Ranganathan, S. & Tew, K.D. (1991). Immunohistochemical localization of glutathione S-transferases alpha, mu, and pi in normal tissue and carcinomas from human colon. *Carcinogenesis*, 12, 2383-7.

Reszka, E. & Wasowicz, W. (2001). Significance of genetic polymorphisms in glutathione S-transferase multigene family and lung cancer risk. *Int J Occup Med Environ Health*, 14, 99-113.

Reszka, E., Wasowicz, W. & Gromadzinska, J. (2007). Antioxidant defense markers modulated by glutathione S-transferase genetic polymorphism: results of lung cancer case-control study. *Genes Nutr*, 2, 287-94.

Romero, R.Z., Morales, R., Garcia, F., Huarriz, M., Bandres, E., De la Haba, J., Gomez, A., Aranda, E. & Garcia-Foncillas, J. (2006). Potential application of GSTT1-null genotype in predicting toxicity associated to 5-fluouracil irinotecan and leucovorin regimen in advanced stage colorectal cancer patients. *Oncol Rep*, 16, 497-503.

Sau, A., Pellizzari Tregno, F., Valentino, F., Federici, G. & Caccuri, A.M. (2010). Glutathione transferases and development of new principles to overcome drug resistance. *Arch Biochem Biophys*, 500, 116-22.

Sheehan, D., Meade, G., Foley, V.M. & Dowd, C.A. (2001). Structure, function and evolution of glutathione transferases: implications for classification of non-mammalian members of an ancient enzyme superfamily. *Biochem J*, 360, 1-16.

Sorensen, M., Raaschou-Nielsen, O., Brasch-Andersen, C., Tjonneland, A., Overvad, K. & Autrup, H. (2007). Interactions between GSTM1, GSTT1 and GSTP1 polymorphisms and smoking and intake of fruit and vegetables in relation to lung cancer. *Lung Cancer*, 55, 137-44.

Sprenger, R., Schlagenhaufer, R., Kerb, R., Bruhn, C., Brockmoller, J., Roots, I. & Brinkmann, U. (2000). Characterization of the glutathione S-transferase GSTT1 deletion: discrimination of all genotypes by polymerase chain reaction indicates a trimodular genotype-phenotype correlation. *Pharmacogenetics*, 10, 557-65.

Steinhoff, C., Franke, K.H., Golka, K., Thier, R., Romer, H.C., Rotzel, C., Ackermann, R. & Schulz, W.A. (2000). Glutathione transferase isozyme genotypes in patients with prostate and bladder carcinoma. *Arch Toxicol*, 74, 521-6.

Stoehlmacher, J., Park, D.J., Zhang, W., Groshen, S., Tsao-Wei, D.D., Yu, M.C. & Lenz, H.J. (2002). Association between glutathione S-transferase P1, T1, and M1 genetic polymorphism and survival of patients with metastatic colorectal cancer. *J Natl Cancer Inst*, 94, 936-42.

Sundberg, K., Johansson, A.S., Stenberg, G., Widersten, M., Seidel, A., Mannervik, B. & Jernstrom, B. (1998). Differences in the catalytic efficiencies of allelic variants of glutathione transferase P1-1 towards carcinogenic diol epoxides of polycyclic aromatic hydrocarbons. *Carcinogenesis*, 19, 433-6.

Sweeney, C., Coles, B.F., Nowell, S., Lang, N.P. & Kadlubar, F.F. (2002). Novel markers of susceptibility to carcinogens in diet: associations with colorectal cancer. *Toxicology*, 182, 83-7.

Tan, K.L. & Board, P.G. (1996). Purification and characterization of a recombinant human Theta-class glutathione transferase (GSTT2-2). *Biochem J*, 315, 727-32.

Tetlow, N. & Board, P.G. (2004). Functional polymorphism of human glutathione transferase A2. *Pharmacogenetics*, 14, 111-6.

Tetlow, N., Coggan, M., Casarotto, M.G. & Board, P.G. (2004). Functional polymorphism of human glutathione transferase A3: effects on xenobiotic metabolism and steroid biosynthesis. *Pharmacogenetics*, 14, 657-63.

Tetlow, N., Liu, D. & Board, P. (2001). Polymorphism of human Alpha class glutathione transferases. *Pharmacogenetics*, 11, 609-17.

Tew, K.D., Manevich, Y., Grek, C., Xiong, Y., Uys, J. & Townsend, D.M. (2011). The role of glutathione S-transferase P in signaling pathways and S-glutathionylation in cancer. *Free Radic Biol Med*, 51, 299-313.

Tew, K.D. & Ronai, Z. (1999). GST function in drug and stress response. *Drug Resist Updat*, 2, 143-147.

Townsend, D.M., Findlay, V.J., Fazilev, F., Ogle, M., Fraser, J., Saavedra, J.E., Ji, X., Keefer, L.K. & Tew, K.D. (2006). A glutathione S-transferase pi-activated prodrug causes kinase activation concurrent with S-glutathionylation of proteins. *Mol Pharmacol*, 69, 501-8.

Townsend, D.M., Findlay, V.L. & Tew, K.D. (2005). Glutathione S-transferases as regulators of kinase pathways and anticancer drug targets. *Methods Enzymol*, 401, 287-307.

Townsend, D.M., Manevich, Y., He, L., Hutchens, S., Pazoles, C.J. & Tew, K.D. (2009). Novel role for glutathione S-transferase pi. Regulator of protein S-Glutathionylation following oxidative and nitrosative stress. *J Biol Chem*, 284, 436-45.

Townsend, D.M. & Tew, K.D. (2003). The role of glutathione-S-transferase in anti-cancer drug resistance. *Oncogene*, 22, 7369-75.

Tsuchida, S. & Sato, K. (1992). Glutathione transferases and cancer. *Crit Rev Biochem Mol Biol*, 27, 337-84.

van der Logt, E.M., Bergevoet, S.M., Roelofs, H.M., van Hooijdonk, Z., te Morsche, R.H., Wobbes, T., de Kok, J.B., Nagengast, F.M. & Peters, W.H. (2004). Genetic polymorphisms in UDP-glucuronosyltransferases and glutathione S-transferases and colorectal cancer risk. *Carcinogenesis*, 25, 2407-15.

Vasieva, O. (2011). The many faces of glutathione transferase pi. *Curr Mol Med*, 11, 129-39.

Villafania, A., Anwar, K., Amar, S., Chie, L., Way, D., Chung, D.L., Adler, V., Ronai, Z., Brandt-Rauf, P.W., Yamaizumii, Z., Kung, H.F. & Pincus, M.R. (2000). Glutathione-S-Transferase as a selective inhibitor of oncogenic ras-p21-induced mitogenic signaling through blockade of activation of jun by jun-N-terminal kinase. *Ann Clin Lab Sci*, 30, 57-64.

Vlaykova, T., Gulubova, M., Vlaykova, D., Cirovski, G., Yovchev, Y., Dimov, D. & Chilingirov, P. (2009). Possible Influence of GSTM1 and GSTT1 null genotype on the risk for development of sporadic colorectal cancer. *Biotechnol & Biotechnol Equip.*, 23, 1084-1089.

Vlaykova, T., Gulubova, M., Vlaykova, D., Yaneva, K., Cirovski, G., Chilingirov, P. & Stratiev, S. (2005). Expression of GST-pi and its impact on the survival of patients treated with chemotherapy for colorectal cancer. . *Trakia J Sci* 3, 39-44.

Vlaykova, T., Miteva, L., Gulubova, M. & Stanilova, S. (2007). Ile(105)Val GSTP1 polymorphism and susceptibility to colorectal carcinoma in Bulgarian population. *Int J Colorectal Dis*, 22, 1209-15.

Wang, T., Arifoglu, P., Ronai, Z. & Tew, K.D. (2001). Glutathione S-transferase P1-1 (GSTP1-1) inhibits c-Jun N-terminal kinase (JNK1) signaling through interaction with the C terminus. *J Biol Chem*, 276, 20999-1003.

Wang, X., Pavelic, Z.P., Li, Y., Gleich, L., Gartside, P.S., Pavelic, L., Gluckman, J.L. & Stambrook, P.J. (1997). Overexpression and amplification of glutathione S-transferase pi gene in head and neck squamous cell carcinomas. *Clin Cancer Res*, 3, 111-4.

Watson, M.A., Stewart, R.K., Smith, G.B., Massey, T.E. & Bell, D.A. (1998). Human glutathione S-transferase P1 polymorphisms: relationship to lung tissue enzyme activity and population frequency distribution. *Carcinogenesis*, 19, 275-80.

Welfare, M., Monesola Adeokun, A., Bassendine, M.F. & Daly, A.K. (1999). Polymorphisms in GSTP1, GSTM1, and GSTT1 and susceptibility to colorectal cancer. *Cancer Epidemiol Biomarkers Prev*, 8, 289-92.

Whitbread, A.K., Masoumi, A., Tetlow, N., Schmuck, E., Coggan, M. & Board, P.G. (2005). Characterization of the omega class of glutathione transferases. *Methods Enzymol*, 401, 78-99.

Whitbread, A.K., Tetlow, N., Eyre, H.J., Sutherland, G.R. & Board, P.G. (2003). Characterization of the human Omega class glutathione transferase genes and associated polymorphisms. *Pharmacogenetics*, 13, 131-44.

Whyatt, R.M., Perera, F.P., Jedrychowski, W., Santella, R.M., Garte, S. & Bell, D.A. (2000). Association between polycyclic aromatic hydrocarbon-DNA adduct levels in maternal and newborn white blood cells and glutathione S-transferase P1 and CYP1A1 polymorphisms. *Cancer Epidemiol Biomarkers Prev*, 9, 207-12.

Wu, Y., Fan, Y., Xue, B., Luo, L., Shen, J., Zhang, S., Jiang, Y. & Yin, Z. (2006). Human glutathione S-transferase P1-1 interacts with TRAF2 and regulates TRAF2-ASK1 signals. *Oncogene*, 25, 5787-800.

Yang, B., Guo, M., Herman, J.G. & Clark, D.P. (2003). Aberrant promoter methylation profiles of tumor suppressor genes in hepatocellular carcinoma. *Am J Pathol*, 163, 1101-7.

Yu, K.D., Fan, L., Di, G.H., Yuan, W.T., Zheng, Y., Huang, W., Chen, A.X., Yang, C., Wu, J., Shen, Z.Z. & Shao, Z.M. (2009). Genetic variants in GSTM3 gene within GSTM4-GSTM2-GSTM1-GSTM5-GSTM3 cluster influence breast cancer susceptibility depending on GSTM1. *Breast Cancer Res Treat*, 121, 485-96.

Zhao, T., Singhal, S.S., Piper, J.T., Cheng, J., Pandya, U., Clark-Wronski, J., Awasthi, S. & Awasthi, Y.C. (1999). The role of human glutathione S-transferases hGSTA1-1 and hGSTA2-2 in protection against oxidative stress. *Arch Biochem Biophys*, 367, 216-24.

3

Distinct Pathologic Roles for Glycogen Synthase Kinase 3β in Colorectal Cancer Progression

Toshinari Minamoto[1], Masanori Kotake[1,3], Mitsutoshi Nakada[2],
Takeo Shimasaki[4], Yoshiharu Motoo[4] and Kazuyuki Kawakami[1]
[1]Division of Translational and Clinical Oncology, Cancer Research Institute,
[2]Department of Neurosurgery, Graduate School of Medical Science,
Kanazawa University, Kanazawa,
[3]Department of Surgery, Ishikawa Prefectural Central Hospital, Kanazawa,
[4]Department of Medical Oncology, Kanazawa Medical University, Uchinada, Ishikawa,
Japan

1. Introduction

Colorectal cancer (CRC) is the third most frequent cancer type and the second leading cause of cancer-related deaths worldwide (Cunningham et al., 2010; Jemal et al., 2010). This is despite the recent trend of stabilizing or declining rates for CRC incidence and mortality in economically developed countries (Center et al., 2009; Edwards et al., 2010; Umar & Greenwald, 2009). Surgical intervention is the initial treatment for most CRC patients. Continuous efforts to optimize surgery for patients with localized CRC has resulted in markedly improved 5-year and 10-year survival rates (Cunningham et al., 2010; Wu & Fazio, 2000). Given the large number of CRC patients who undergo curative surgery, there is now a substantial number who are susceptible to recurrent or metastatic tumors and could therefore benefit from additional systemic therapies. An increasing array of options and protocols for chemotherapies and biologically targeted therapies is now available for use in the adjuvant setting and for the treatment of recurrent and metastatic CRC.

Based on a more detailed knowledge of the molecular characteristics of CRC (Markowitz et al., 2009; Walther et al., 2009), biologically-based therapeutics have been developed for the treatment of advanced stage CRC patients. Currently approved agents for the treatment of advanced and metastatic CRC include therapeutic monoclonal antibodies that target vascular endothelial growth factor (VEGF) and epidermal growth factor receptor (EGFR). Despite a substantial biological rationale for the use of these new classes of therapeutic agents, large-scale clinical trials have observed only incremental clinical benefits for overall patient populations. Clearly, not all patients with recurrent and metastatic CRC benefit from these therapies. This is due to inherent and acquired resistance of tumors to the chemotherapeutic and biologically-based agents. Moreover, there are few reliable markers for predicting the therapeutic and adverse effects of these agents and that would allow patients who benefit from these systemic treatments to be identified. Therefore, new therapeutic targets are urgently required to further improve the survival of patients with recurrent and metastatic CRC. One such target may be glycogen synthase kinase 3β (GSK3β), a serine/threonine protein kinase that has recently been implicated in various human cancers.

In this Chapter, we briefly summarize the scientific basis and current status of systemic treatments for CRC, including combinations of surgery, chemotherapy and molecular target-directed therapy. Based on our published and ongoing studies, we then focus on GSK3β as an emerging therapeutic target in CRC and other cancer types. We describe the underlying biological mechanism that allows exploration of a novel therapeutic strategy for CRC involving the targeting of aberrant GSK3β.

2. Molecular basis of colorectal cancer

2.1 Multistep and multiple molecular alterations

Colorectal carcinogenesis displays all the major biological hallmarks of cancer (Hanahan & Weinberg, 2011). CRC evolves and develops through orchestrated, multistep genetic and epigenetic alterations in oncogenes, tumor suppressor genes and DNA mismatch repair genes. These include frequent aberrations in certain chromosomes, such as allelic imbalance at several chromosomal loci (e.g., chromosome 5q, 8p, 17p, 18q) and chromosome amplification and translocation. Various combinations of somatic and germ-line alterations in these genes and chromosomes characterize the different genotypes and phenotypes of sporadic and hereditary forms of CRC (Cunningham et al., 2010; Markowitz & Bertagnolli, 2009; Walther et al., 2009). Among the genes involved in the molecular process of CRC development, several genetic markers have been reported to harbor diagnostic and prognostic information and to predict the benefit from or resistance to systemic therapy (Ellis & Hicklin, 2009; Markowitz & Bertagnolli, 2009; Walther et al., 2009).

Recent advances in DNA sequencing technology have allowed sequencing of the entire coding genome of human cancer to become a reality. The high throughput, next-generation sequencing of 18,000 genes in the Reference Sequence data-base of the National Center for Biotechnology Information in the USA has identified cancer-associated somatic mutations in 848 genes. Amongst these, 140 are considered as candidate genes responsible for the development and phenotype of CRC (Sjöblom et al., 2006; Wood et al., 2007).

2.2 Oncogene addiction

The unrestrained survival and proliferation of cancer cells relies on distinct oncogenic signalling pathways in which various oncoproteins, growth factor receptors and their ligands are aberrantly activated, leading to the concept of "oncogene addiction" (Sharma & Settleman, 2007; Weinstein, 2002; Weinstein & Joe, 2006). In theory, acute ablation of oncogene function should lead to the rapid dissipation of its pro-survival signal in cancer cells, thus resulting in apoptotic cell death. This "oncogenic shock" concept underlies the strategy of molecular targeting in cancer therapy (Sharma et al., 2006). The scientific rationale behind the development and application of therapeutic monoclonal antibodies targeting VEGF and EGFR for the treatment of CRC is based on these concepts. Intriguingly, however, the EGFR expression level in primary CRC determined by immunohistochemistry was not observed to correlate with the efficacy of therapeutic anti-EGFR antibodies in clinical trials of metastatic CRC (Hecht et al., 2010; commented by Grothey, 2010).

3. Systemic treatment: An overview

Surgery remains the cornerstone for the cure of localized CRC (Cunningham et al., 2010; Wu & Fazio, 2000). For colon cancer, total resection of the primary tumor with ample surgical margins and regional lymphadenectomy are the requisites for curative surgery. For rectal cancer, curative resection includes total excision of the mesorectum with adequate circumferential and distal surgical margins (R0) and lymphadenectomy along the inferior mesenteric vessels. Laparoscopic surgery has now become prevalent and safe, with long-term oncological outcomes of CRC patients undergoing this surgery reported as comparable to those treated by the open surgical approach (Lacy et al., 2008; The Clinical Outcomes of Surgical Therapy Study Group, 2004). Within 5 years after curative surgical resection, disease relapse (tumor recurrence or metastasis) occurs in 40 to 50% of patients with stage III CRC and in 20% of those with stage II CRC (Midgley & Kerr, 1999). Systemic therapy with

	Chemotherapeutic agents			Therapeutic monoclonal antibodies		
	5-FU Capecitabine	Irinotecan	Oxaliplatin	Bevacizumab	Cetuximab	Panitumumab
Target	TS	Topo-isomerase I	DNA cross-link	VEGF	EGFR	EGFR
Indication	PO adjuvant metastatic	metastatic	PO adjuvant metastatic	metastatic	metastatic	metastatic
Combination						
FOLFOX	+ LV		+	combined	combined	combined
FOLFIRI	+ LV	+		combined	combined	combined
FOLFOXIRI	+ LV	+	+			
Predictive markers	TS, DPD, TP	UGT1A1*	ERCC-1	VEGF? Tumor micro-vessels?	EGFR copy number**, K-ras, B-raf, PI3CA, AREG, EREG	K-ras, B-raf, PI3CA

Table 1. Key agents and their combinations presently used for the treatment of CRC

Abbreviations: AREG, amphyregulin; DPD, dihydropyrimidine dehydrogenase; EGFR, epidermal growth factor receptor; ERCC-1, excision-repair cross-complementing-1; EREG, epiregulin; 5-FU, 5-fluorouracil; FOLFIRI, folinate, 5-FU and irinotecan; FOLFOX, folinate, 5-FU and oxaliplatin; FOLFOXIRI, FOLFOX and irinotecan; LV, leukovorin; PI3KCA, phosphoinositide 3 kinase (PI3K) p110 catalytic subunit gene; PO, postoperative; TP, thymidine phosphorylase; TS, thymidylate synthase; UGT1A1, uridine diphosphate (UDP)-glucuronosyltransferase 1A1; VEGF, vascular endothelial growth factor.

* The number of TA repeats in the TATA element in UGT1A1 gene predicts the drug toxicity and resultant adverse effects.

** EGFR copy number is measured by fluorescence in-situ hybridization (FISH).

either chemotherapy and/or targeted therapies have been demonstrated to provide benefit to these CRC patients in both the post-operative adjuvant and advanced disease settings (Inoue et al., 2006; Midgley et al., 2009). Table 1 summarizes the key chemotherapeutic agents and therapeutic monoclonal antibodies targeting VEGF and EGFR and the combinations currently prescribed as adjuvant therapy for relapse-prone CRC patients and patients with metastatic tumors (reviewed in Cunningham et al., 2010; Meyerhardt & Mayer, 2005; Midgley et al., 2009; Wolpin et al., 2007; Wolpin & Mayer, 2008). The putative predictive markers for response to the respective agents are also shown in Table 1 (Walther et al., 2009).

3.1 Adjuvant chemotherapy

The purpose of postoperative adjuvant chemotherapy for stage II or III CRC is to destroy residual tumor cells and/or micrometastatic foci that are latent at the time of curative surgery. The chemotherapeutic mainstay for CRC, 5-fluorouracil (5-FU), exerts its anti-tumor effect by inhibiting thymidylate synthase (TS), a critical enzyme for nucleic acid synthesis. Folinic acid (leucovorin: LV) is frequently used to enhance the anti-tumor effect of 5-FU. The clinical and pharmacological rationale for this combination derives from the biological role of LV in stabilizing the ternary complex between TS and fluoro-deoxyuridine monophosphate (dUMP), an active metabolite of 5-FU, thereby enhancing TS inhibition. Adjuvant treatment regimens consist of oral (capecitabine) or infusional fluoropyrimidine-based chemotherapy as a single agent with LV, or in combination with irinotecan (a topoisomerase I inhibitor), oxaliplatin (a DNA cross-linker) or both (Table 1) (Midgley et al., 2009; Wolpin et al., 2007; Wolpin & Mayer, 2008).

Adjuvant fluoropyrimidine-based chemotherapy reduces the risk of cancer-related mortality by 30% and increases the 5-year survival rate by 5-12% in patients with stage III (node-positive) CRC. Adjuvant chemotherapy for stage II (node-negative) CRC patients is controversial because it increases the 5-year survival rate by just 3-4%. It has been proposed that "high-risk" stage II CRC patients characterized by T4 tumor, luminal stenosis or obstruction, poor histological differentiation, extramural vessel invasion, inadequate lymphadenectomy or surgical margins (R1) should preferentially undergo adjuvant chemotherapy (Cunningham et al., 2010; Midgley et al., 2009). Tumor relapse after curative resection occurs mostly within 3 years, irrespective of adjuvant chemotherapy (Sargent et al., 2007). Several clinical trials have failed to show a survival benefit from combining molecular target-directed agents (e.g., bevacizumab, cetuximab) with adjuvant chemotherapy (reviewed in Cunningham et al., 2010). Improvement in the survival of patients at high risk of tumor relapse therefore depends on intensive surveillance for early diagnosis of metastatic lesions, as well as identification of patients who are susceptible to tumor recurrence and who could thus benefit from more aggressive adjuvant treatment.

3.2 Treatment of metastatic CRC

A series of systemic, fluoropyrimidine-based combinatorial chemotherapies (Table 1) has substantially improved tumor response to treatment and increased the duration of progression-free and overall survival in patients with metastatic CRC. The remarkable advance in treating metastatic CRC in recent years has been due to the emergence and clinical application of molecular targeted therapeutics (Cunningham et al., 2010; Midgley et al., 2009). As stated above, a number of therapeutic monoclonal antibodies that target relevant oncogenic pathways have been tested in clinical trials for CRC. Among them, the most widely used agents are bevacizumab, a recombinant humanized monoclonal antibody against VEGF (Ellis & Hicklin, 2008a; Li & Saif, 2009), cetuximab, a chimeric monoclonal antibody against EGFR (Balko et al, 2010) and panitumumab, a fully humanized monoclonal antibody against EGFR (Davis & Jimeno, 2010). These therapeutic antibodies have been used as monotherapy for the treatment of patients with metastatic CRC, or in combination with systemic chemotherapy (Table 1). Many clinical trials have demonstrated the additive effect of these antibodies on tumor response rate and progression-free survival (reviewed in Cunningham et al., 2010; Midgley et al., 2009). However, the combination of each therapeutic antibody with systemic chemotherapy regimens produced incremental but not always robust benefits to overall survival when compared to chemotherapy alone (Fojo & Parkinson, 2010).

3.3 Obstacles to systemic therapy
3.3.1 Drug resistance and predictive markers
The major obstacles to systemic therapy for CRC include drug resistance (both inherent and acquired) and the lack of reliable biomarkers for predicting response or resistance to drugs in clinical use (Ellis & Hicklin, 2009). This has led to the recent trend of using intensive combinatorial regimens for advanced CRC patients. Surprisingly, some recent clinical trials have shown that combinatorial target-directed therapies resulted in decreased survival, inferior quality of life and unexpected detrimental effects (Douillard et al., 2010; Hecht et al., 2009; Li & Saif, 2009; Tol et al., 2009).

Understanding the molecular mechanisms that underlie drug resistance and identifying predictive markers for drug sensitivity are *one and the same thing*. Pharmacogenomic approaches (Furuta et al., 2009; Walther et al., 2009) have identified a number of factors involved in drug metabolism and secretion, some of which (e.g., *UGT1A1* polymorphism) have been tested in clinical practice (Table 1). Several studies have suggested various biological mechanisms of resistance to VEGF-targeted cancer therapies (Bergers & Hanahan, 2008; Ebos et al., 2008; Ellis & Hicklin, 2008b), but to date there are no clinically useful predictive markers. Mutational activation of oncogenic pathways that lie downstream of EGFR signaling is known to cause intrinsic resistance to therapies that target this receptor. This has led to the identification of predictive markers (e.g., K-*ras*, B-*raf*, *PIK3CA*) that allow better patient selection for such treatments (Banck & Grothey, 2009; Cantwell-Dorris et al., 2011; De Roock et al., 2010a; Sartore-Bianchi et al., 2009). However, the complex pathways involved in tumor progression are often intercalated and therefore single markers cannot accurately predict the efficacy or outcome of CRC patients undergoing molecular targeted therapies (Baldus et al., 2010; De Roock et al., 2010b; Hecht et al., 2010).

Research into the mechanisms of acquired resistance to molecular targeted agents has generated new therapeutic strategies and agents aimed at counteracting the resistance mechanism (Bowles & Jimeno, 2011; Cidón, 2010; Dasari & Messersmith, 2010; Presen et al., 2010). Thus, improving the anti-tumor effects of molecular targeted therapies will depend on the identification of novel molecular pathways, development of new classes of rationally designed biological agents, and identification of predictive markers for response and resistance.

3.3.2 Economic issues
The high cost of developing the biologically-based therapeutic agents shown in Table 1 is a major issue in light of the modest clinical benefits, acquired drug resistance and lack of

suitable predictive markers. A recent study reported significantly higher hospital costs for CRC patients with recurrence compared to those without (Macafee et al., 2009). Outside of the United States, the high cost of molecular targeted drugs has restricted their use to patients with sufficient income and/or health insurance. This issue highlights the importance of accurate predictive markers that allow identification of patients who are most likely to benefit from targeted agents, thus improving the cost effectiveness.

4. GSK3β as an emerging therapeutic target

4.1 GSK3β biology

GSK3 was identified as a serine/threonine protein kinase that phosphorylates and inhibits glycogen synthase (GS), a rate-limiting enzyme in the regulation of glucose/glycogen metabolism in response to insulin-mediated signaling (Embi et al., 1980). In contrast to its original name and depending on its substrates and binding partners (Table 2) (Medina & Wandosell, 2011; Xu et al., 2009), GSK3 has been found to participate in many fundamental cellular pathways including proliferation, differentiation, motility, cell cycle and apoptosis (Doble & Woodgett, 2003; Harwood, 2001; Jope & Johnson, 2004; Nakada et al., 2011). The two isoforms of this kinase, GSK3α and GSK3β, are encoded by their respective genes. Their functions do not always overlap (Rayasam et al., 2009) and much recent attention has been directed towards the function of GSK3β.

Unlike most protein kinases, GSK3β is active in normal cells and this activity is controlled by its subcellular localization, differential phosphorylation at serine 9 (S9) and tyrosine 216 (Y216) residues, and different binding partners. A consensus motif and context-based computational analysis of *in vivo* protein phosphorylation sites indicate that GSK3β is one of the kinases with the most substrates (Linding et al., 2007). In normal cells, multiple signaling pathways mediated by phosphoinositide 3 kinase (PI3K)-Akt, Wnt and mitogen-activated protein kinase (MAPK) are known to negatively regulate the activity of GSK3β via S9 phosphorylation (Medina & Wandosell, 2011). The molecular structure and details of the functional and regulatory machinery of GSK3β have been thoroughly described in many excellent reviews cited in this section and are not the focus of this Chapter.

4.2 GSK3β in common chronic diseases

Accumulating evidence suggests pathological roles for GSK3β in glucose intolerance due to inhibition of GS and other signaling cascades involved in the regulation of glucose homeostasis (Frame & Zheleva, 2006; Lee & Kim, 2007) and in neurodegenerative changes through accumulation of the neurotoxic substances amyloid Aβ and tau protein (Annaert & De Strooper, 2002; Bhat & Budd, 2002). Recognition that GSK3β promotes inflammation also implicates this molecule in a broad spectrum of common diseases including type 2 diabetes mellitus and neuropsychiatric disorders involving an inflammatory reaction (Jope et al., 2007). GSK3β has therefore emerged as a therapeutic target in these prevalent diseases (Cohen & Goedert, 2004; Kypta, 2005; Meijer et al., 2004; Phukan et al., 2010). Another line of studies has demonstrated an osteogenic function for the Wnt/β-catenin signaling pathway (Hartman, 2006; Krishnan et al., 2006; Ralston & de Crombrugghe, 2006). This suggests that GSK3β may be a putative therapeutic target for osteoporotic bone disease, since under physiological conditions it is a well established member of a complex that destroys β-catenin

Categories	Substrates
Metabolism	glycogen synthase, ATP citrate lyase, PKA, PDH, acetyl-CoA, carboxylase, PP1, PP2A, PP2A inhibitor, cyclin D1, eIF2B, NGF receptor, axin, APP, Bax, VDAC, hexokinase II, presenilin, LRP5/6
Cell structure	tau, MAP1B, NCAM, neurofilament, CRMP2, dynein, dynein-like protein, maltose binding protein, APC, kinesin light chain
Signaling & Transcription	
Wnt	β-catenin, snail, smad1, Hath1, smad 3
Akt	SRC-3, B-cell lymphoma (BCL)-3, p21
PI3K-Akt	Mcl-1, c-Jun, phosphatase and tensin homologue (PTEN)
Ras-PI3K-Akt	c-Myc, cyclin D1
TNFα	nuclear factor (NF)-κB
Hedgehog	Ci (citrus interruptus), Gli-2
hypoxia	hypoxia inducible factor (HIF)-1α
insulin	glycogen synthase, SREBP
undetermined & others	cyclin E, AP-1, CREB, C/EBP, cdc25A, Notch, p53, p27[Kip1], NFAT, GR, HSF-1, FGD-1, FGD-3, c-Myb, mCRY2, NACα, MafA, IPF1/PDX1, presenilin 1 C-terminal fragment

Table 2. Known substrates for phosphorylation by GSK3β

Abbreviations: AP-1, activator protein 1; APC, adenomatous polyposis coli; APP, amyloid precursor protein; ATP, adenosine triphosphate; C/EBP, CCAAT (cytidine-cytidine-adenosine-adenosine-thymidine)-enhancer-binding protein; CREB, cyclic adenosine monophosphate (cAMP) response element binding protein; CRMP2, collapsin response mediator protein 2; eIF2B, eukaryotic protein synthesis initiation factor-2B; FGD, FYVE, RhoGEF and PH domain-containing protein; GR, glucocorticoid receptor; HSF-1, heat shock factor protein 1; IPF1, insulin promoter factor 1; LRP5/6, low-density lipoprotein (LDL) receptor-related protein 5/6; MafA, musculoaponeurotic fibrosarcoma oncogene homolog A: MAP1B, microtubule-associated protein 1B; mCRY2, mouse cryptochrome 2; NACα, nascent polypeptide-associated complex α subunit; NCAM, neural cell adhesion molecule; NFAT, nuclear factor of activated T-cells; NGF, nerve growth factor; PDH, pyruvate dehydrogenase; PDX1, pancreatic and duodenal homeobox 1; PKA, protein kinase A; PP, protein phosphatase; SREBP, sterol regulatory element-binding protein; TNFα, tumor necrosis factor α; VDAC, voltage-dependent anion channel.

(Fuchs et al., 2005). In this context, an orally bioavailable GSK3α/β dual inhibitor was generated and tested as a new drug for the treatment of osteoporosis (Kulkarni et al., 2006).

4.3 GSK3β in cancer

An increasing number of cellular structural and functional proteins have been identified as targets for GSK3β phosphorylation-dependent regulation (Table 2). However, this has also generated results that show conflicting roles for the signaling pathways regulated by GSK3β in either suppressing or promoting cancer.

4.3.1 GSK3β suppresses cancer

In physiologically normal cells, many of the substrates for GSK3β-mediated phosphory-lation and subsequent ubiquitin-mediated degradation include oncogenic signaling and transcription factors, cell cycle regulators and proto-oncoproteins (Table 2). A previous study showed that GSK3β phosphorylates and stabilizes a major cell cycle regulator, p27[Kip1] (Surjit & Lal, 2007). Recent studies have shown that inhibition of GSK3β stabilizes snail and induces epithelial-mesenchymal transition (EMT), a morphological and phenotypic change closely associated with tumor cell invasion and metastasis (Bachelder et al., 2005; Zhou et al., 2004; reviewed in Doble & Woodgett, 2007; Schlessinger & Hall, 2004; Zhou & Hung, 2005). These findings are mostly observed in normal but not neoplastic cells and have led to the hypothesis that GSK3β functions as a tumor suppressor (reviewed in Luo, 2009; Manoukian & Woodgett, 2003; Patel & Woodgett, 2008).

Consistent with this hypothesis, a number of studies in breast, lung and non-melanoma skin cancers have shown that GSK3β is inactivated in tumor cells, but that its activation induces apoptosis (reviewed in Luo, 2009; Patel & Woodgett, 2008). It has been reported in several studies that GSK3β renders cancer cells resistant to chemotherapeutic agents (reviewed in Luo, 2009). However, in contrast to the observations described in the next section (**4.3.2**), including our own, none of these studies addressed differences in the expression, activity and biological properties of GSK3β between tumor cells and their normal cell counterparts. Furthermore, these studies did not investigate the direct consequences of GSK3β inhibition for tumor cell survival, proliferation and chemotactic migration and invasion.

4.3.2 Deregulated GSK3β promotes cancer

Wnt signaling plays a crucial role in embryonic development, the regeneration of adult tissues and in many other cellular processes. Aberrant activation of the Wnt pathway due to mutation or deregulated expression of its components mediates the multistep process of colorectal tumorigenesis (Kikuchi, 2007; Klaus & Birchmeier, 2008; Lustig & Behrens, 2003; Willert & Jones, 2006). Over 90% of CRC develops following activation of the Wnt signaling pathway in which β-catenin plays a central role (Fuchs et al., 2005; Giles et al., 2003). GSK3β interrupts activation of the canonical Wnt pathway by phosphorylating β-catenin and recruiting it to ubiquitin-mediated degradation. GSK3β is therefore believed to antagonize tumorigenesis that involves active Wnt signaling (Bienz & Clevers, 2000; Manoukian & Woodgett, 2002; Polakis P, 1999), as represented for example by CRC development. This notion is also supported by the frequent mutational activation of Ras and PI3K-Akt signaling (Markowitz & Bertagnolli, 2009; Parsons et al., 2005), since it is well established that Akt kinase phosphorylates the S9 residue of GSK3β and inhibits its activity (Medina & Wandosell, 2011). However, few studies had focused on the biological properties of GSK3β in cancer until we investigated a putative pathological role for this kinase in CRC, as described below.

Most CRC cell lines and primary CRC tumors in our studies have shown increased expression and activity of GSK3β and deregulation of its activity due to imbalance in the differential phosphorylation of S9 (inactive) and Y216 (active) residues. This is in comparison to non-neoplastic cells (e.g., HEK293) and normal colon mucosa in which GSK3β activity appears to be regulated by the differential phosphorylation. These tumor cell features are unrelated to the activation of β-catenin or Akt (Mai et al., 2009; Shakoori et al., 2005). A non-radioisotopic, *in vitro* kinase assay demonstrated an increased ability of GSK3β derived from most CRC cell lines and primary CRC tumors to phosphorylate its substrate, as compared to non-neoplastic counterparts (Mai et al., 2006, 2009). These observations suggest that, in contrast to having hypothetical tumor suppressor function, GSK3β may actually promote cancer.

A putative pathological role for GSK3β in cancer was demonstrated by subsequent observations that inhibition of GSK3β activity using pharmacological (small-molecule) agents and of its expression by RNA interference reduced the survival and proliferation of CRC cells. Such inhibition also predisposed the cells to apoptosis *in vitro* and in tumor xenografts, suggesting that CRC cells depend on aberrant GSK3β for their survival and proliferation (Mai et al., 2006, 2009; Shakoori et al., 2005, 2007). A series of studies by our group led us to propose that aberrant GSK3β is a novel and potentially important therapeutic target in cancer (Miyashita et al., 2009b; Motoo et al., 2011; Nakada et al., 2011), thus allowing us to apply for domestic and international patents in this field (Minamoto).

Following our studies on the antitumor effects of GSK3β inhibition, similar observations were reported for CRC by other groups (Ghosh & Altieri, 2005; Rottmann et al., 2005; Tan et al., 2005; Tsuchiya et al., 2007) (Table 3). Similar results were also published for other cancer types with underlying biological mechanisms that included GSK3β inhibition of several pathways involved in tumorigenesis (reviewed in Miyashita et al., 2009b; Nakada et al., 2011). A putative role for GSK3β in cancer is still being debated (Luo, 2009; Manoukian & Woodgett, 2003; Patel & Woodgett, 2008) and was discussed in section **4.3.1**. However, the overall results to date indicate that aberrant expression and activity of GSK3β is likely to be a common and fundamental characteristic of a broad spectrum of human cancers.

4.3.3 Oncogene addiction and the effect of GSK3β inhibition against cancer

As stated in section **2.2**, the hypothesis of oncogene addiction has been proposed as a rationale for molecular targeting in cancer treatment. It refers to the observation that a cancer cell, despite its plethora of genetic alterations, seemingly exhibits dependence on a single oncoprotein or oncogenic pathway for its sustained survival and/or proliferation (Sharma & Settleman, 2007; Weinstein, 2002; Weinstein & Joe, 2006). This unique state of dependence by cancer cells is highlighted by the fact that inactivation of the normal counterpart of such proto-oncogene products in non-neoplastic cells is tolerated without obvious consequence. A profound implication of this hypothesis is that acute interruption of the critical oncogenic pathways upon which cancer cells are dependent should have a major detrimental effect (oncogene shock), while sparing normal cells that are not similarly addicted to these pathways (Sharma et al, 2006). In our series of studies, inhibition of GSK3β had little effect on cell survival, growth, apoptosis or senescence in non-neoplastic cells (e.g., HEK293) and on major vital organs in rodents (Mai et al., 2006, 2009; Shakoori et al., 2005, 2007). This concurs with previous reports showing that GSK3β inhibition does not influence the survival or growth of human mammary epithelial cells, embryonic lung fibroblasts (WI38) and mouse embryonic fibroblasts (NIH-3T3) (Kunnimalaiyaan et al., 2007; Ougolkov et al., 2005). With respect to the oncogene addiction hypothesis (Sharma & Settleman, 2007; Weinstein, 2002; Weinstein & Joe, 2006), the selective therapeutic effect of GSK3β inhibition against cancer can be explained by differences in biological properties of GSK3β between neoplastic and non-neoplastic cells (Mai et al., 2006, 2009; Shakoori et al., 2005).

5. GSK3β and the hallmarks of colorectal cancer

Understanding the molecular mechanism behind a pathogenic role for GSK3β in cancer is important for the development of treatment strategies that target this kinase. A current review highlights 8 hallmarks of cancer in which phenotypic properties are progressively

Authors	Study design	Types of GSK3β inhibitors	Pathological roles of GSK3β and underlying mechanism
Shakoori et al, 2005	*in vitro*	AR-A014418, SB-216763, siRNA	Deregulated GSK3β expression and activity are associated with CRC cell survival and proliferation by mechanism independent of activation of Wnt/β-catenin signaling and Akt. GSK3β inhibition attenuates survival and proliferation of colon cancer cells.
Mai et al, 2006	*in vitro*	AR-A014418, SB-216763, siRNA	NRIKA detected higher activity of GSK3β for phosphorylating its substrate (β-catenin) in gastrointestinal cancer cells including CRC cells than non-neoplastic HEK293 cells.
Shakoori et al, 2007	tumor xenograft	AR-A014418, SB-216763	GSK3β inhibition attenuates survival and proliferation of SW480 colon cancer cell xenografts with no detrimental effects on the major vital organs in the rodents.
Mai et al, 2009	*in vitro*, tumor xenograft	AR-A014418, SB-216763, siRNA	GSK3β inhibition attenuates survival and proliferation of colon cancer cells by decreasing hTERT expression and telomerase activity and inducing cell senescence.
Ghosh et al, 2005	*in vitro*	LiCl, TDZD8, SB-216763, siRNA	GSK3β functions against activation of p53-dependent apoptosis in colon cancer cells.
Tan et al, 2005	*in vitro*	LiCl, SB-216763, SB415286, LY2119301	GSK3β functions against activation of p53-dependent apoptosis through a direct Bax-mediated mitochondrial pathway in colon cancer cells.
Rottmann et al, 2005	*in vitro*, tumor xenograft	LiCl, siRNA	GSK3β functions against colon cancer cell apoptosis by inhibiting a TRAIL receptor-dependent synthetic lethal relationship between *Myc* activation and *FBW7* loss of function.
Tsuchiya et al, 2007	*in vitro*	BIO, LiCl, keupaullone	GSK3β inhibits colonocyte differentiation by destabilizing the transcription factor, Hath1.

Table 3. Pathological roles and functions of GSK3β in colorectal cancer

Abbreviations: hTERT, human telomerase reverse transcriptase; NRIKA, non-radioisotopic *in vitro* kinase assay; siRNA, small interfering RNA; TRAIL, tumor necrosis factor (TNF)-related apoptosis-inducing ligand.

acquired during multistep pathogenesis, thus allowing cancer cells to become tumorigenic and ultimately malignant (Hanahan & Weinberg, 2011). These hallmarks are sustained proliferative signaling, evasion of growth suppressors, resistance to cell death, enabling of replicative immortality, induction of angiogenesis, activation of invasion and metastasis, reprogramming of energy metabolism and evasion of immune destruction. The development of each hallmark involves multiple signaling pathways. In this section, we address how GSK3β modulates some of these hallmark characteristics of CRC by referring to the studies shown in Table 3, including our own work.

5.1 Cell proliferation
Unrestrained cell proliferation is the most prominent feature of cancer. Our previous study showed that the effect of GSK3β inhibition against the proliferative capacity of CRC cells was associated with decreased expression of cyclin D1 and cyclin-dependent kinase (CDK) 6 and phosphorylation of the Rb protein (Mai et al., 2009). These observations suggest that Rb function was restored, leading to the binding and inhibition of E2F transcription factor (reviewed in Classon & Harlow, 2002; Knudsen & Knudsen, 2008). This is consistent with a subsequent report that forced expression of exogenous GSK3β promotes the proliferation of ovarian cancer cells by inducing cyclin D1 expression (Cao et al., 2006). Together, the results suggest that suppression of excess cancer cell proliferation via the inhibition of GSK3β is partly due to negative regulation of cell cycling by cyclin D1. In normal or non-neoplastic cells, cyclin D1 is one of the primary targets of GSK3β for phosphorylation and subsequent degradation in the ubiquitin-proteasome system (Diehl et al., 1998) (Table 2). The opposing role of GSK3β in cyclin D1 expression may explain the lack of effect of GSK3β inhibition on cell survival and growth of non-neoplastic cells found in earlier studies (Kunnimalaiyaan et al., 2007; Mai et al., 2009; Ougolkov et al., 2005; Shakoori et al., 2005).

5.2 Resistance to cell death via tumor suppressor pathways
A major mechanism by which cancer cells evade cell death is via the inactivation of tumor suppressor pathways mediated by p53 (Royds & Iacopetta B, 2006; Vousden & Lane, 2007; Zilfou & Lowe, 2009) and Rb (Classon & Harlow, 2002; Knudsen & Knudsen, 2008). The studies listed in Table 3 showed that inhibition of GSK3β induced apoptosis in human CRC cell lines. This effect was associated with increased expression of p53 and of p21 in colon cancer cells with wild-type p53, and decreased Rb phosphorylation in colon cancer cells irrespective of their p53 status (Ghosh & Altieri, 2005; Mai et al., 2009; Tan et al., 2005). Another study showed that GSK3β suppresses the apoptosis of colon cancer cells by inhibiting a tumor necrosis factor (TNF)-related apoptosis-inducing ligand (TRAIL) receptor-dependent synthetic lethal relationship between c-*Myc* activation and *FBW7* (a gene encoding a ubiquitin ligase receptor) loss of function (Rottmann et al., 2005). These studies suggest a putative pathological role for aberrant GSK3β in mediating CRC cell resistance to apoptosis induced by a pathway involving tumor suppressor proteins, TRAIL and c-Myc.

One of the representative pathways for cell survival is mediated by nuclear factor-κB (NF-κB) (Inoue et al., 2007; Karin, 2006, 2009). Based on previous studies showing the potential involvement of GSK3β in NF-κB-mediated cell survival during mouse embryonic development (Hoeflich et al., 2000; Schwabe & Brenner, 2002), it was reported that GSK3β sustains pancreatic cancer cell survival by maintaining transcriptional activity of NF-κB (Ougolkov et al., 2005; Wilson & Baldwin, 2008). While these studies examined the activity of exogenous (transfected) NF-κB, we previously observed no effect of GSK3β inhibition on endogenous NF-κB transcriptional activity in gastrointestinal cancer cells (including CRC) and glioblastoma cells (Mai et al., 2009; Miyashita et al., 2009a). Therefore, a role for GSK3β in regulating NF-κB activity in cancer is controversial.

5.3 Replicative cell immortality

Another critical mechanism used by cancer cells to evade cell death is replicative cell immortality. A close relationship exists in cancer cells between the molecular mechanisms for immortality and escape from replicative senescence (Finkel et al., 2007). Cancer cells acquire constitutive expression and activity of human telomerase reverse transcriptase (hTERT) and telomerase in order to circumvent telomere-dependent pathways of cell mortality (Harley, 2008).

We recently observed a decreased level of hTERT mRNA in colon cancer cells following inhibition of either the activity or expression of GSK3β. Inhibition of GSK3β attenuates telomerase activity and increases the β-galactosidase-positive (senescent) population in colon cancer cells. These effects were associated with increased expression of p53, p21 and c-Jun N-terminal kinase 1 (JNK1) and decreases in CDK6 expression and Rb phosphorylation (Mai et al., 2009). The findings are consistent with the known relationship between these proteins and cell senescence (reviewed in Kiyono, 2007) and with GSK3β activity (Ghosh & Altieri, 2005; Kulikov et al., 2005; Liu et al., 2004; Mai et al., 2009; Qu et al., 2004; Rössig et al., 2002). Consistent with our observation, a recent study found that inhibition of GSK3β suppressed hTERT expression and telomerase activity and shortened the telomere length in various cancer cell lines including HCT116 colon cancer cells, and attenuated cell proliferation and hTERT expression in ovarian cancer xenografts (Bilsland et al., 2009). The putative role for GSK3β in protecting cancer cells from telomere-dependent senescence and mortality is attributed to its effects on hTERT expression and telomerase activity.

5.4 Influence on the cancer microenvironment and tumor invasion

In cancer, various events are orchestrated to produce a distinct tumor microenvironment that dictates the malignant potential. These include depletion of nutrients involved in cell proliferation, tumor cell invasion, tumor neovascularization in response to hypoxic condition, as well as stromal, inflammatory and immune reactions in the host (Joyce, 2005). The promotion of inflammation and immune response by GSK3β (Jope et al, 2007) suggests a broad pathological role for this kinase in the cancer microenvironment.

The pro-invasive phenotype of cancer cells is characterized by EMT, enhanced cell motility and their ability to induce neovascularization. As discussed in section **4.3.1**, inhibition of GSK3β stabilizes snail and induces EMT (Bachelder et al., 2005; Zhou et al., 2004; reviewed in Doble & Woodgett, 2007; Schlessinger & Hall, 2004; Zhou & Hung, 2005). A hypoxic tumor microenvironment induces the expression of hypoxia-inducible factor-1α (HIF-1α), a transcription factor that controls oxygen homeostasis by regulating target genes involved in angiogenesis, glycolysis and cell proliferation (reviewed in Semenza, 2009). A previous study showed that under physiological conditions, GSK3β inhibits angiogenesis by negatively regulating endothelial cell survival and migration in response to PI3K-, MAPK- and protein kinase A (PKA)-dependent signaling pathways (Kim et al., 2002). Another study demonstrated that hypoxia induces a biphasic effect on HIF-1α stabilization in liver cancer cells. Accumulation of HIF-1α occurs in early hypoxia and is dependent on an active PI3K/Akt pathway and inactive GSK3β. In contrast, prolonged hypoxia results in the inactivation of Akt and activation of GSK3β. This negatively regulates HIF-1α activity by inhibiting its accumulation (Mottet et al., 2003). Collectively, it thus appears unlikely that GSK3β participates in cancer cell EMT and in tumor angiogenesis.

Formation of lamellipodia, the characteristic cellular microarchitecture, is responsible not only for cell migration under physiological conditions (e.g., embryonic development, wound healing) but also for cancer cell migration and invasion (Machesky, 2008; Small et al., 2002; Yilmaz & Christofori, 2009). A member of the Rho-GTPase family, Rac1, is known to participate in the formation of lamellipodia and may thus play an important role in cancer progression (Raftpoulou & Hall, 2004; Sahai & Marshall, 2002). It has been reported that GSK3β participates in cell motility by facilitating the formation of lamellipodia (Koivisto et al., 2003) and by activating Rac1 (Farooqui et al., 2006; Kobayashi et al., 2006; Vaidya et al., 2006). Focal adhesion kinase (FAK) is also known to play a key role in regulating cell motility and migration and to be deregulated in cancer (McLean et al., 2005). Earlier studies reported that FAK is one of the downstream effectors in GSK3β-mediated pathways (Kobayashi et al., 2006) and also regulates Rac1 (McLean et al., 2005). Consistent with a recent study for glioblastoma (Nowicki et al., 2008), our preliminary study has shown that inhibition of GSK3β attenuates pancreatic cancer cell migration and invasion by negatively regulating FAK and Rac1 activities (unpublished observation). Therefore, in regard to cancer treatments that target GSK3β, it is important to explore a possible role for GSK3β in CRC cell invasion by investigating its effects on cellular microarchitecture, motility and migration.

5.5 Cancer cell stemness and metabolic traits

Cell stemness and the reprogramming of energy metabolism are primary cell characteristics that share distinct molecular pathways and allow cancer cells to survive, proliferate, invade their host tissues, metastasize and resist treatment. Here, we address future directions in our approach towards ascertaining the potential of GSK3β as a therapeutic target in cancers including CRC.

5.5.1 Cancer cell stemness and GSK3β

Arising from the concept of tissue stem cells, the notion of cancer stem cells has emerged and proposes that cancer initiating cells are a distinct subpopulation within a tumor that have the ability to self-renew and differentiate (Clarke et al., 2006; O'Brien et al., 2010). Similar to other cancer types, a small population of cancer initiating cells has been identified and characterized in CRC (Dalerba et al., 2007; O'Brien et al., 2007; Ricci-Vitiani et al., 2007; reviewed in Yeung & Mortensen, 2009). Current cancer treatments assume that all cancer cells in tumors are homogeneous and have a similar capacity to proliferate, invade and metastasize, as well as having similar susceptibility to chemotherapy and radiation. However, accumulating evidence suggests that cancer stem cells and cancer cells that are undergoing EMT share various biological traits (Polyak & Weinberg, 2009). These cells are also strongly resistant to current forms of therapeutics, thereby identifying this subpopulation of cancer cells as the ultimate target for cancer treatment (Lou & Dean, 2007). Consistent with the physiological roles of GSK3β in Wnt, Hedgehog and Notch signaling (Foltz et al., 2002; Manoukian & Woodgett, 2002; Takenaka et al., 2007), GSK3β inhibition by pharmacological means promotes embryonic stem cell pluripotency (Sato et al., 2004) and hematopoietic stem cell reconstitution (Trowbridge et al., 2006). Conversely, recent studies have demonstrated that GSK3β sustains the respective molecular pathways leading to tumor cell stemness in a specific type of leukemia and in glioblastoma (Korur et al., 2009; Wang et al., 2008). Although the underlying molecular mechanisms are not well understood, these differential roles for GSK3β in normal and cancer stem cells could ultimately benefit cancer treatment strategies by allowing this kinase to be targeted with little harm to patients. As addressed in the next section (5.5.2), anaerobic glycolysis and the presence of a distinct niche are thought to be characteristics of cancer stem cells, in addition to their extreme resistance to drug treatment. Therefore, clarification of a putative role for GSK3β in regulating CRC cell stemness is of great interest. This could lead to a new strategy for treatment that targets the biology of cancer cell stemness.

5.5.2 Distinct metabolic traits of cancer cells and GSK3β

Production of excess energy is thought to provide an intrinsic and selective pressure that allows cancer cells to expand clonally and to acquire immortalized and destructive phenotypes. Even under normoxic conditions, most cancer cells depend on increased glucose uptake and aerobic glycolysis to produce their energy source, adenosine triphosphates (ATP) (Kim & Dang, 2006; Vander Heiden & Cantley, 2010). This is known as the Warburg effect and involves truncated oxidative phosphorylation in the tricarboxylic acid (TCA) cycle, thus resulting in mitochondrial uncoupling (Samudio et al., 2009). These properties allow cancer cells to survive and invade host tissues in a microenvironment where the supply of both oxygen and nutrients is deficient, as well as conferring resistance to apoptosis-inducing therapeutic stimuli (Smallbone et al., 2007). Therefore, the glycolytic phenotype of cancer cells is a potential target for cancer diagnosis and treatment (Gatenby & Gillies, 2007; Kroemer & Pouyssegur, 2008). For example, enhanced glucose uptake by cancer cells can be used to visualize cancer by positron emission tomography (PET) using the radioisotope-labeled glucose analogue 2-[^{18}F]-fluoro-2-deoxy-D-glucose (FDG). FDG-PET in combination with computed tomography (PET-CT) enables the detection of metastatic lesions for most cancers with sensitivity and specificity both greater than 90% (Mankoff et al., 2007).

The association between a glycolytic phenotype (i.e., TCA cycle defects) and resistance to apoptosis is attributed to decreased mitochondrial hydrogen peroxide production and cytochrome C release (Samudio et al., 2009; Vander Heiden & Cantley, 2010). Pyruvate dehydrogenase (PDH) plays a crucial role in triggering the TCA cycle by converting pyruvate to citric acid. PDH kinase 1 (PDK1), which phosphorylates and inactivates PDH, is frequently over-activated in cancer cells, resulting in an impaired TCA cycle and mitochondrial hyperpolarization. Thus, inhibition of PDK1 would re-activate PDH and restore mitochondrial membrane polarity, thereby facilitating cancer cell apoptosis in response to chemotherapeutic agents and radiation. Dichloroacetate (DCA), an orally bio-available small molecule, is a well characterized PDK1 inhibitor. The ability of DCA to inhibit lactate production by stimulating PDH and the TCA cycle has long been used to treat lactic acidosis, which is a complication of inherited mitochondrial disorders (Stacpoole, 2003, 2006). A recent study demonstrated that DCA induces cancer cell apoptosis by selectively inhibiting PDK1 in cancer cells, leading to metabolic remodeling from glycolysis to glucose oxidation and the normalization of mitochondrial function (Bonnet et al., 2008). A clinical trial of oral DCA in children with congenital lactic acidosis reported that DCA was well tolerated and safe (Stacpoole, 2006). Thus, orally administered DCA is a promising and selective anticancer agent.

The primary role of GSK3β is to control GS activity (Table 2). It thus acts as a checkpoint at the bifurcation between glycogenesis and glycolysis, the two major pathways of glucose/glycogen metabolism (Lee & Kim, 2007). We recently found that inhibition of GSK3β in colon cancer cells increased GS expression and decreased its S640 phosphorylation (unpublished observation), suggesting that GSK3β inhibition may switch cancer cells from a glycolytic to a glycogenic phenotype. It was previously reported that GSK3β phosphorylates and inactivates PDH (Hoshi et al., 1996) (Table 2), a key enzyme for the TCA cycle in mitochondria. This suggests that deregulated GSK3β contributes to truncation of the TCA cycle and mitochondrial uncoupling in cancer cells, resulting in resistance to chemotherapy and radiation. It has also been reported that the distinct metabolism of cancer cells involves not only anaerobic glycolysis but also other metabolic pathways such as the pentose phosphate pathway, amino acid and nucleic acid synthesis and glutaminolysis (DeBerardinis et al., 2008). GSK3β has a number of key metabolic enzymes as substrates (Table 2), suggesting this molecule could have broad control over various pathological metabolic pathways in cancer cells.

6. Perspectives

Biologically-based therapy of cancer holds great promise, particularly for patients who are refractory to existing forms of therapy. Current paradigms reviewed in the earlier part of this Chapter (**3. Systemic treatment: an overview**) include the targeting of growth factor receptor-type protein tyrosine kinases and angiogenic factors. Such therapies are directed against cancer cell survival, proliferation and tumor angiogenesis; however they are unable to completely eradicate cancer, as demonstrated by most large-scale clinical trials.

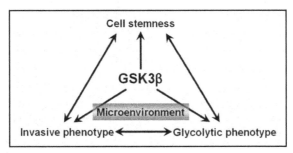

Fig. 1. GSK3β promotes cell stemness, invasive capacity and excess glucose metabolism that interact to produce a distinct cancer microenvironment.

The distinct pathologic properties of GSK3β in cancer described here highlight its potential to be an innovative target for the radical treatment of this disease, including CRC. GSK3β can potentially promote cancer cell stemness, invasive capacity and glucose metabolism, thus creating the selective pressures that allow cancer cells to persist in a distinct microenvironment (Figure 1). Understanding the complex biological mechanisms for the multiple roles of GSK3β in promoting cancer should allow elucidation of novel molecular pathways that lead to cancer development and progression. This will also provide a detailed scientific basis for the development of cancer treatment strategies that target aberrant GSK3β.

Concerns regarding the therapeutic use of GSK3β inhibitors remain because these may activate oncogenic (e.g., Wnt) signaling, thus promoting cell proliferation (Manoukian & Woodgett, 2003). However, this issue has not deterred preclinical studies of GSK3β inhibitors for the treatment of many cancer types (reviewed in Miyashita et al., 2009b) or Phase II clinical trials for the treatment of neurological diseases (Chico et al., 2010). Currently, two clinical trials are being undertaken to test a pharmacological GSK3β inhibitor (LY2090314) for enhancement of the anti-tumor effect of chemotherapeutic agents for advanced solid cancer (phase I: http://clinicaltrials.gov/ct2/show/study/NCT01287520) and leukemia (phase II: http://clinicaltrials.gov/ct2/show/study/NCT01214603). Such trials targeting GSK3β should complement, enhance or substitute the current front line therapies that target growth factor receptors and angiogenic factors in refractory colorectal cancer.

7. Acknowledgments

This study was supported in part by Grants-in-Aid for Scientific Research from the Japanese Ministry of Education, Science, Sports, Technology and Culture (to KK, TM); from the Ministry of Health, Labour and Welfare (to TM); from the Japan Society for the Promotion of Science (to KK, TM); and from the Japan Society for Technology (to KK and TM).

8. References

Annaert, W. & De Strooper, B. (2002). A cell biological perspective on Alzheimer's disease. *Annu Rev Cell Dev Biol.* Vol. 18, pp. 25-51, ISSN: 1081-0706 (Print, Linking), 1530-8995 (Electronic)

Bachelder, R.E., Yoon, S., Franci, C., de Herreros, A.G. & Mercurio, A.M. (2005). Glycogen synthase kinase-3 is an endogenous inhibitor of Snail transcription: implications for the epithelial-mesenchymal transition. *J Cell Biol.* Vol. 168, No. 1, pp. 29-33, ISSN: 0021-9525 (Print, Linking), 1540-8140 (Electronic)

Baldus, S.E., Schaefer, K-L., Engers, R., Hartleb, D., Stoecklein, N.H. & Gabbert, H.E. (2010). Prevalence and heterogeneity of *KRAS, BRAF,* and *PIK3CA* mutations in primary colorectal adenocarcinomas and their corresponding metastases. *Clin Cancer Res.* Vol. 16, No. 3, pp. 790-799, ISSN: 1078-0432 (Print, Linking)

Balko, A.L., Black, E.P. & Balko, J.M. (2010). First-line treatment of metastatic cancer: focus on Cetuximab in combination with chemotherapy. *Clin Med Rev Oncol.* Vol. 2, pp. 319-327, ISSN: 1179-2531 (Electronic, Linking)

Banck, M.S. & Grothey, A. (2009). Biomarkers of resistance to epidermal growth factor receptor monoclonal antibodies in patients with metastatic colorectal cancer. *Clin Cancer Res.* Vol. 15, No. 24, pp. 7492-7501, ISSN: 1078-0432 (Print, Linking)

Bergers, G. & Hanahan, D. (2008). Modes of resistance to anti-angiogenic therapy. *Nat Rev Cancer.* Vol. 8, No. 8, pp. 592-603, ISSN: 1474-175X (Print, Linking), 1474-1768 (Electronic)

Bhat, R.V. & Budd, S.L. (2002). GSK3β signalling: casting a wide net in Alzheimer's disease. *Neurosignals.* Vol. 11, No. 5, pp. 251-261, ISSN: 1424-862X (Print, Linking), 1424-8638 (Electronic)

Bienz, M. & Clevers, H. (2000). Linking colorectal cancer to Wnt signaling. *Cell.* Vol. 103, No. 2, pp. 311-320, ISSN: 0092-8674 (Print, Linking), 1097-4172 (Electronic)

Bilsland, A.E., Hoare, S., Stevenson, K., Plumb, J., Gomez-Roman, N., Cairney, C., Burns, S., Lafferty-Whyte, K., Roffey, J., Hammonds, T. & Keith, W.N. (2009). Dynamic telomerase gene suppression via network effects of GSK3 inhibition. *PLoS One.* Vol. 4, No. 7, pp. e6459, ISSN: 1932-6203 (Electronic, Linking)

Bonnet, S., Archer, S.L., Allalunis-Turner, J., Haromy, A., Beaulieu, C., Thompson, R., Lee, C.T., Lopaschuk, G.D., Puttagunta, L., Bonnet, S., Harry, G., Hashimoto, K., Porter, C.J., Andrade, M.A., Thebaud, B. & Michelakis, E.D. (2007). A mitochondria-K+ channel axis is suppressed in cancer and its normalization promotes apoptosis and inhibits cancer growth. *Cancer Cell.* Vol. 11, No. 1, pp. 37-51, ISSN: 1535-6108 (Print, Linking), 1878-3686 (Electronic)

Bowles, D.W. & Jimeno, A. (2011). New phosphatidylinsitol 3-kinase inhibitors for cancer. *Expert Opin Investig Drugs.* Vol. 20, No. 4, pp. 507-518, ISSN: 1354-3784 (Print, Linking), 1744-7658 (Electronic)

Cantwell-Dorris, E.R., O'Leary, J.J. & Sheils, O.M. (2011). BRAF[V600E]: implications for carcinogenesis and molecular therapy. *Mol Cancer Ther.* Vol. 10, No. 3, pp. 385-394, ISSN: 1535-7163 (Print, Linking), 1538-8514 (Electronic)

Cao, Q., Lu, X. & Feng, Y. (2006). Glycogen synthase kinase-3β positively regulates the proliferation of human ovarian cancer cells. *Cell Res.* Vol. 16, No. 7, pp. 671-677, ISSN: 1001-0602 (Print, Linking), 1748-7838 (Electronic)

Center, M.M., Jemal, A. & Ward, E. (2009). International trends in colorectal cancer incidence rates. *Cancer Epidemiol Biomarkers Prev.* Vol. 18, No. 6, pp. 1688-1694, ISSN: 1055-9965 (Print, Linking), 1538-7755 (Electronic)

Chico, L.K., Van Eldik, L.J. & Watterson, D.M. (2009). Targeting protein kinases in central nervous system disorders. *Nat Rev Drug Discov.* Vol. 8, No. 11, pp. 892-909, ISSN: 1474-1776 (Print, Linking), 1474-1784 (Electronic)

Cidón, E.U. (2010). The challenge of metastatic colorectal cancer. *Clin Med Insights Oncol.* Vol. 4, pp. 55-60, ISSN: 1179-5549 (Electronic)

Clarke, M.F., Dick, J.E., Dirks, P.B., Eaves, C.J., Jamieson, C.H., Jones, D.L., Visvader, J., Weissman, I.L. & Wahl, G.M. (2006). Cancer stem cells—perspectives on current status and future directions: AACR Workshop on Cancer Stem Cells. *Cancer Res.* Vol., 66, No. 19, pp. 9339-9344, ISSN: 0008-5472 (Print, Linking), 1538-7445 (Electronic)

Classon, M. & Harlow, E. (2002). The retinoblastoma tumor suppressor in development and cancer. *Nat Rev Cancer.* Vol. 2, No. 12, pp. 910-917, ISSN: 1474-175X (Print, Linking), 1474-1768 (Electronic)

Cohen, P. & Goedert, M. (2004). GSK3 inhibitors: development and therapeutic potential. *Nat Rev Drug Discov.* Vol. 3, No. 6, pp. 479-487, ISSN: 1474-1776 (Print, Linking), 1474-1784 (Electronic)

Cunningham, D., Atkin, W., Lenz, H.J., Lynch, H.T., Minsky, B., Nordlinger, B. & Starling, N. (2010). Colorectal cancer. *Lancet.* Vol. 375, No. 9719, pp. 1030-1047, ISSN: 0140-6736 (Print, Linking), 1474-547X (Electronic)

Dalerba, P., Dylla, S.J., Park, I.K., Liu, R., Wang, X., Cho, R.W., Hoey, T., Gurney, A., Huang, E.H., Simeone, D.M., Shelton, A.A., Parmiani, G., Castelli, C. & Clarke, M.F. (2007). Phenotypic characterization of human colorectal cancer stem cells. *Proc Natl Acad Sci U S A.* Vol. 104, No. 24, pp. 10158-10163, ISSN: 0027-8424 (Print, Linking), 1091-6490 (Electronic)

Dasari, A. & Messersmith, W.A. (2010). New strategies in colorectal cancer: biomarkers of response to epidermal growth factor receptor monoclonal antibodies and potential therapeutic targets in phosphoinositide 3-kinase and mitogen-activated protein kinase pathways. *Clin Cancer Res.* Vol. 16, No. 15, pp. 3811-3818, ISSN: 1078-0432 (Print, Linking)

Davis, S.L. & Jimeno, A. (2010). Metastatic colorectal cancer: focus on panitumumab. *Clin Med Rev Oncol.* Vol. 2, pp. 109-121, ISSN: 1179-2531 (Electronic, Linking)

DeBerardinis, R.J., Sayed, N., Ditsworth, D. & Thompson, C.B. (2008). Brick by brick: metabolism and tumor cell growth. *Curr Opin Genet Dev.* Vol. 18, No. 1, pp. 54-61, ISSN: 0959-437X (Print, Linking), 1879-0380 (Electronic)

De Roock, W., Claes, B., Bernasconi, D., De Schutter, J., Biesmans, B., Fountzilas, G., Kalogeras, K.T., Kotoula, V., Papamichael, D., Laurent-Puig, P., Penault-Llorca, F., Rougier, P., Vincenzi, B., Santini, D., Tonini, G., Cappuzzo, F., Frattini, M., Molinari, F., Saletti, P., De Dosso, S., Martini, M., Bardelli, A., Siena, S., Sartore-Bianchi, A., Tabernero, J., Macarulla, T., Di Fiore, F., Gangloff, A.O., Ciardiello, F., Pfeiffer, P., Qvortrup, C., Hansen, T.P., Van Cutsem, E., Piessevaux, H., Lambrechts, D., Delorenzi, M. & Tejpar, S. (2010a). Effects of *KRAS, BRAF, NRAS,* and *PIK3CA* mutations on the efficacy of cetuximab plus chemotherapy in chemotherapy-refractory metastatic colorectal cancer: a retrospective consortium analysis. *Lancet Oncol.* Vol. 11, No. 8, pp. 753-762, ISSN: 1470-2045 (Print, Linking), 1474-5488 (Electronic)

De Roock, W., Jonker, D.J., Di Nicolantonio, F., Sartore-Bianchi, A., Tu, D., Siena, S., Lamba, S., Arena, S., Frattini, M., Piessevaux, H., Van Cutsem, E., O'Callaghan, C.J., Khambata-Ford, S., Zalcberg, J.R., Simes, J., Karapetis, C.S., Bardelli, A. & Tejpar, S. (2010b). Association of KRAS p.G13D mutation with outcome in patients with chemotherapy-refractory metastatic colorectal cancer treated with cetuximab. *JAMA.* Vol. 304, No. 16, pp. 1812-1820, ISSN: 0098-7484 (Print, Linking), 1538-3598 (Electronic)

Diehl, J.A., Cheng, M., Roussel, M.F. & Sherr, C.J. (1998). Glycogen synthase kinase-3β regulates cyclin D1 proteolysis and subcellular localization. *Genes Dev.* Vol. 12, No. 22, pp. 3499-3511, ISSN: 0890-9369 (Print, Linking), 1549-5477 (Electronic)

Doble, B.W. & Woodgett, J.R. (2003). GSK-3: tricks of the trade for a multi-tasking kinase. *J Cell Sci.* Vol. 116, No. Pt7, pp. 1175-1186, ISSN: 0021-9533 (Print, Linking), 1477-9137 (Electronic)

Doble, B.W. & Woodgett, J.R. (2007). Role of glycogen synthase kinase-3 in cell fate and epithelial-mesenchymal transition. *Cells Tissues Organs.* Vol. 185, No. 1-3, pp. 73-84, ISSN: 1422-6405 (Print, Linking), 1422-6421 (Electronic)

Douillard, J.Y., Siena, S., Cassidy, J., Tabernero, J., Burkes, R., Barugel, M., Humblet, Y., Bodoky, G., Cunningham, D., Jassem, J., Rivera, F., Kocákova, I., Ruff, P., Błasińska-Morawiec, M., Šmakal, M., Canon, J.L., Rother, M., Oliner, K.S., Wolf, M. & Gansert, J. (2010). Randomized, phase III trial of panitumumab with infusional fluorouracil, leucovorin, and oxaliplatin (FOLFOX4) versus FOLFOX4 alone as first-line treatment in patients with previously untreated metastatic colorectal cancer: the PRIME study. *J Clin Oncol.* Vol. 28, No. 31, pp. 4697-4705, ISSN: 0732-183X (Print, Linking), 1527-7755 (Electronic)

Ebos, J.M.L., Lee, C.R. & Kerbel, R.S. (2009). Tumor and host-mediated pathways of resistance and disease progression in response to antiangiogenic therapy. *Clin Cancer Res.* Vol. 15, No. 16, pp. 5020-5025, ISSN: 1078-0432 (Print, Linking)

Edwards, B.K., Ward, E., Kohler, B.A., Eheman, C., Zauber, A.G., Anderson, R.N., Jemal, A., Schymura, M.J., Lansdorp-Vogelaar, I., Seeff, L.C., van Ballegooijen, M., Goede, S.L. & Ries, L.A.G. (2010). Annual report to the nation on the status of cancer, 1975-2006, featuring colorectal cancer trends and impact of interventions (risk factors, screening, and treatment) to reduce future rates. *Cancer.* Vol. 116, No. 3, pp. 544-573, ISSN: 0008-543X (Print, Linking), 1097-0142 (Electronic)

Ellis, L.M. & Hicklin, D.J. (2008a). VEGF-targeted therapy: mechanisms of anti-tumor activity. *Nat Rev Cancer.* Vol. 8, No. 8, pp. 579-591, ISSN: 1474-175X (Print, Linking), 1474-1768 (Electronic)

Ellis, L.M. & Hicklin, D.J. (2008b). Pathways mediating resistance to vascular endothelial growth factor–targeted therapy. *Clin Cancer Res.* Vol. 14, No. 20, pp. 6371-6375, ISSN: 1078-0432 (Print, Linking)

Ellis, L.M. & Hicklin, D.J. (2009). Resistance to targeted therapies: refining anticancer therapy in the era of molecular oncology. *Clin Cancer Res.* Vol. 15, No. 24, pp. 7471-7478, ISSN: 1078-0432 (Print, Linking)

Embi, N., Rhylatt, D.B. & Cohen, P. (1980). Glycogen synthase kinase-3 from rabbit skeletal muscle. Separation from cyclic-AMP-dependent protein kinase and phosphorylase kinase. *Eur J Biochem.* Vol. 107, No. 2, pp. 519-527, ISSN: 0014-2956 (Print, Linking), 1432-1033 (Electronic)

Farooqui, R., Zhu, S. & Fenteany, G. (2006). Glycogen synthase kinase-3 acts upstream of ADP-ribosylation factor 6 and Rac1 to regulate epithelial cell migration. *Exp Cell Res.* Vol. 312, No. 9, pp. 1514-1525, ISSN: 0014-4827 (Print, Linking), 1090-2422 (Electronic)

Finkel, T., Serrano, M. & Blasco, M.A. (2007). The common biology of cancer and ageing. *Nature.* Vol. 448, No. 7155, pp. 767-774, ISSN: 0028-0836 (Print, Linking), 1476-4687 (Electronic)

Fojo, T. & Parkinson, D.R. (2010). Biologically targeted cancer therapy and marginal benefits: are we making too much of too little or are we achieving too little by giving too much? *Clin Cancer Res.* Vol. 16, No. 24, pp. 5972-5980, ISSN: 1078-0432 (Print, Linking)

Foltz, D.R., Santiago, M.C., Berechid, B.E. & Nye, J.S. (2002). Glycogen synthase kinase-3β modulates Notch signaling and stability. *Curr Biol.* Vol. 12, No. 12, pp. 1006-1011, ISSN: 0960-9822 (Print, Linking), 1879-0445 (Electronic)

Frame, S. & Zheleva, D. (2006). Targeting glycogen synthase kinase-3 in insulin signalling. *Expert Opin Ther Targets.* Vol. 10, No. 3, pp. 413-428, ISSN: 1472-8222 (Print, Linking), 1744-7631 (Electronic)

Fuchs, S.Y., Ougolkov, A.V., Spiegelman, V.S. & Minamoto, T. (2005). Oncogenic β-catenin signaling networks in colorectal cancer. *Cell Cycle.* Vol. 4, No. 11, pp. 1522-1539, ISSN: 1538-4101 (Print), 1551-4005 (Electronic, Linking)

Furuta, T. (2009). Pharmacogenomics in chemotherapy for GI tract cancer. *J Gastroenterol.* Vol. 44, No. 10, pp. 1016-1025, ISSN: 0944-1174 (Print, Linking), 1435-5922 (Electronic)

Gatenby, R.A. & Gillies, R.J. (2007). Glycolysis in cancer: a potential target for therapy. *Int J Biochem Cell Biol.* Vol. 39, No. 7-8, pp. 1358-1366, ISSN: 1357-2725 (Print, Linking), 1878-5875 (Electronic)

Ghosh, J.C. & Altieri, D.C. (2005). Activation of p53-dependent apoptosis by acute ablation of glycogen synthase kinase-3β in colorectal cancer cells. *Clin Cancer Res.* Vol. 11, No. 12, pp. 4580-4588, ISSN: 1078-0432 (Print, Linking)

Giles, R.H., van Es, J.H. & Clevers, H. (2003). Wnt storm: Wnt signaling in cancer. *Biochim Biophys Acta.* Vol. 1653, No. 1, pp. 1-24, ISSN: 0006-3002 (Print, Linking)

Grothey, A. (2010). EGFR antibodies in colorectal cancer: where do they belong? *J Clin Oncol.* Vol. 28, No. 31, pp. 4668-4670, ISSN: 0732-183X (Print, Linking), 1527-7755 (Electronic)

Hanahan, D. & Weinberg, R.A. (2011). Hallmarks of cancer: the next generation. *Cell.* Vol. 144, No. 5, pp. 646-673, ISSN: 0092-8674 (Print, Linking), 1097-4172 (Electronic)

Harley, C.B. (2008). Telomerase and cancer therapeutics. *Nat Rev Cancer.* Vol. 8, No. 3, pp. 167-179, ISSN: 1474-175X (Print, Linking), 1474-1768 (Electronic)

Hartman, C.A. (2006). A Wnt canon orchestrating osteoblastogenesis. *Trends Cell Biol.* Vol. 16, No. 3, pp. 151-158, ISSN: 0962-8924 (Print, Linking), 1879-3088 (Electronic)

Harwood, A.J. (2001). Regulation of GSK-3: a cellular multiprocessor. *Cell.* Vol. 105, No. 7, pp. 821-824, ISSN: 0092-8674 (Print, Linking), 1097-4172 (Electronic)

Hecht, J. R., Mitchell, E., Chidiac, T., Scroggin, C., Hagenstad, C., Spigel, D., Marshall, J., Cohn, A., McCollum, D., Stella, P., Deeter, R., Shahin, S. & Amado, R.G. (2009). A randomized phase IIIB trial of chemotherapy, bevacizumab, and panitumumab compared with chemotherapy and bevacizumab alone for metastatic colorectal cancer. *J Clin Oncol.* Vol. 27, No. 5, pp. 672-680, ISSN: 0732-183X (Print, Linking), 1527-7755 (Electronic)

Hecht, J.R., Mitchell, E., Neubauer, M.A., Burris, H.A. 3rd, Swanson, P., Lopez, T., Buchanan, G., Reiner, M., Gansert J. & Berlin, J. (2010). Lack of correlation between epidermal growth factor receptor status and response to Panitumumab monotherapy in metastatic colorectal cancer. *Clin Cancer Res.* Vol. 16, No. 7, pp. 2205-2213, ISSN: 1078-0432 (Print, Linking)

Hoeflich, K.P., Luo, J., Rubie, E.A., Tsao, M.S., Jin, O. & Woodgett, J.R. (2000). Requirement for glycogen synthase kinase-3β in cell survival and NF-κB activation. *Nature.* Vol. 406, No. 6791, pp. 86-90, ISSN: 0028-0836 (Print, Linking), 1476-4687 (Electronic)

Hoshi, M., Takashima, A., Noguchi, K., Murayama, M., Sato, M., Kondo, S., Saitoh, Y., Ishiguro, K., Hoshino, T. & Imahori K. (1996). Regulation of mitochondrial pyruvate dehydrogenase activity by tau protein kinase I/glycogen synthase kinase 3β in brain. *Proc Natl Acad Sci U S A.* Vol. 93, No. 7, pp. 2719-2723, ISSN: 0027-8424 (Print, Linking), 1091-6490 (Electronic)

Inoue, Y., Miki, C. & Kusunoki, M. (2006). Current directions in chemotherapy for colorectal cancer. *J Gastroenterol.* Vol. 41, No. 9, pp. 821-831, ISSN: 0944-1174 (Print, Linking), 1435-5922 (Electronic)

Inoue, J-I., Gohda, J., Akiyama, T. & Semba, K. (2007). NF-κB activation in development and progression of cancer. *Cancer Sci.* Vol. 98, No. 3, pp. 268-274, ISSN: 1347-9032 (Print, Linking), 1349-7006 (Electronic)

Jemal, A., Siegel, R., Xu, J. & Ward, E. (2010). Cancer statistics, 2010. *CA Cancer J Clin.* Vol. 60, No. 5, pp. 277-300, ISSN: 0007-9235 (Print, Linking), 1542-4863 (Electronic)

Jope, R.S. & Johnson, G.V. (2004). The glamour and gloom of glycogen synthase kinase-3. *Trends Biochem Sci.* Vol. 29, No. 2, pp. 95-102, ISSN: 0968-0004 (Print, Linking)

Jope, R.S., Yuskaitis, C.J. & Beurel, E. (2007). Glycogen synthase kinase-3 (GSK3): inflammation, diseases, and therapeutics. *Neurochem Res.* Vol. 32, No. 4-5, pp. 577-595, ISSN: 0364-3190 (Print, Linking), 1573-6903 (Electronic)

Joyce, J.A. (2005). Therapeutic targeting of the tumor microenvironment. *Cancer Cell.* Vol. 7, No. 6, pp. 513-520, ISSN: 1535-6108 (Print, Linking), 1878-3686 (Electronic)

Karin, M. (2006). Nuclear factor-κB in cancer development and progression. *Nature.* Vol. 441, No. 7092, pp. 431-436, ISSN: 0028-0836 (Print, Linking), 1476-4687 (Electronic)

Karin, M. (2009). NF-κB as a critical link between inflammation and cancer. *Cold Spring Harb Perspect Biol.* Vol. 1, pp. a000141, ISSN: 1943-0264 (Electronic)

Kikuchi, A. (2007). Tumor formation by genetic mutations in the components of the Wnt signaling pathway. *Cancer Sci.* Vol. 94, No. 3, pp. 225-229, ISSN: 1347-9032 (Print, Linking), 1349-7006 (Electronic)

Kim, H.S., Skurk, C., Thomas, S.R., Bialik, A., Suhara, T., Kureishi, Y., Birnbaum, M., Keaney, J.F. Jr. & Walsh, K. (2002). Regulation of angiogenesis by glycogen synthase kinase-3β. *J Biol Chem.* Vol. 277, No. 44, pp. 41888-41896, ISSN: 0021-9258 (Print, Linking), 1083-351X (Electronic)

Kim, J. & Dang, C.V. (2006). Cancer's molecular sweet tooth and the Warburg effect. *Cancer Res.* Vol. 66, No. 18, pp. 8927-8930, ISSN: 0008-5472 (Print, Linking); 1538-7445 (Electronic)

Korur, S., Huber, R.M., Sivasankaran, B., Petrich, M., Morin, P., Jr., Hemmings, B.A., Merlo, A. & Lino, M.M. (2009). GSK3β regulates differentiation and growth arrest in glioblastoma. *PLoS One.* Vol. 4, No. 10, pp. e7443, ISSN: 1932-6203 (Linking)

Kiyono, T. (2007). Molecular mechanisms of cellular senescence and immortalization of human cells. *Expert Opin Ther Targets.* Vol. 11, No. 12, pp. 1623-1637, ISSN: 1472-8222 (Print, Linking), 1744-7631 (Electronic)

Klaus, A. & Birchmeier, W. (2008). Wnt signalling and its impact on development and cancer. *Nat Rev Cancer.* Vol. 8, No. 5, pp. 387-398, ISSN: 1474-175X (Print, Linking), 1474-1768 (Electronic)

Knudsen, E. & Knudsen, K. (2008). Tailoring to RB: tumour suppressor status and therapeutic response. *Nat Rev Cancer.* Vol. 8, No. 9, pp. 714-724, ISSN: 1474-175X (Print, Linking), 1474-1768 (Electronic)

Kobayashi, T., Hino, S., Oue, N., Asahara, T., Zollo, M., Yasui, W. & Kikuchi, A. (2006). Glycogen synthase kinase 3 and h-prune regulate cell migration by modulating focal adhesions. *Mol Cell Biol.* Vol. 26, No. 3, pp. 898-911, ISSN: 0270-7306 (Print, Linking), 1098-5549 (Electronic)

Koivisto, L., Alavian, K., Hakkinen, L., Pelech, S., McCulloch, C. & Larjava, H. (2003). Glycogen synthase kinase-3 regulates formation of long lamellipodia in human keratinocytes. *J Cell Sci.* Vol. 116, No. Pt 18, pp. 3749-3760, ISSN: 0021-9533 (Print, Linking), 1477-9137 (Electronic)

Krishnan, V., Bryant, H.U. & MacDougald, O.A. (2006). Regulation of bone mass by Wnt signaling. *J Clin Invest.* Vol. 116, No. 5, pp. 1202-1209, ISSN: 0021-9738 (Print, Linking), 1558-8238 (Electronic)

Kroemer, G. & Pouyssegur, J. (2008). Tumor cell metabolism: Cancer's Achilles' heel. *Cancer Cell.* Vol. 13, No. 6, pp. 472-482, ISSN: 1535-6108 (Print, Linking), 1878-3686 (Electronic)

Kulikov, R., Boehme, K.A. & Blattner, C. (2005). Glycogen synthase kinase 3-dependent phosphorylation of Mdm2 regulates p53 abundance. *Mol Cell Biol.* Vol. 25, No. 16, pp. 7170-7180, ISSN: 0270-7306 (Print, Linking), 1098-5549 (Electronic)

Kulkarni, N.H., Onyia, J.E., Zeng, Q., Tian, X., Liu, M., Halladay, D.L., Frolik, C.A., Engler, T., Wei, T., Kriauciunas, A., Martin, T.J., Sato, M., Bryant, H.U. & Ma, Y.L. (2006). Orally bioavailable GSK-3α/β dual inhibitor increases markers of cellular differentiation *in vitro* and bone mass *in vivo*. *J Bone Miner Res*. Vol. 21, No. 6, pp. 910-920, ISSN: 0884-0431 (Print, Linking), 1523-4681 (Electronic)

Kunnimalaiyaan, M., Vaccaro, A.M., Ndiaye, M.A. & Chen, H. (2007). Inactivation of glycogen synthase kinase-3β, a downstream target of the raf-1 pathway, is associated with growth suppression in medullary thyroid cancer cells. *Mol Cancer Ther*. Vol. 6, No. 3, pp. 1151-1158, ISSN: 1535-7163 (Print, Linking), 1538-8514 (Electronic)

Kypta, R.M. (2005). GSK-3 inhibitors and their potential in the treatment of Alzheimer's disease. *Expert Opin Ther Patents*. Vol. 15, No. 10, pp. 1315-1331, ISSN: 1354-3776 (Print, Linking), 1744-7674 (Electronic)

Lacy, A.M., Delgado, S., Castells, A., Prins, H.A., Arroyo, V., Ibarzabal, A. & Pique, J.M. (2008). The long-term results of a randomized clinical trial of laparoscopy-assisted versus open surgery for colon cancer. *Ann Surg*. Vol. 248, No. 1, pp. 1-7, ISSN: 0003-4932 (Print, Linking), 1528-1140 (Electronic)

Lee, J. & Kim, M-S. (2007). The role of GSK3 in glucose homeostasis and the development of insulin resistance. *Diabetes Res Clin Pract*. Vol. 77, No. suppl 1, pp. S49-S57, ISSN: 1572-1671 (Print, Linking)

Li, J. & Saif, M.W. (2009). Current use and potential role of bevacizumab in the treatment of gastrointestinal cancers. *Biologics Targets Ther*. Vol. 3, pp. 429-441, ISSN: 1177-5475 (Print, Linking), 1177-5491 (Electronic)

Linding, R., Jensen, L.J., Ostheimer, G.J., van Vugt, M.A., Jorgensen, C., Miron, I.M., Diella, F., Colwill, K., Taylor, L., Elder, K., Metalnikov, P., Nguyen, V., Pasculescu, A., Jin, J., Park, J.G., Samson, L.D., Woodgett, J.R., Russell, R.B., Bork, P., Yaffe, M.B. & Pawson, T. (2007). Systemic discovery of in vivo phosphorylation networks. *Cell*. Vol. 129, No. 7, pp. 1415-1426, ISSN: 0092-8674 (Print, Linking), 1097-4172 (Electronic)

Liu, S., Yu, S., Hasegawa, Y., LaPushin, R., Xu, H.J., Woodgett, J.R., Mills, G.B. & Fang, X. (2004). Glycogen synthase kinase 3β is a negative regulator of growth factor-induced activation of the c-Jun N-terminal kinase. *J Biol Chem*. Vol. 279, No. 49, pp. 51075-51081, ISSN: 0021-9258 (Print, Linking), 1083-351X (Electronic)

Lou, H. & Dean, M. (2007). Targeted therapy for cancer stem cells: the patched pathway and ABC transporters. *Oncogene*. Vol. 26, No. 9, pp. 1357-1360, ISSN: 0950-9232 (Print, Linking), 1476-5594 (Electronic)

Luo, J. (2009). Glycogen synthase kinase 3β (GSK3β) in tumorigenesis and cancer chemotherapy. *Cancer Lett*. Vol. 273, No. 2, pp. 194-200, ISSN: 0304-3835 (Print, Linking), 1872-7980 (Electronic)

Lustig, B. & Behrens, J. (2003). The Wnt signalling pathway and its role in tumor development. *J Cancer Res Clin Oncol*. Vol. 129, No. 4, pp. 199-221, ISSN: 0171-5216 (Print, Linking), 1432-1335 (Electronic)

Macafee, D.A.L., West, J., Scholefield, J.H. & Whynes, D.K. (2009). Hospital costs of colorectal cancer care. *Clin Med Oncol*. Vol. 3, pp. 27-37, ISSN: 1177-9314 (Electronic, Linking)

Machesky, L.M. (2008). Lamellipodia and filopodia in metastasis and invasion. *FEBS Lett*. Vol. 582, No. 14, pp. 2102-2111, ISSN: 0014-5793 (Print, Linking), 1873-3468 (Electronic)

Mai, W., Miyashita, K., Shakoori, A., Zhang, B., Yu, Z.W., Takahashi, Y., Motoo, Y., Kawakami, K. & Minamoto, T. (2006). Detection of active fraction of GSK3β in cancer cells by non-radioisotopic *in vitro* kinase assay. *Oncology*. Vol. 71, No. 3-4, pp. 297-305, ISSN: 0030-2414 (Print, Linking), 1423-0232 (Electronic)

Mai, W., Kawakami, K., Shakoori, A., Kyo, S., Miyashita, K., Yokoi, K., Jin, M., Shimasaki, T., Motoo, Y. & Minamoto, T. (2009). Deregulated GSK3β sustains gastrointestinal cancer cells survival by modulating human telomerase reverse transcriptase and telomerase. *Clin Cancer Res*. Vol. 15, No. 22, pp. 6810-6819, ISSN: 1078-0432 (Print, Linking)

Mankoff, D.A., Eary, J.F., Link, J.M., Muzi, M., Rajendran, J.G., Spence, A.M. & Krohn, K.A. (2007). Tumor-specific positron emission tomography imaging in patients: [18F] fluorodeoxyglucose and beyond. *Clin Cancer Res*. Vol. 13, No. 12, pp. 3460-3469, ISSN: 1078-0432 (Print, Linking)

Manoukian, S.S. & Woodgett, J. (2002). Role of GSK-3 in cancer: regulation by Wnts and other signaling pathways. *Adv Cancer Res*. Vol. 84, pp. 203-229, ISSN: 0065-230X (Print, Linking)

Markowitz, S.D. & Bertagnolli, M.M. (2009). Molecular basis of colorectal cancer. *N Engl J Med*. Vol. 361, No. 25, pp. 2449-2460, ISSN: 0028-4793 (Print, Linking), 1533-4406 (Electronic)

McLean, G.W., Carragher, N.O., Avizienyte, E., Evans, J., Brunton, V.G. & Frame, M.C. (2005). The role of focal adhesion kinase in cancer - a new therapeutic opportunity. *Nat Rev Cancer*. Vol. 5, No. 7, pp. 505-515, ISSN: 1474-175X (Print, Linking), 1474-1768 (Electronic)

Medina, M. & Wandosell, F. (2011). Deconstructing GSK-3: the fine regulation of its activity. *Int J Alzheimers Dis*. Vol. 2011, Article ID 479249, ISSN: 2090-0252 (Electronic)

Meijer, L., Flajolet, M. & Greengard, P. (2004). Pharmacological inhibitors of glycogen synthase kinase 3. *Trends Pharmacol Sci*. Vol. 25, No. 9, pp. 471-480, ISSN: 0165-6147 (Print, Linking), 1873-3735 (Electronic)

Meyerhardt, J.A. & Mayer, R.J. (2005). Systemic therapy for colorectal cancer. *N Engl J Med*. Vol. 352, No. 5, pp. 476-487, ISSN: 0028-4793 (Print, Linking), 1533-4406 (Electronic)

Midgley, R. & Kerr, D. (1999). Seminar on colorectal cancer. *Lancet*. Vol. 353, No. 9150, pp. 391-399, ISSN: 0140-6736 (Print, Linking), 1474-547X (Electronic)

Midgley, R.S., Yanagisawa, Y. & Kerr, D. (2009). Evolution of nonsurgical therapy for colorectal cancer. *Nat Clin Pract Gastroenterol Hepatol*. Vol. 6, No. 2, pp. 108-120, ISSN: 1743-4378 (Print, Linking), 1743-4386 (Electronic)

Minamoto, T., inventor; National University Corporation Kanazawa University; assignee. Suppression of cancer and method for evaluating anticancer agent based on the effect of inhibiting GSK3β. International patent WO2006/073202. 2006 Jul 13. United States patent US 11/794,716. 2006 Jan 4. European patent EP1845094 2007 Oct 17. Japan patent 2006-550915 2007 Jun 21.

Miyashita, K., Kawakami, K., Mai, W., Shakoori, A., Fujisawa, H., Nakada, M., Hayashi, Y., Hamada, J. & Minamoto, T. (2009a). Potential therapeutic effect of glycogen synthase kinase 3β inhibition against human glioblastoma. *Clin Cancer Res*. Vol. 15, No. 3, pp. 887-897, ISSN: 1078-0432 (Print, Linking)

Miyashita, K., Nakada, M., Shakoori, A., Ishigaki, Y., Shimasaki, T., Motoo, Y., Kawakami, K. & Minamoto, T. (2009b). An emerging strategy for cancer treatment targeting aberrant glycogen synthase kinase 3β. *Anticancer Agents Med Chem*. Vol. 9, No. 10, pp. 1114-1122, ISSN: 1871-5206 (Print, Linking), 1875-5992 (Electronic)

Motoo, Y., Shimasaki, T., Ishigaki, Y., Nakajima, H., Kawakami, K. & Minamoto, T. (2011). Metabolic disorder, inflammation, and deregulated molecular pathways converging in pancreatic cancer development: implications for new therapeutic strategies. *Cancers.* Vol. 3, No. 1, pp. 446-460, ISSN: 2072-6694 (Electronic, Linking)

Mottet, D., Dumont, V., Deccache, Y., Demazy, C., Ninane, N., Raes, M. & Michiels, C. (2003). Regulation of hypoxia-inducible factor-1α protein level during hypoxic conditions by the phosphatidylinositol 3-kinase/Akt/glycogen synthase kinase 3β pathway in HepG2 cells. *J Biol Chem.* Vol. 278, No. 33, pp. 31277-31285, ISSN: 0021-9258 (Print, Linking), 1083-351X (Electronic)

Nakada, M., Minamoto, T., Pyko, I.V., Hayashi, Y. & Hamada, J.I. (2011). The pivotal role of GSK3β in glioma biology, In: *Brain Tumor / Book 2*, Miklos Garami, InTech, ISBN: 978-953-307-587-7, in press

Nowicki, M., Dmitrieva, N., Stein, A.M., Cutter, J.L., Godlewski, J., Saeki, Y., Nita, M., Berens, M.E., Sander, L.M., Newton, H.B., Chiocca, E.A. & Lawler, S. (2008). Lithium inhibits invasion of glioma cells; possible involvement of glycogen synthase kinase-3. *Neuro Oncol.* Vol. 10, No. 5, pp. 690-699, ISSN: 1522-8517 (Print, Linking), 1523-5866 (Electronic)

O'Brien, C.A., Kreso, A. & Jamieson, C.H.M. (2010). Cancer stem cells and self-renewal. *Clin Cancer Res.* Vol. 16, No. 12, pp. 3113-3120, ISSN: 1078-0432 (Print, Linking)

O'Brien, C.A., Pollet, A., Gallinger, S. & Dick, J.E. (2007). A human colon cancer cell capable of initiating tumour growth in immunodeficient mice. *Nature.* Vol. 445, No. 7123, pp. 106-115, ISSN: 0028-0836 (Print, Linking), 1476-4687 (Electronic)

Ougolkov, A.V., Fernandez-Zapico, M.E., Savoy, D.N., Urrutia, R.A. & Billadeau, D.D. (2005). Glycogen synthase kinase-3β participates in nuclear factor κB-mediated gene transcription and cell survival in pancreatic cancer cells. *Cancer Res.* Vol. 65, No. 6, pp. 2076-2081, ISSN: 0008-5472 (Print, Linking), 1538-7445 (Electronic)

Parsons, D.W., Wang, T.L., Samuels, Y., Bardelli, A., Cummins, J.M., DeLong, L., Silliman, N., Ptak, J., Szabo, S., Willson, J.K., Markowitz, S., Kinzler, K.W., Vogelstein, B., Lengauer, C. & Velculescu, V.E. (2005). Colorectal cancer: mutations in a signalling pathway. *Nature.* Vol. 436, No. 7052, pp. 792, ISSN: 0028-0836 (Print, Linking), 1476-4687 (Electronic)

Patel, S. & Woodgett, J. (2008). Glycogen synthase kinase-3 and cancer: good cop, bad cop? *Cancer Cell.* Vol. 14, No. 5, pp. 351-353, ISSN: 1535-6108 (Print, Linking), 1878-3686 (Electronic)

Phukan, S., Babu, V.S., Kannoji, A., Hariharan, R. & Balaji, V.N. (2010). GSK3β: role in therapeutic landscape and development of modulators. *Br J Pharmacol.* Vol. 160, No. 1, pp. 1-19, ISSN: 0007-1188 (Print, Linking), 1476-5381 (Electronic)

Polakis, P. (1999). The oncogenic activation of β-catenin. *Curr Opin Genet Dev.* Vol. 9, No. 1, pp. 15-21, ISSN: 0959-437X (Print, Linking), 1879-0380 (Electronic)

Polyak, K., Weiberg, R.A. (2009). Transitions between epithelial and mesenchymal states: acquisition of malignant and stem cell traits. *Nat Rev Cancer.* Vol. 9, No. 4, pp. 265-273, ISSN: 1474-175X (Print, Linking), 1474-1768 (Electronic)

Prenen, H., Tejpar, S. & Van Cutsem, E. (2010). New strategies for treatment of KRAS mutant metastatic colorectal cancer. *Clin Cancer Res.* Vol. 16, No. 11, pp. 2921-2926, ISSN: 1078-0432 (Print, Linking)

Qu, L., Huang, S., Baltzis, D., Rivas-Estilla, A.M., Pluquet, O., Hatzoglou, M., Koumenis, C., Taya, Y., Yoshimura, A. & Koromilas, A.E. (2004). Endoplasmic reticulum stress induces p53 cytoplasmic localization and prevents p53-dependent apoptosis by a pathway involving glycogen synthase kinase-3β. *Genes Dev.* Vol. 18, No. 3, pp. 261-277, ISSN: 0890-9369 (Print, Linking), 1549-5477 (Electronic)

Raftpoulou, M. & Hall, A. (2004). Cell migration: Rho GTPases lead the way. *Dev Biol.* Vol. 265, No. 1, pp. 23-32, ISSN: 0012-1606 (Print, Linking), 1095-564X (Electronic)

Ralston, S.H. & de Crombrugghe, B. (2006). Genetic regulation of bone mass and susceptibility to osteoporosis. *Genes Dev.* Vol. 20, No. 18, pp. 2492-2506, ISSN: 0890-9369 (Print, Linking), 1549-5477 (Electronic)

Rayasam, G.V., Tulasi, V.K., Sodhi, R., Davis, J.A. & Ray, A. (2009). Glycogen synthase kinase-3: more than a namesake. *Br J Pharmacol.* Vol. 156, No. 6, pp. 885-898, ISSN: 0007-1188 (Print, Linking), 1476-5381 (Electronic)

Ricci-Vitiani, L., Lombardi, D.G., Pilozzi, E., Biffoni, M., Todaro, M., Peschle, C. & De Maria, R. (2007). Identification and expansion of human colon-cancer-initiating cells. *Nature.* Vol. 445, No. 7123, pp. 106-115, ISSN: 0028-0836 (Print, Linking), 1476-4687 (Electronic)

Rössig, L., Badorff, C., Holzmann, Y., Zeiher, A.M. & Dimmeler, S. (2002). Glycogen synthase kinase-3 couples AKT-dependent signaling to the regulation of p21[Cip1] degradation. *J Biol Chem.* Vol. 277, No. 22, pp. 9684-9689, ISSN: 0021-9258 (Print, Linking), 1083-351X (Electronic)

Rottmann, S., Wang, Y., Nasoff, M., Deveraux, Q.L. & Quon, K.C. (2005). A TRAIL receptor-dependent synthetic lethal relationship between *Myc* activation and GSK3β/FBW7 loss of function. *Proc Natl Acad Sci USA.* Vol. 102, No. 42, pp. 15195-15200, ISSN: 0027-8424 (Print, Linking), 1091-6490 (Electronic)

Royds, J.A. & Iacopetta, B. (2006). p53 and disease: when the guardian angel fails. *Cell Death Diff.* Vol. 13, No. 6, pp. 1017-1026, ISSN: 1350-9047 (Print, Linking), 1476-5403 (Electronic)

Sahai, E. & Marshall, C.J. (2002). Rho-GTPases and cancer. *Nat Rev Cancer.* Vol. 2, No. 2, pp. 133-142, ISSN: 1474-175X (Print, Linking), 1474-1768 (Electronic)

Samudio, I., Fiegl, M. & Andreeff, M. (2009). Mitochondrial uncoupling and the Warburg effect: molecular basis for the reprogrammimg of cancer cell metabolism. *Cancer Res.* Vol. 69, No. 6, pp. 2163-2166, ISSN: 0008-5472 (Print, Linking), 1538-7445 (Electronic)

Sargent, D. J, Patiyil, S., Yothers, G., Haller, D.G., Gray, R., Benedetti, J., Buyse, M., Labianca, R., Seitz, J.F., O'Callaghan, C.J., Francini, G., Grothey, A., O'Connell, M., Catalano, P.J., Kerr, D., Green, E., Wieand, H.S., Goldberg, R.M., de Gramont, A. & ACCENT Group. (2007). End points for colon cancer adjuvant trials: observations and recommendations based on individual patient data from 20,898 patients enrolled onto 18 randomized trials from the ACCENT Group. *J Clin Oncol.* Vol. 25, No. 29, pp. 4569-4574, ISSN: 0732-183X (Print, Linking), 1527-7755 (Electronic)

Sartore-Bianchi, A., Martini, M., Molinari, F., Veronese, S., Nichelatti, M., Artale, S., Di Nicolantonio, F., Saletti, P., De Dosso, S., Mazzucchelli, L., Frattini, M., Siena, S. & Bardelli, A. (2009). PI3CA mutations in colorectal cancer are associated with clinical resistance to EGFR-targeted monoclonal antibodies. *Cancer Res.* Vol. 69, No. 5, pp. 1851-1857, ISSN: 0008-5472 (Print, Linking), 1538-7445 (Electronic)

Sato, N., Meijer, L., Skaltsounis, L., Greengard, P. & Brivanlou, A.H. (2004). Maintenance of pluripotency in human and mouse embryonic stem cells through activation of Wnt signaling by a pharmacological GSK-3-specific inhibitor. *Nat Med.* Vol. 10, No. 1, pp. 55-63, ISSN: 1078-8956 (Print, Linking), 1546-170X (Electronic)

Schlessinger, K. & Hall, A. (2004). GSK-3β sets Snail's pace. *Nat Cell Biol.* Vol. 6, No. 10, pp. 913-915, ISSN: 1465-7392 (Print, Linking), 1476-4679 (Electronic)

Schwabe, R.F. & Brenner, D.A. (2002). Role of glycogen synthase kinase-3 in TNF-α-induced NF-κB activation and apoptosis in hepatocytes. *Am J Physiol Gastrointest Liver Physiol.* Vol. 283, No. 1, pp. G204-211, ISSN: 0193-1857 (Print, Linking), 1522-1547 (Electronic)

Semenza, G.L. (2009). Regulation of oxygen homeostasis by hypoxia-inducible factor 1. *Physiology (Bethesda).* Vol. 24, pp. 97-106, ISSN: 1548-9213 (Print), 1548-9221 (Electronic, Linking)

Shakoori, A., Ougolkov, A., Yu, Z.W., Zhang, B., Modarressi, M.H., Billadeau, D.D., Mai, M., Takahashi, Y. & Minamoto, T. (2005). Deregulated GSK3β activity in colorectal cancer: its association with tumor cell survival and proliferation. *Biochem Biophys Res Commun.* Vol. 334, No. 4, pp. 1365-1373, ISSN: 0006-291X (Print, Linking), 1090-2104 (Electronic)

Shakoori, A., Mai, W., Miyashita, K., Yasumoto, K., Takahashi, Y., Ooi, A., Kawakami, K. & Minamoto, T. (2007). Inhibition of GSK3β attenuates proliferation of human colon cancer cells in rodents. *Cancer Sci.* Vol. 98, No. 9, pp. 1388-1393, ISSN: 1347-9032 (Print, Linking), 1349-7006 (Electronic)

Sharma, S.V., Fischbach, M.A., Haber, D.A. & Settleman, J. (2006). "Oncogenic shock": explaining oncogene addiction through differential signal attenuation. *Clin Cancer Res.* Vol. 12, No. 14 Suppl, pp. 4392s-4395s, ISSN: 1078-0432 (Print, Linking)

Sharma, S.V. & Settleman, J. (2007). Oncogene addiction: setting the stage for molecularly targeted cancer therapy. *Genes Dev.* Vol. 21, No. 24, pp. 3214-3231, ISSN: 0890-9369 (Print, Linking), 1549-5477 (Electronic)

Sjöblom, T., Jones, S., Wood, L.D., Parsons, D.W., Lin, J., Barber, T.D., Mandelker, D., Leary, R.J., Ptak, J., Silliman, N., Szabo, S., Buckhaults, P., Farrell, C., Meeh, P., Markowitz, S.D., Willis, J., Dawson, D., Willson, J.K., Gazdar, A.F., Hartigan, J., Wu, L., Liu, C., Parmigiani, G., Park, B.H., Bachman, K.E., Papadopoulos, N., Vogelstein, B., Kinzler, K.W. & Velculescu, V.E. (2006). The consensus coding sequences of human breast and colorectal cancers. *Science.* Vol. 314, No. 5797, pp. 268-274. ISSN: 0193-4511 (Print, Linking)

Small, J.V., Stradal, T., Vignal, E. & Rottner, K. (2002). The lamellipodium: where motility begins. *Trends Cell Biol.* Vol. 12, No. 3, pp. 112-120, ISSN: 0962-8924 (Print, Linking), 1879-3088 (Electronic)

Smallbone, K., Gatenby, R.A., Gillies, R.J., Maini, P.K. & Gavaghan, D.J. (2007). Metabolic changes during carcinogenesis: potential impact on invasiveness. *J Theor Biol.* Vol. 244, No. 4, pp. 703-713, ISSN: 0022-5193 (Print, Linking), 1095-8541 (Electronic)

Stacpoole, P.W., Nagaraja, N.V. & Hutson, A.D. (2003). Efficacy of dichloroacetate as a lactate-lowering drug. *J Clin Pharmacol.* Vol. 43, No. 7, pp. 683-691, ISSN: 0091-2700 (Print, Linking), 1552-4604 (Electronic)

Stacpoole, P.W., Kerr, D.S., Barnes, C., Bunch, S.T., Carney, P.R., Fennell, E.M., Felitsyn, N.M., Gilmore, R.L., Greer, M., Henderson, G.N., Hutson, A.D., Neiberger, R.E., O'Brien, R.G., Perkins, L.A., Quisling, R.G., Shroads, A.L., Shuster, J.J., Silverstein,

J.H., Theriaque, D.W. & Valenstein, E. (2006). Controlled clinical trial of dichloroacetate for treatment of congenital lactic acidosis in children. *Pediatrics.* Vol. 117, No. 5, pp. 1519-1531, ISSN: 0031-4005 (Print, Linking), 1098-4275 (Electronic)

Surjit, M. & Lal, S.K. (2007). Glycogen synthase kinase-3 phosphorylates and regulates the stability of p27[kip1] protein. *Cell Cycle.* Vol. 6, No. 5, pp. 580-588, ISSN: 1538-4101 (Print), 1551-4005 (Electronic, Linking)

Takenaka, K., Kise, Y. & Miki, H. (2007). GSK3β positively regulates Hedgehog signaling through Sufu in mammalian cells. *Biochem Biophys Res Commun.* Vol. 353, No. 2, pp. 501-508, ISSN: 0006-291X (Print, Linking), 1090-2104 (Electronic)

Tan, J., Zhuang, L., Leong, H., Iyer, N.G., Liu, E.T. & Yu, Q. (2005). Pharmacologic modulation of glycogen synthase kinase-3β promotes p53-dependent apoptosis through a direct Bax-mediated mitochondrial pathway in colorectal cancer cells. *Cancer Res.* Vol. 65, No. 19, pp. 9012-9020, ISSN: 0008-5472 (Print, Linking), 1538-7445 (Electronic)

The Clinical Outcomes of Surgical Therapy Study Group. (2004). A comparison of laparoscopically assisted and open colectomy for colon cancer. *N Engl J Med.* Vol. 350, No. 20, pp. 2050-2059, ISSN: 0028-4793 (Print, Linking), 1533-4406 (Electronic)

Tol, J., Koopman, M., Cats, A., Rodenburg, C.J., Creemers, G.J., Schrama, J.G., Erdkamp, F.L., Vos, A.H., van Groeningen, C.J., Sinnige, H.A., Richel, D.J., Voest, E.E., Dijkstra, J.R., Vink-Börger, M.E., Antonini, N.F., Mol, L., van Krieken, J.H., Dalesio, O. & Punt, C.J. (2009). Chemotherapy, bevacizumab, and cetuximab in metastatic colorectal cancer. *N Engl J Med.* Vol. 360, No. 6, pp. 563-572, ISSN: 0028-4793 (Print, Linking), 1533-4406 (Electronic)

Trowbridge, J.J., Xenocostas, A., Moon, R.T. & Bhatia, M. (2006). Glycogen synthase kinase-3 is an in vivo regulator of hematopoietic stem cell repopulation. *Nat Med.* Vol. 12, No. 1, pp. 89-98, ISSN: 1078-8956 (Print, Linking), 1546-170X (Electronic)

Tsuchiya, K., Nakamura, T., Okamoto, R., Kanai, T. & Watanabe, M. (2007). Reciprocal targeting of Hath1 and β-catenin by Wnt glycogen synthase kinase 3β in human colon cancer. *Gastroenterology.* Vol. 132, No. 1, pp. 208-220, ISSN: 0016-5085 (Print, Linking), 1528-0012 (Electronic)

Umar, A. & Greenwald, P. (2009). Alarming colorectal cancer incidence trends: a case for early detection and prevention. *Cancer Epidemiol Biomarkers Prev.* Vol. 18, No. 6, pp. 1672-1673, ISSN: 1055-9965 (Print, Linking), 1538-7755 (Electronic)

Vaidya, R.J., Ray, R.M. & Johnson, L.R. (2006). Akt-mediated GSK-3β inhibition prevents migration of polyamine-depleted intestinal epithelial cells via Rac1. *Cell Mol Life Sci.* Vol. 63, No. 23, pp. 2871-2879, ISSN: 1420-682X (Print, Linking), 1420-9071 (Electronic)

Vander Heiden, M.G., Cantley, L.C. & Thompson, C.B. (2010). Understanding the Warburg effect: the metabolic requirements of cell proliferation. *Science.* Vol. 324, No. 5630, pp. 1029-1033, ISSN: 0193-4511 (Print, Linking)

Vousden, K.H. & Lane, D.P. (2007). p53 in health and disease. *Nat Rev Mol Cell Biol.* Vol. 8, No. 4, pp. 275-283, ISSN: 1471-0072 (Print, Linking), 1471-0080 (Electronic)

Walther, A., Johnstone, E., Swanton, C., Midgley, R., Tomlinson, I. & Kerr, D. (2009). Genetic prognostic and predictive markers in colorectal cancer. *Nat Rev Cancer.* Vol. 9, No. 7, pp. 489-499, ISSN: 1474-175X (Print, Linking), 1474-1768 (Electronic)

Wang, Z., Smith, K.S., Murphy, M., Piloto, O., Somervaille, T.C.P. & Cleary, M.L. (2008). Glycogen synthase kinase 3 in *MLL* leukaemia maintenance and targeted therapy.

Nature. Vol. 455, No. 7217, pp. 1205-1209, ISSN: 0028-0836 (Print, Linking), 1476-4687 (Electronic)

Weinstein, I.B. (2002). Cancer: addiction to oncogene—the Achilles' heal of cancer. *Science.* Vol. 297, No. 5578, pp. 63-64, ISSN: 0193-4511 (Print, Linking)

Weinstein, I.B. & Joe, A.K. (2006). Mechanisms of disease: oncogene addiction—a rationale for molecular targeting in cancer therapy. *Nat Clin Pract Oncol.* Vol. 3, No. 8, pp. 448-457, ISSN: 1743-4254 (Print, Linking); 1743-4262 (Electronic)

Willert, K. & Jones, K.A. (2006). Wnt signaling: is the party in the nucleus? *Gene Dev.* Vol. 20, No. 11, pp. 1394-1404, ISSN: 0890-9369 (Print, Linking), 1549-5477 (Electronic)

Wilson, W. 3rd. & Baldwin, A.S. (2008). Maintenance of constitutive IκB kinase activity by glycogen synthase kinase-3α/β in pancreatic cancer. *Cancer Res.* Vol. 68, No. 19, pp. 8156-8163, ISSN: 0008-5472 (Print, Linking), 1538-7445 (Electronic)

Wolpin, B.M., Meyerhardt, J.A., Mamon, H.J. & Mayer, R.J. (2007). Adjuvant treatment of colorectal cancer. *CA Cancer J Clin.* Vol. 57, No. 3, pp. 168-185, ISSN: 0007-9235 (Print, Linking), 1542-4863 (Electronic)

Wolpin, B.M. & Mayer, R.J. (2008). Systemic treatment of colorectal cancer. *Gastroenterology.* Vol. 134, No. 5, pp. 1296-1310, ISSN: 0016-5085 (Print, Linking), 1528-0012 (Electronic)

Wood, L.D., Parsons, D.W., Jones, S., Lin, J., Sjöblom, T., Leary, R.J., Shen, D., Boca, S.M., Barber, T., Ptak, J., Silliman, N., Szabo, S., Dezso, Z., Ustyanksky, V., Nikolskaya, T., Nikolsky, Y., Karchin, R., Wilson, P.A., Kaminker, J.S., Zhang, Z., Croshaw, R., Willis, J., Dawson, D., Shipitsin, M., Willson, J.K., Sukumar, S., Polyak, K., Park, B.H., Pethiyagoda, C.L., Pant, P.V., Ballinger, D.G., Sparks, A.B,, Hartigan, J., Smith, D.R., Suh, E., Papadopoulos, N., Buckhaults, P., Markowitz, S.D., Parmigiani, G., Kinzler, K.W., Velculescu, V.E. & Vogelstein, B. (2007). The genomic landscapes of human breast and colorectal cancers. *Science.* Vol. 318, No. 5853, pp. 1108-1113. ISSN: 0193-4511 (Print, Linking)

Wu, J.S. & Fazio, V.W. (2000). Colon cancer. *Dis Colon Rectum.* Vol. 43, No. 11, pp. 1473-1486, ISSN: 0012-3706 (Print, Linking), 1530-0358 (Electronic)

Xu, C., Kim, N.G. & Gumbiner, B.M. Regulation of protein stability by GSK3 mediated phosphorylation. (2009). *Cell Cycle.* Vol. 8, No. 24, pp. 4032-4039, ISSN: 1538-4101 (Print), 1551-4005 (Electronic, Linking)

Yeung, T.M. & Mortensen, N.J. (2009). Colorectal cancer stem cells. *Dis Colon Rectum.* Vol. 52, No. 10, pp. 1788-1796, ISSN: 0012-3706 (Print, Linking), 1530-0358 (Electronic)

Yilmaz, M. & Christofori, G. (2009). EMT, the cytoskeleton, and cancer cell invasion. *Cancer Metastasis Rev.* Vol. 28, No. 1-2, pp. 15-33, ISSN: 0167-7659 (Print, Linking), 1573-7233 (Electronic)

Zhou, B.P., Deng, J., Xia, W., Xu, J., Li, Y.M., Gunduz, M. & Hung, M.C. (2004). Dual regulation of Snail by GSK-3β-mediated phosphorylation in control of epithelial-mesenchymal transition. *Nat Cell Biol.* Vol. 6, No. 10, pp. 931-940, ISSN: 1465-7392 (Print, Linking), 1476-4679 (Electronic)

Zhou, B.P. & Hung, M.C. (2005). Wnt, hedgehog and β-Trcp in the regulation of metastasis. *Cell Cycle.* Vol. 4, No. 6, pp. 772-776, ISSN: 1538-4101 (Print), 1551-4005 (Electronic, Linking)

Zilfou, J.T. & Lowe, S.W. (2009). Tumor suppressive functions of p53. *Cold Spring Harb Perspect Biol.* Vol. 1, No. 5, pp. a001883, ISSN: 1943-0264 (Electronic)

4

Growth Factors and the Redox State as New Therapeutic Targets for Colorectal Cancer

Teodoro Palomares, Marta Caramés,
Ignacio García-Alonso and Ana Alonso-Varona
University of the Basque Country,
Spain

1. Introduction

Colorectal cancer (CRC) is an important health problem in many western countries due to its significant morbidity/mortality. Despite advances in its diagnosis and treatment, survival associated with this cancer when it has extended to adjacent organs, lymphatic nodules or distal organs is drastically reduced. The liver is the most common site of CRC metastasis, since it represents a unique microenvironment for the formation of metastases, not only due to its sinusoidal endothelium (Barberá-Guillén et al., 1989), but also due to its abundant expression of growth factors (GFs) (Stoeltzing et al., 2003).

At present, curative treatment of localized metastases is possible via partial liver resection. However, this surgical procedure is only potentially curative, since 65% of patients subjected to resection of liver metastases experience relapse within 5 years (Sun & Tang, 2003; Allendorf et al., 2004). In the light of this frequent recurrence, it is essential to develop new preventive therapeutic strategies, which require a detailed knowledge of the biological events that occur following hepatectomy. In this sense, we have previously demonstrated the tumor-enhancing effect associated with liver resection in a mouse tumor model; in addition, we showed that hepatectomized rat serum increased cell proliferation *in vitro*, when compared with laparotomized rat serum or fetal calf serum (García-Alonso et al., 2003; García-Alonso et al., 2008a, 2008b). These findings indicated that GFs produced by the liver promote the development of metastases.

At present, CRC treatment includes various active drugs, either as individual agents or in combination: 5-fluorouracil (5-FU), capecitabine, irinotecan and oxaliplatin, among others. Despite this wide array of anti-tumor agents, relapse often occurs in CRC patients, due in large part to the resistance of the tumor cells to these anti-neoplastic agents. Various different mechanisms have been reported as being responsible for the development of chemoresistance and, though each may be important in itself, they take on an even greater significance if we consider how they may be interrelated.

One of these mechanisms of resistance to anti-neoplastic agents is the presence of GFs, which may be able to protect certain tumor cells against cytotoxic cell death. For this reason, one of the most promising cell targets nowadays are these GFs and their receptors. Thus, since 2004, three new agents have been approved which in combination with cytotoxic agents are administered in cases of advanced and metastatic CRC: bevacizumab, a monoclonal antibody to vascular endothelial growth factor (VEGF) (Hurwitz et al., 2004), and cetuximab and panitumumab, which are monoclonal antibodies to the epidermal growth factor receptor (EGFR) (Cunningham et al., 2004; Odom et al., 2011).

An increasing amount of evidence indicates that the intracellular redox state plays an essential role in the mechanisms underlying the actions of GFs. In particular, GFs have been reported to generate reactive oxygen species (ROS) which can function as second messengers, mediating important cellular functions, such as proliferation and programmed cell death. Intracellular redox homeostasis is sustained primarily by glutathione (GSH), which has long been known to be an important factor in cancer chemoresistance.

In the present chapter, we analyze three important concerns in relation to CRC chemoresistance:

- The influence of GFs in CRC biology and in the response to current cytotoxic therapies.
- The involvement of the redox state in the mechanisms of action of GFs in CRC cells.
- The exogenous modulation of the redox state as a new pharmacological strategy to improve the response to chemotherapeutic agents.

2. Growth factors and colorectal cancer

GFs play a fundamental role in CRC biology, mediating critical functions in cancerous cells, such as proliferation, angiogenesis and the inhibition of cell death. The recurrence of cancer after excision surgery is still a major clinical problem. Accumulating clinical and experimental evidence has indicated that specific factors involved in liver regeneration may influence the growth patterns of residual or dormant micrometastases after resection, suggesting that the process of hepatic regeneration has a significant proliferative effect on tumor cells. In this regard, GFs appear to be involved in tumor recurrence and in metastasis formation. Thus, after partial resection of liver metastases, various types of GFs, which are responsible for liver regeneration, are locally released. However, these may also stimulate the proliferation of undetected tumor cells in the remaining liver, i.e. highly metastatic colon cancer cells can respond to liver regeneration associated mitogens, whose expression is induced after hepatectomy. GFs such as hepatocyte growth factor (HGF), epidermal growth factor (EGF), transforming growth factor alpha (TGF-α), transforming growth factor beta (TGF-β), basic-fibroblastic growth factor (b-FGF), insulin growth factor–I (IGFI) and vascular endothelial growth factor (VEGF) have been reported to be associated with tumor progression and metastasis (Christophi et al., 2008).

Hepatocyte Growth Factor (HGF) is essential for the process of hepatic regeneration. It is a potent mitogenic agent produced by stellate, endothelial and Kupffer sinusoidal cells, which binds to a receptor of the tyrosine kinase (TK) family. This family of genes is encoded by the proto-oncogene c-Met which is expressed in hepatocytes, as well as in other cell types, including tumor cells (Di Renzo et al., 1991). It has a pro-angiogenic effect and stimulates cell motility as well as the secretion of matrix metalloproteinases (MMPs) by pericytes, suggesting an important role in tumor invasion. In the case of CRC, the co-expression of HGF and its receptor is correlated with tumor pathogenesis and with the metastatic phenotype, and for this reason, it has been proposed as a possible molecular marker to be incorporated into CRC staging procedures (Kammula et al., 2007). Moreover, it is known that epithelial tumor metastases undergo an epithelial to mesenchymal transition (EMT) before becoming invasive. The stimuli which promote this transition include HGF and other

GFs such as b-FGF, EGF, TGF-β, as well as extracellular matrix (ECM) constituents including MMPs (Kalluri & Zeisberg, 2006; Christophi et al., 2008). For these reasons, HGF is considered to be a potentially valuable new therapeutic target for different tumors. Studies using NK4, a HGF antagonist, have shown an inhibitory effect on proliferation, invasion and angiogenesis in cell lines of gastric and pancreatic carcinoma, and of CRC (Hirao et al., 2002; Wen et al., 2007). In addition, anti-HGF monoclonal antibodies have been developed, thereby blocking binding to its receptor (Cao et al., 2001). Other developments include anti c-Met antibodies (Jin et al., 2008), and strategies aimed at silencing the expression of c-Met or HGF via antisense oligonucleotides (Stabile et al., 2004), o iRNA (Shinomiya et al., 2004).

Epidermal Growth Factor Receptor (EGFR) ligands, the most physiologically relevant of which include EGF, TGF-α, and Amphiregulin (AR). All of these bind to the extracellular domain of EGFR, which is a member of the ErbB transmembrane TK receptor family (Hynes & Lane, 2005). Binding of these ligands to the receptor activates the Ras/Raf/MAPK and PI3K-AKT signaling pathways which are involved in tumor cell proliferation, inhibition of apoptosis, invasion, migration and angiogenesis (Le Golvan & Resnick, 2010; Wanebo & Berz, 2010). Abnormal expression of these ligands has been demonstrated in many advanced tumors, including breast cancers, gliomas, and lung cancer. In the case of CRC, EGFR overexpression has been detected in 60-80% of cases (Le Golvan & Resnick, 2010) and a correlation has been reported with early tumor recurrence and extra-hepatic metastasis (Christophi et al., 2008). However, its exact role in the CRC metastatic cascade has not yet been characterized due to controversial results obtained with anti-EGFR antibody therapy. In this regard, the therapeutic use of two monoclonal antibody agents (cetuximab and panitumumab) has been authorized in patients with metastatic CRC; although they have a modest effect when used as single agents, they have been found to be beneficial in some patients when used in combination with conventional chemotherapeutic agents (Wanebo & Berz, 2010; Tol & Punt, 2010). In fact, it has been shown that the response to this therapy is independent of EGFR expression in tumor tissue (Chung et al., 2005). Thus, some studies suggest that EGFR expression in the primary tumor does not necessarily correspond with the same level of expression in metastatic tissue, while other studies have reported 78-100% concordance in EGFR expression in both tissue compartments (Tol & Punt, 2010). These discrepancies may partially be due to differences in the detection techniques employed. Nevertheless, recent studies have demonstrated that the therapeutic efficacy of the anti-EGFR antibody is limited to patients in whom the K-Ras oncogene is not mutated, since mutation of this oncogene can induce constitutive activation of the Ras/Raf/MAPK signaling pathway, which is independent of the activation of EGFR via ligand binding (Benvenuti et al., 2007; Tol & Punt, 2010).

Transforming Growth Factor β (TGF-β) acts as a tumor suppressor due to its inhibition of growth and its activation of apoptosis. However, in CRC, this suppressor activity is lost due to the existence of mutations in the genes which encode TGF-β, the type II receptor (TGFR β 2), or SMAD proteins, in such a way that the antiproliferative signal associated with this factor is interrupted (Markowitz & Bertagnolli, 2009). On the other hand, TGF-β has a pro-tumor effect due to its effect on the stroma, promoting angiogenesis, and on the tumor cells themselves, stimulating their motility and their invasive capacity (Blobe & Gordon, 2000). Thus, TGF-β, whose serum values are correlated with a poor CRC prognosis, acts as a tumor promoter, inducing the development of hepatic metastasis (Shim et al., 1999).

Insulin Growth Factor I (IGF-I) and its TK receptor are implicated in the development and progression of CRC due to their induction of proliferation. A correlation has been found between serum levels of IGF-I, high levels of IGF-IR expression in tumor cells and the development of hepatic metastasis. This pro-tumor effect is due to the fact that the signal induced by the binding of IGF-I to its receptor promotes the migration of endothelial cells, invasion and the formation of new blood vessels following the stimulation of VEGF production by endothelial cells (Wu et al., 2002), suggesting that IGF-I is an important contributor to tumor growth and hepatic metastatic development after hepatectomy (Christophi et al., 2008).

Vascular Endothelial Growth Factor (VEGF) is an endothelial cell mitogen which induces cell migration, proliferation, invasion and increased vascular permeability and has a potent pro-angiogenic activity. It has been shown that a large percentage of tumors which produce high levels of VEGF are associated with a high density of vessels in the tumor, metastasis, chemoresistance and poor prognosis (Sullivan & Brekken, 2010).

The VEGF family is made up of six growth factors. These exert their effects via binding to one of the three VEGFRs which belong to the tyrosine kinase receptor (TKR) family. These are localized predominantly on endothelial cells and angioblasts (Tol & Punt, 2010). In addition, in solid tumors, it is postulated that the production of VEGF is increased following liberation of hypoxia-inducible factor 1α (HIF-1α) (Kaur et al., 2005), EGF (Niu et al., 2002) and HGF (Dong et al., 2001). In turn, VEGF induces the synthesis of other factors related to tumor development, such as stroma-derived factor 1 (SDF-1) which induces an increase in the population of cancer-associated fibroblasts (CAFs) (Kalluri & Zeisberg, 2006, Christophi et al., 2008).

The risk of developing hepatic metastasis associated with CRC may be related to the expression of different VEGF isoforms which bind to the different VEGFRs. Thus, it has been shown that in 50% of CRCs, VEGFR-2 is expressed on the surface of the tumor cells (Duff et al., 2006). This extensive expression, which reflects the dependence of some solid tumors on neoangiogenesis, has led to the proposal that VEGF and VEGFR may be therapeutic targets in the treatment of CRC. Bevacizumab is a humanized monoclonal antibody which binds to VEGFA blocking the binding of this GF to VEGFR, thereby avoiding the corresponding intracellular signal transduction. Although parameters which allow a prediction of the efficacy of this monoclonal antibody have not been reported, bevacizumab has been approved as a first and second-line therapy for the treatment of metastatic CRC, enhancing survival, stabilizing the disease and achieving partial regression when used with chemotherapy. Two recent and complete reviews by Tol & Punt (2010) and Wanebo & Berz, (2010) analyze randomized and non-randomized trials of neo-adjuvant therapy using bevacizumab in metastatic CRC.

3. The role of the redox state in the mechanism of action of growth factors

The redox state is a key characteristic which influences important cell biological processes including enzymatic reactions, cell signaling, cell proliferation and apoptosis. The term redox signaling refers to a regulatory process in which the signal is transmitted through redox reactions. The intra- and extracellular redox levels allow the carrying out of different extra and intracellular signaling (intra-cytoplasmic and nuclear), which subsequently give rise to the cascade of effector signals that regulate diverse cellular activities such as cell proliferation.

GF signals are transmitted from the cell surface by means of the activation of TK-type transmembrane receptors and the induction of the corresponding intracellular effects.

Among these signal transduction pathways, protein phosphorylation plays a fundamental role. This process is reversible and dynamic, being controlled by the opposing actions of protein tyrosine kinases (PTKs) and protein tyrosine phosphatases (PTPs). As a consequence of the binding of GF to its specific receptor, dimerization occurs followed by the autophosphorylation of tyrosine residues in the intracellular domain of the receptor (Cadena & Gill, 1992). These residues are key sites of interaction with cytoplasmic proteins which contain SH2 (*Src homology type* 2) domains; these mediate the signal transduction of GFs, such as PLC- γ, GAP-ras (*GTP-ase-activating protein of ras*), PIK3 and Grb2 (Johnson & Vaillancourt, 1994). The action of all these proteins, via different mechanisms, converges to activate the Ras protein, which in its turn, activates the Raf tyrosine. Subsequently, a phosphorylation cascade is produced in such a manner that Raf phosphorylates another kinase, the MAPK kinase which phosphorylates members of a family of serine/threonine kinases, the MAP kinases. Finally, MAP kinases phosphorylate the transcription factors which promote the transcription of genes necessary for the final cellular response (Davis, 1993).

Many studies have demonstrated that the cellular redox status plays a key role in GF-mediated signaling systems (Thannickal & Fanburg, 2000). Although there is evidence that GFs generate ROS, it is not yet clear how ROS activate these cell signaling pathways. One plausible mechanism is that ROS could act as second messengers which participate in phosphorylation/dephosphorylation processes (Storz, 2005). ROS, such as hydrogen peroxidase (H_2O_2), induce the phosphorylation and activation of some PTKs, such as the kinases implicated in the MAP kinase cascade (Rao, 1996). In contrast, PTPs have a cysteine residue in their catalytic domain, which must be in its reduced form for total activity of the receptor. It has been shown that in cell signaling phenomena, ROS may induce the inactivation of PTPs (Rhee et al., 2000). Interestingly, ROS play a crucial role in vascular angiogenesis, not only due to their induction of VEGF (Sen et al., 2002), but also to their implication in the VEGF signaling pathway. Thus, VEGF stimulates ROS production via the activation of nicotinamide adenine dinucleotide phosphate (NADPH) oxidase, which is essential for the satisfactory propagation of the angiogenic signal (Roy et al., 2008); in fact, NADPH oxidase has been proposed as a target for anticancer therapy (Ushio-Fukai & Nakamura, 2008).

Similarly, it has been demonstrated that EGF stimulates ROS production in cells and that inhibition of this production leads to a weakening of the signaling system of the corresponding factor (Mills et al., 1998). A ROS mediated signaling cascade has also been reported to be activated following stimulation of the c-Met/HGF system; this cascade has been found to be associated with the crucial role of the receptor in the development of metastasis (Ferraro et al., 2006).

All of these biological effects occur at low to moderate concentrations of ROS. For this reason, redox regulation is essential for the maintenance of an optimal level of oxidation which permits precise signal transduction and the appropriate cellular response.

4. Glutathione metabolism in colorectal cancer

Cells are exposed to oxidative stress which is generated by normal metabolism and also by exogenous factors, such as ionizing radiation, some chemotherapeutic drugs and xenobiotics. The oxidative modification of cell components via ROS is one of the most potentially damaging processes for normal cellular activity (Halliwell, 1991). However, ROS are well recognized for playing a dual role. Thus, a number of studies have provided convincing evidence that, depending on the level of oxidative stress, ROS can function as pro-life signals in certain contexts (as mentioned above, low or mild increases in ROS play a pivotal role in many physiological reactions, such as the regulation of transcription factors and cellular signaling pathways) (Maellaro et al., 2000) and pro-death signals in others (high concentrations of ROS can induce apoptosis) (Le Bras et al., 2005). Consequently, the maintenance of the redox status is a key factor for cell survival, in the case of both normal and cancer cells.

In order to maintain redox balance and also to protect themselves from oxidative stress, cells possess powerful redox regulation systems, known as the "redox buffer", including GSH and thioredoxin (TRX), as well as antioxidant enzymes, such as superoxide dismutase (SOD), catalase, GSH peroxidase (GPx) and thioredoxin reductase (TrxR). In addition, cells also have available other non-enzymatic antioxidants which are obtained via the diet, among which are ascorbic acid (vitamin C), α-tocopherol (vitamin E), flavonoids, carotenoids and selenium.

Intracellular redox homeostasis is sustained primarily by GSH, the most prevalent intracellular non-protein thiol. In fact, the ratio between its reduced and oxidized states (GSH/GSSG) is considered to be an indicator of the redox status of the cell. GSH is intracellularly synthesized from the three amino acids glutamic acid, cysteine and glycine; it possesses an unusual γ peptide bond between glutamic acid and cysteine, and has a thiol group on the latter aminoacid. The biosynthesis and degradation of GSH occurs within the γ-glutamyl cycle, in which GSH is transported to the extracellular space and γ-glutamyl-aminoacids are transported to the intracellular space. GSH is synthesized from glutamate by two consecutive reactions which are catalyzed by the γ-glutamylcysteine synthetase (γ-GCS) and GSH synthetase enzymes. GSH can be exported outside the cell, although its constituent aminoacids can be reincorporated into the cell, thanks to a transpeptidation reaction catalyzed by the γ-glutamyl transpeptidase (γ-GT) enzyme, which is a glycoprotein localized on the outer surface of the plasma membrane. Transpeptidation occurs in the presence of aminoacids, giving rise to γ-glutamyl-aminoacids and cysteinylglycine (Cys-Gly). The γ-glutamyl-aminoacids are transported into the cell, whereas in the case of cysteinylglycine, bond breakage by means of a dipeptidase is first required. This dipeptidase is present on the outer surface of the plasma membrane, thereby allowing the incorporation of the peptides into the cell. The γ-glutamyl-aminoacids are the substrate of the γ-glutamyl cyclotransferase enzyme, which transforms the glutamyl residue into 5-oxoproline, liberating the remaining aminoacids. Next, by means of the 5-oxo-L-prolinase (5-OPase) enzyme, 5-oxoproline is transformed into glutamate and this reaction involves the consumption of ATP. The cycle is completed with the action again of γ-GCS and GSH synthetase (Fig. 1) (Meister & Anderson, 1983).

Due to its structural characteristics, GSH participates in numerous processes which are essential for cell physiology. GSH and its related enzymes are involved in cell proliferation and participate in the cell cycle, in the synthesis of proteins and in DNA synthesis and repair (Higuchi, 2004). In addition, its capacity as a reducing and antioxidant agent renders GSH an essential component for the maintenance of the integrity of the protein and lipid components of the cell, as well as a substrate for antioxidant GSH peroxidase enzymes, a selenium-dependent system. As indicated previously, another of its important functions consists in the protection of the cell from free radicals, endogenous and exogenous toxic substances, and carcinogens. GSH also defends the cell against the effects produced by radiation and some chemotherapeutic drugs, such as alkylating agents. The formation of GSH S-conjugated products generated during intracellular detoxification may occur due to the non-enzymatic reaction of exogenous electrophilic compounds or to the action of GSH S-transferase (GST) enzymes. GST conjugates can then be eliminated via an ATP-dependent GS-X pump.

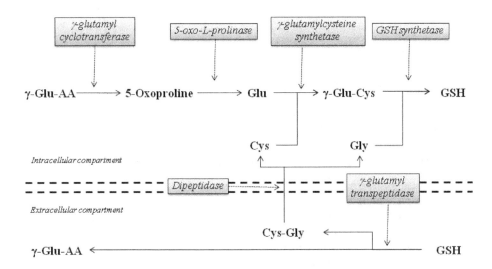

Fig. 1. The γ-glutamyl cycle. Abbreviations: γ-glu-AA, γ-glutamyl-aminoacids; Glu, glutamic acid; Cys, cysteine; Gly, glycine.

In addition to its essential role in normal growth, GSH is also involved in cell differentiation. Thus, it has been reported that as the cell progresses from proliferation to differentiation, cellular GSH content decreases. For example, it has been observed that butyrate-induced differentiation of the HT-29 human colon cell line is associated with reduced levels of cellular GSH (Bernard & Balasubramanian, 1997). These findings led to the notion that thiol status may be dependent on cellular energy metabolism. In this regard, the tumor cells have a very high cellular metabolism and, consequently, they generate high levels of ROS. Here, we should underline the importance of regulation of redox balance for the survival of malignant cells; the activation of redox regulatory systems, in which GSH plays an important role, could be considered to be the first line of adaptation of cancerous cells to oxidative stress. In fact it has been reported that non-differentiated and highly metastatic melanoma cells have a significantly higher GSH content than non-tumorigenic melanocytes (Thrall et al., 1991). Moreover, it has been demonstrated that whereas elevation of intracellular GSH is associated with mitogenic stimulation (Palomares et al., 1997), GSH depletion decreases the rate of cell proliferation and inhibits cancer growth (Del Olmo et al., 2000).

Increased levels of ROS in cancerous cells may have profound consequences, including enhanced cell proliferation, increased incidence of mutations and genetic instability, and reduced sensitivity of cells to anticancer agents, leading to resistance. In the case of CRC, intense oxidative stress and significant oxidative DNA adducts have been found during all stages of colorectal carcinogenesis (Schmid, et al., 2000). In fact, these DNA adducts, as well as GST polymorphisms, have been suggested as molecular biomarkers for the detection of early CRC and the prediction of the clinical effectiveness of chemopreventive drugs (Garcea et al., 2003). Elevated GST expression (Naidu et al., 2003) and a significant increase in GSH levels (Balendiran et al., 2004) have been found in CRC; these are often associated with an increased resistance to cancer chemotherapy drugs via GSH conjugation. Elevated GSH levels may also be related to γ-GCS, another GSH-related enzyme whose levels have also been found to be elevated in CRC (Tatebe et al., 2002). Finally, it should be remembered that GSH and its related enzymes is only one of the redox regulation systems which are implicated in CRC, since an increased expression of TRX-1 in human CRC has been found to be associated with reduced survival times of patients (Raffel et al., 2003).

In summary, the GSH system involves complex and dynamic processes in which several related enzymes participate. Although it may be difficult to know *a priori* what type of GSH metabolism a given CRC may have, the fact that some CRC cells contain high levels of GSH has led to the suggestion that it may be an important factor in limiting the therapeutic efficiency of conventional cancer treatment.

5. The influence of glutathione metabolism in the response to chemotherapy

A common cause of treatment failure in CRC is chemoresistance. This resistance to current cytotoxic therapies limits their success in the majority of advanced cancer patients. This is particularly true in the case of liver metastases.

GSH is able to modulate cell susceptibility to chemotherapy. In particular, GSH plays an important role in the protection against cell injury caused by various anticancer agents (see Balendiran et al., 2004 for review), and elevated GSH levels render tumor cells resistant to chemotherapeutic drugs. In the particular case of CRC, there is also evidence that the GSH status of colon cancer cells is a critical determinant of cell damage by various agents. Indeed, it has been proposed that elevated intracellular GSH levels may be a cause of acquired resistance to 5-FU, platinum agents and camptothecins. In this regard, it has been suggested that the increased levels of antioxidant enzymes in response to the generation of ROS by 5-FU, a standard drug for the treatment of this disease, may underlie the acquired resistance to this anti-tumor agent (Hwang et al., 2007). In *in vitro* studies, we have shown that treatment with 5-FU produced the greatest antiproliferative effect after 24 hours of incubation and that later, once drug treatment had been stopped, the growth of tumor cells rebounded (Palomares et al., 2009). This finding may be due to the recovery of GSH levels after the initial 5-FU-induced reduction, which has also been suggested by other authors (Chen et al., 1995).

It has also been reported that GSH may modulate the cytotoxicity of platinum agents (Sadowitz et al., 2002). However, intracellular GSH levels do not appear to influence the cell growth-inhibiting activity of these compounds in cells not previously exposed to platinum complexes (Boubakari et al., 2004), suggesting that GSH may be more relevant in acquired resistance. Furthermore, several authors have reported the influence of GSH on sensitivity to camptothecins (Yoshida et al., 2006).

In order to decrease the resistance of tumor cells to chemotherapeutic drugs, many GSH-based therapeutic strategies have focused on lowering GSH levels, principally via the use of agents which reduce this tripeptide or inhibit its synthesis. The agent which is most frequently used to reduce the levels of this thiol, not only in basic research but also in clinical assays, is L-buthionine-[S,R]-sulfoximine (BSO) (Fig. 2). We found that this potent inhibitor of γ-GCS enhances the sensitivity of tumor cells to treatment with ionizing radiation and cytostatic drugs, such as alkylating agents (Palomares et al., 1999). We have also found that the reduction in GSH content (around 52%) produced by BSO significantly inhibits the proliferation of colon cancer WiDr cells (Palomares et al., 2009).

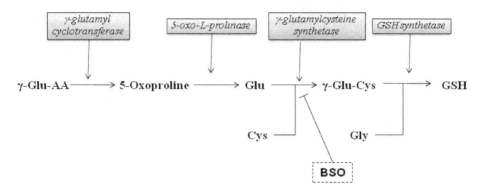

Fig. 2. Inhibition of γ-glutamylcysteine synthetase by L-buthionine-[S,R]-sulfoximine (BSO).

However, the anti-tumor efficacy of BSO is accompanied by increased toxicity, due to the fact that BSO exerts its effects in a non-selective manner. In fact, it reduces GSH levels in both tumor and normal cells and thus sensitizes both cell populations to the toxic effect of anticancer agents. This finding has been reported in clinical studies, such as that of Bailey et al. (1998), who upon combining BSO and melphalan, found an important increase in medullar toxicity with respect to that produced by the administration of the alkylating agent alone. Thus, BSO treatment produces toxicity at the level of the immune, gastrointestinal, urinary and central nervous systems. This toxicity limits, *de facto*, the therapeutic potential of BSO and of other non-selective GSH reducing agents.

One of the principal reasons for the limited effects of chemotherapy is the insufficient therapeutic index of available drugs. This index could be increased by regimes which protect healthy tissues against toxicity and at the same time enhance the sensitivity of tumor tissue to anticancer drugs. Since GSH is highly relevant in protecting both normal and tumor cells, one way of achieving this objective would be to selectively modulate GSH levels. An increase in GSH levels or in the capacity of normal cells to synthesize GSH, would enhance their resistance, leading to a protector effect. In contrast, a reduction in GSH content or in the capacity of tumor cells to synthesize this tripeptide would enhance sensitivity to the effects of anti-tumor agents. In this regard, it was suggested many years ago that agents which induce a selective modulation in GSH levels could be beneficially added to conventional treatments in order to enhance the anti-tumor efficacy of radiotherapy and/or chemotherapy (Russo et al., 1986).

Selective modulation of GSH as a therapeutic strategy requires an in-depth knowledge of the physiological differences in GSH synthesis and metabolism between healthy and tumor cells, as well as of the level of expression of GSH-related enzymes. In this regard, lower expression of the 5-OPase enzyme has been found in some tumor cell lines in comparison to healthy cells, leading to the suggestion that this enzyme may be a key player in obtaining the required selective modulation of GSH (Chen & Batist, 1998).

Within the γ-glutamyl cycle, 5-OPase catalyses the hydrolysis of 5-oxo-L-proline to L-glutamate, one of the three aminoacids which participate in GSH synthesis, joining in this way the reactions of GSH synthesis and metabolism in this cycle (see Fig. 1). It has also been observed that L-2-oxothiazolidine-4-carboxylate (OTZ) –an analog of 5-oxo-proline– also acts as a substrate of 5-OPase, thereby converting this cysteine prodrug into S-carboxycysteine, hydrolyzing it subsequently to cysteine and CO_2 (Fig. 3).

Some studies have found that in contrast to BSO, OTZ treatment is selective, increasing GSH levels in healthy tissue and reducing it paradoxically in tumor tissue (Chen & Batist, 1998). These authors have suggested that OTZ, by competing with 5-oxo-L-proline for 5-OPase, could exert two different effects on GSH levels, depending on the level of expression of the 5-OPase enzyme and on the quantity of aminoacids necessary for the synthesis of the said tripeptide. In this way, OTZ would increase intracellular levels of GSH in healthy cells by means of increasing the contribution of cysteine – in normal conditions, the limiting aminoacid in GSH synthesis in these cells - (Meister A, 1983), but would reduce GSH content in tumor cells by means of the inhibition of glutamate synthesis from 5-oxo-L-proline. In fact, it has been observed that in tumor cells and in other cells under conditions of oxidative stress, glutama`te is the limiting factor in GSH synthesis (Kang, 1993)

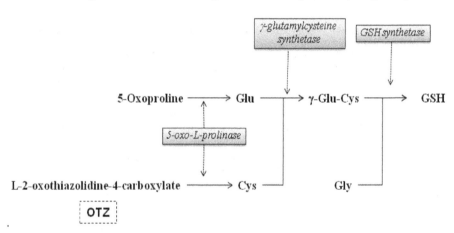

Fig. 3. Metabolism of L-2-oxothiazolidine-4-carboxylate (OTZ) and of 5-oxo-L-proline by means of the 5-OPase enzyme.

In *in vitro* studies, OTZ has been found to be useful as a protector in human lymphocytes against toxicity due to nitrogenated mustard, or in cultures of human fibroblasts against radio-induced toxicity. In *in vivo* studies using mouse models, OTZ has demonstrated its efficacy in protecting against liver damage produced by alcohol, by reducing the degree of cystitis induced by cyclophosphamide (CY) or of hepatotoxicity produced by acetaminophen, among others. OTZ has been used in diverse clinical assays for the treatment of a variety of pathologies associated with ROS generation and with reduced GSH levels. Diseases in which OTZ treatment has been successfully employed include acute respiratory distress syndrome (Morris et al., 2008), amyotrophic lateral sclerosis (Cudkowicz et al., 1999) and atherosclerosis (Vita et al., 1998). Patients subjected to peritoneal dialysis (Moberly et al., 1998) and patients infected with the AIDS virus (Barditch-Crovo et al., 1998) have also benefited from this treatment.

Paradoxically, in contrast to the effect produced in healthy tissue, OTZ reduces GSH levels in some human tumor cell lines including breast adenocarcinoma and ovary adenocarcinoma (Chen & Batist, 1998). In the same way, we have also demonstrated the selective character of GSH modulation by OTZ, *in vitro* as well as *in vivo*. Thus, OTZ was found to reduce the intracellular content of GSH in melanoma cells, producing reduced proliferation and increased chemosensitivity, whereas it increased GSH levels in peripheral blood mononuclear cells, exhibiting a corresponding cytoprotector effect (Del Olmo et al., 2000, 2006; Bilbao et al., 2002).

Several authors have pointed to the usefulness of GSH modulating agents as an adjuvant in chemotherapy treatments for CRC. Regarding 5-FU, a number of studies support the therapeutic use of antioxidant compounds in combination with this drug. Thus, therapy with high doses of antioxidants such as pyrrolidine dithiocarbamate (PDTC) and N-acetylcysteine (NAC) seem to enhance the therapeutic efficacy of 5-FU (Bach et al., 2001).

NAC is a prodrug of cysteine, which is an essential element for GSH synthesis. It was developed to avoid the important toxicity produced as a consequence of the direct administration of this aminoacid. The mechanisms of protection of this thiol against mutagenesis and carcinogenesis are related to a large number of biological effects, including antioxidant activity, involvement in DNA repair mechanisms, modulation of gene expression and of signal transduction, immunological activity, regulation of cell survival and of apoptosis, inhibition of cell transformation, of invasion and metastasis and of angiogenic activity, among others (Morini et al., 1999). However, some authors have reported contradictory effects of NAC in its anticancer action. Moreover, it has been demonstrated that antioxidant protection therapy in cancer patients should be used with caution, since it can give rise to counterproductive effects (Brizel & Overgaard, 2003). The reduction in the concentration of free radicals due to the excessive administration of antioxidants can stimulate the survival of damaged cells, enhancing the neoplastic stage, thereby promoting carcinogenesis more than inhibiting it. Furthermore, we and others have demonstrated that the increase in GSH levels induced by NAC is not specific to normal cells; rather, this can also occur in tumor cells, such as melanoma, increasing its proliferative capacity and protecting it against the cytotoxic effects of acrolein, one of the active metabolites of CY (Del Olmo et al., 2000).

It has also been found that the reduced levels of GSH induced by BSO and OTZ, lead to an increased cytotoxic effect of 5-FU in different human CRC cells (Meurette et al., 2005; Palomares et al., 2009). It has also been observed that BSO enhances the activity of SN-38 (an active metabolite of the anticancer drug irinotecan) in WiDr colon cancer cells (Caramés et al., 2010), and in cell lines of ovary cancer resistant to cisplatin, as well as of breast cancer. BSO is also capable of reverting resistance to SN-38 in leukemia cells with increased GSH levels (Yoshida et al., 2006). This increased anti-tumor effect of SN-38 may be related to the reduced activity of the transcription factor NF-κB, which is dependent on the intracellular redox status and thus sensitive to a reduced content of intracellular GSH. In fact, SN-38 is known to activate NF-κB and so the pharmacological inhibition of this NF-κB signaling pathway can enhance the anti-tumor activity of SN-38 in colon cancer cells *in vitro* and of irinotecan *in vivo* (Lagadec et al., 2008).

Regarding platinum compounds, various authors have demonstrated that GSH participates in the detoxification of these agents and that reduced GSH levels sensitize cancer cells to the cytotoxic effects of these anti-tumor agents (Jansen et al., 2002). We have found that both BSO and OTZ increase the efficacy of oxaliplatin in the WiDr human colon cancer cell line

(Caramés et al., 2010). Thus, reduced GSH levels mediated by BSO or OTZ lead to an increase in cytotoxicity induced by drugs which are more frequently used nowadays for CRC therapy, with an additive effect being observed in the antiproliferative effects of these combinations.

6. The influence of growth factors in the sensitivity of tumor cells to chemotherapy

Research on the phenomenon of chemotherapy resistance has traditionally focused on the tumor cells themselves. However, it has become apparent that the tumor microenvironment may also influence chemoresistance in an important way. In this regard, it is necessary to underline the fundamental role of GFs in cancer biology and in the formation of metastasis, since they control critical functions in cancer cells, such as proliferation, angiogenesis and the inhibition of apoptosis. Thus, GFs, due to their capacity to modulate the sensitivity of tumor cells to cytotoxic drugs, have become important targets for the development of new anti-cancer therapies, either as individual agents or in combination with conventional chemotherapy, with the aim of enhancing the efficacy of anti-cancer drugs.

It has been demonstrated that the presence of GFs significantly reduces the cytotoxic activity of a number of commonly used drugs. In this regard, some authors have pointed out that HGF protects tumor cells against the cytotoxicity and apoptosis induced by DNA-damaging agents, such as ionizing radiation or adriamycin (Shen et al., 2007), and that it may contribute to the resistance of RMS cells to conventional treatment (Jankowski et al., 2003). Similarly, it has been suggested that this factor could induce resistance to cisplatin in lung cancer cells (Chen et al., 2008). Nevertheless, in contrast to expectations, it has also been observed that HGF sensitizes ovary cancer cells to the drugs paclitaxel and cisplatin (Bardella et al., 2007). These findings indicate that HGF effects depend on the targeted tumor type. Indeed, various other studies have reported the effect of VEGF in reducing the efficacy of endocrine therapy in breast cancer (Qu et al., 2008). It has also been found that VEGF diminishes the response to drugs in myeloid leukemia (De Jonge et al., 2008) and that doxorubicin exerts a milder inhibitory effect in the presence of VEGF overexpression in soft-tissue sarcoma (Zhang et al., 2006). Regarding EGF, it has been widely demonstrated that this GF reduces the response of tumors, such as human breast carcinoma, to cytotoxic compounds and to radiotherapy (Schmidt & Lichtner, 2002).

In the case of CRC, we (Palomares et al., 2009) and others (Sun & Tang, 2003; Allendorf et al., 2004) have demonstrated that HGF, EGF and VEGF significantly reduce the efficacy of drugs currently used in CRC. In particular, the increased expression of HGF and VEGF results in fluoropyrimidine-based adjuvant chemotherapy being less effective, increasing the risk of recurrence. In relation to EGF, it has been shown that its receptor, EGFR, increases resistance to 5-FU. Moreover, 5-FU itself induces the activation of EGFR, which protect colon cancer cells against chemotherapy (Hiro et al., 2008). Moreover, it has been reported that SN-38, through a mechanism involving ROS, induces the activation of EGF and EGFR, and this could contribute to resistance to irinotecan (Kishida et al., 2005). These data suggest that inhibition of the EGFR signaling pathway could revert resistance to treatment with the fluoropyrimidines and irinotecan. On the basis of this hypothesis, some authors have carried out assays using tyrosine kinase inhibitors of EGFR, such as gefitinib (Stebbing et al., 2008), as well as inhibitors of the Src tyrosine kinase (Ischenko et al., 2008).

The molecular mechanisms underlying GF-mediated resistance continue to be largely unknown. On the one hand, GFs induce cell proliferation and the activation of anti-apoptotic signaling pathways, via proteins such as Bcl-XL, thereby contributing to the resistance to apoptosis in CRC cells following treatment with 5-FU, oxaliplatin and irinotecan (Schulze-Bergkamen et al., 2008). In addition, it has also been suggested that GFs may also induce an increase in the repair of damaged DNA (Hiro et al., 2008). On the other hand, it has been observed that the EGFR-Src-STAT3 oncogenic signaling pathway plays an important role in CRC, contributing to proliferation, cell survival and treatment resistance (Hbibi et al., 2008). In fact, it has been demonstrated that this pathway is activated in response to treatment with topoisomerase I inhibitors, such as camptothecins, reducing DNA damage and enhancing cell survival (Vigneron et al, 2008).

Moreover, as we have recently shown, GFs give rise to an increase in GSH levels which, as mentioned earlier, is an important mechanism of cell defense against oxidative stress and against the effects produced by radiation and by some chemotherapeutic agents; this increase in GSH levels has been correlated with diminished 5-FU anti-tumor activity in colon cancer cells (Palomares et al., 2009). In this regard, it has been reported that the combination of an EGFR inhibitor with doxorubicin leads to enhanced cytotoxic effects via the generation of oxidative stress, due to ROS induction and reduced GSH content in rat hepatoma cells (Ortiz et al., 2008).

Additionally, it has been suggested that GF-induced increases in intracellular GSH levels and the activation of the redox-sensitive transcription factor NF-κB could play a major role in inducible chemoresistance. This cell survival transcription factor, which is subject to regulation by GSH (Lou & Kaplowitz, 2007), has been shown to be constitutively activated in many colon cancer cells. NF-κB has been shown to be associated with the proliferation of tumor cells, with invasion, angiogenesis and the production of metastasis (Bours et al., 1994). It has been demonstrated that HGF, via the PI3K/Akt signaling pathway, leads to the activation of NF-κB, by means of which cells are protected against adriamycin and irinotecan (Fan et al., 2005). In the same way, the transmission of the proliferative signal induced by EGF is also mediated by the activation of NF-κB (Sethi et al., 2007), which plays an important role in the regulation of EGFR ligands via a ROS-mediated mechanism (Murillo et al., 2007). Moreover, NF-κB activation in response to exposure to anti-cancer drugs has been shown to be one of the mechanisms of tumor resistance to chemotherapy, as has been reported in the cases of 5-FU and irinotecan (Ahn et al., 2008). In contrast, inhibition of NF-κB has been shown to enhance the sensitivity of colon cancer tumor cells to HT-29 and 5-FU (Voboril et al., 2004).

Overall, these data indicate that GFs play a critical role in the resistance of colon cancer cells to chemotherapeutic agents. In consequence, these factors are potential therapeutic targets for increasing the anti-tumor activity of cytotoxic drugs.

7. New therapeutic strategies to enhance the response of CRC to chemotherapy by reversion of the growth factor pro-tumour effects

Based on the aforementioned data, GFs have been identified as important targets to be considered in the development of new anticancer drugs and, consequently, many experimental studies have been carried out to evaluate the effects of blocking GF effects on tumor cells. These attempts could be classified into three categories, according to the mechanism chosen to avoid the GF stimulation of these cells. The first approach was to administer monoclonal antibodies (MoAb) against one or several GFs, and the results have been quite exciting. Another idea was to produce MoAb against the membrane receptors for different GFs, and again the results have been very promising. In fact, several of these MoAb have already entered the armamentarium for cancer therapy and others are currently at different stages of clinical trials. The third exciting arm of these GF-based therapies consists of the so-called "small molecules" which block the activation of the intracellular part of GF receptors.

The combination of conventional cytotoxic drugs with new agents that specifically interfere with GF signaling pathways presents the advantage of avoiding crossed resistance, since these approaches are directed against different cell targets and have different underlying mechanisms of action. In this regard, many studies have indicated that inhibitors of GFs or of their receptors enhance the efficacy of conventional cytotoxic agents (Wanebo & Berz, 2010). The GF inhibitors bevacizumab and cetuximab are particularly noteworthy. Currently, bevacizumab is used in combination with regimes which contain 5-FU (FOLFOX or FOLFIRI) as a first line therapy in advanced or metastatic CRC (Giantonio et al., 2007; Tol & Punt, 2010). On the other hand, combined therapy consisting of irinotecan and cetuximab is indicated after progression in patients who have previously received 5-FU based therapy (Cunningham et al., 2004).

Other agents, such as gefitinib, have been found in preclinical studies to exhibit synergistic inhibitory effects when administered in combination with different cytotoxic drugs. For example, some authors have observed that gefitinib and irinotecan act synergistically in WiDr cells, as a result of the inhibition of the survival signal induced by irinotecan via the phosphorylation of EGFR (Koizumi et al., 2004). Similarly, *in vitro* studies have shown that the combination of gefitinib and oxaliplatin has a synergistic effect in colon cancer cells due, at least in part, to the fact that the EGFR inhibitor reduces the activity of γ-GT. This enzyme, which participates in the γ-glutamyl cycle, helps to salvage extracellular GSH and contributes to redox control by providing a substrate for GSH synthesis during oxidative stress, thereby preventing apoptosis, as we have showed previously (Castro et al., 2002). Reduced γ-GT activity thereby leads to increased cellular oxaliplatin accumulation and platinum-DNA adducts (Xu et al., 2003).

However, these anti-tumor agents also have their inconveniences. They induce diverse side effects which complicates their clinical use (Mulder et al., 2011). Also, as happens with other chemotherapeutic agents, the development of resistance to these GF-based agents has already been reported (Giaccone & Wang, 2011). For these reasons, it is important to continue the search for new therapeutic strategies which could be used in combination in order to enhance the efficacy of GF-related targeted agents. In this sense, the therapeutic biomodulation of GSH metabolism may hold promise for the improvement of the efficacy of anticancer treatments. Many lines of evidence indicate that this may be an effective approach to treating cancer: i) the fact that tumor cells are under high levels of oxidative stress may represent a great opportunity given that it means they are particularly vulnerable to further increases in ROS levels; ii) colon cancer cells contain particularly high levels of GSH; iii) GF-induced signal transduction pathways are redox sensitive, and accordingly, alterations in cellular GSH content may affect the growth of GF-sensitive cells; and iv) the fact that NF-κB is involved in GF-dependent proliferation and that the activity of this transcription factor might also be subject to regulation by GSH suggests that depletion of cellular GSH could interrupt NF-κB activity and consequently lead to growth inhibition.

In this regard, we have recently demonstrated that GSH-induced depletion by BSO or OTZ abrogated the growth-promoting effects of GFs in WiDr colon cancer cells (Palomares et al., 2009). Similarly, other authors have demonstrated that BSO inhibits GSH upregulation induced by HGF, thereby blocking its mitogenic effect (Yang et al., 2008) and the protection against apoptosis afforded by this factor. It has likewise been reported that BSO interferes with EGF-induced proliferation and that extended exposure (for 48 h or more) of cells to BSO induces cell death, probably via a necrotic mechanism (Carmona-Cuenca et al., 2006). Regarding VEGF, it has also been reported that BSO treatment reverts increased GSH activity induced by this factor and, in this way, its vasculoprotective function (Kuzuya et al., 2001). In contrast, decreased GSH levels produced by BSO have been shown to promote the autocrine secretion of VEGF (Sreekumar et al., 2006).

Thus, the two effects derived from the biomodulation of GSH intracellular content with BSO or OTZ, i.e. i) the reversion of the pro-tumor effect of GFs and ii) the enhanced efficacy of chemotherapy, may contribute to enhancing the therapeutic benefit of chemotherapy treatment. In fact, we have shown that, in the presence of GFs, the combination of either of the GSH modulators with chemotherapeutic drugs produced greater anti-tumor activity than the cytotoxic drugs alone. Thus, we found that both BSO and OTZ completely reverted the resistance (due to the presence of GFs) of WiDr colon cancer cells to 5-FU, a finding which holds promise for more successful anticancer treatment, particularly after surgical resection of hepatic metastases (Palomares et al., 2009). Indeed, 5-FU activity was enhanced by 40% following the addition of GSH modulators. The activity of oxaliplatin was also found to be significantly enhanced (by nearly 25%). Moreover, combined therapy with SN-38 was found to produce the optimal chemotherapeutic combination; thus, OTZ pretreatment combined with SN-38 resulted in an increase of almost 70% in the cytotoxic activity of SN-38 (Caramés et al., 2010). To this benefit, we must also add the advantage of OTZ with respect to BSO, i.e. the selective reduction of GSH levels in tumor cells, protecting healthy cells, as mentioned above.

Other interesting approaches to the GF problem in cancer therapy have been developed. Thus, as cell proliferation and differentiation are deregulated in tumor cells, the induction of cell differentiation with retinoids could help to neutralize the pro-tumor effect of GFs. The mechanisms of action which underlie the effects of retinoids include the activation of nuclear retinoic acid receptors (RAR), but also, curiously, the induction of enhanced ROS levels (Palomares et al. , 2006) and a direct interaction of retinoids with the GSH-dependent protein kinase C, a key regulatory enzyme in signal transduction (Radominska-Pandya et al., 2000). In this sense, we have analyzed the effect of all-trans-retinoic acid (ATRA), a well known pro-differentiating agent, on the growth-promoting effect of GFs in two tumor models. This drug was found to reduce the proliferative rate of RMS (García-Alonso et al., 2005) and CRC cells (Martínez-Astorquiza et al., 2008), and hindered or completely abolished the stimulus produced by serum obtained from hepatectomized rats, and by a wide variety of GFs (HGF, VEGF, PDGF, EGF, bFGF). Furthermore, we also found that cells cultured in medium containing ATRA do not develop resistance to the drug, and these ATRA-preexposed cells responded to subsequent ATRA treatments in the same manner as non-treated cells. However, we observed that the antiproliferative effect of ATRA *in vitro* is not permanent: forty eight hours after removing the drug from the culture medium the cells recovered their normal proliferative rate (Díaz et al., 2009). Nevertheless, in *in vitro* studies, we found that ATRA did not interfere with the antiproliferative effect of chemotherapeutics drugs, such as 5-FU; moreover, when both drugs were administered together, an additive effect was observed (García-Alonso et al., 2010).

In order to corroborate these findings *in vivo*, we designed an experimental model in which daily intraperitoneal doses of ATRA were administered for two weeks, starting three days before a partial hepatectomy was performed in animals bearing liver metastases. These *in vivo* experiments confirmed the efficacy of ATRA in reducing the proliferative rate of tumor cells. In rats bearing RMS S4MH liver metastases, the mean number of liver metastases, as well as their mean size, were significantly reduced and significantly longer survival was achieved. Using this tumor model, we also analyzed the synergistic effect of ATRA with commonly used chemotherapeutic agents such as CY. Once again, animals treated with ATRA+CY presented a significant reduction in the mean number of liver metastases and also an increase in survival compared to animals treated with CY alone. Similar experiments were carried out with the murine CC-531 colon cancer cell line, and similar, albeit not so dramatic, results were found (unpublished data). Thus, the mean number of liver metastases was unmodified by ATRA, but the mean size of the liver foci was significantly reduced, suggesting that tumor progression had been retarded. However, survival remained unaltered. Regarding drug tolerance, ATRA was well tolerated by the animals, with no repercussion on hematological cell counts, serum enzymes or weight gain. These findings point to the need to enhance ATRA effects via other mechanisms. In this regard, it has recently been shown that the selective COX-2 inhibitor celecoxib, increased the expression of RARbeta in human colon cancer cells, as well as sensitivity to ATRA through COX-2-independent mechanisms (Liu et al., 2010).

Novel synthetic derivatives of ATRA have been developed recently and examined in clinical trials (Sogno et al, 2010). However, these trials involve administration of the drug as a conventional chemotherapeutic agent (Kummar et al, 2011). In the light of the above, it is apparent that retinoids (or pro-differentiating agents in general) should be tested as a complementary treatment, and administered as part of a combined therapy during the early postoperative period, when their action would be most effective. Otherwise, it is unlikely that significant improvements will be found in patients treated with these agents in monotherapy.

Overall, and in the light of the important role of GFs in tumor recurrence following surgical resection of hepatic metastases, the use of GSH modulators and pro-differentiating agents seems to hold promise as a novel therapeutic strategy for metastatic CRC, by reversing GF pro-tumor effects and improving the efficacy of chemotherapy.

8. Conclusion

Growth factors play a pivotal role in the regulation of CRC progression and metastasis. They are involved not only in promoting tumor growth, but also in reducing the responsiveness of tumor cells to cytotoxic compounds. The mechanisms of action underlying GF effects include the redox state of the tumor, in particular GSH metabolism, and the level of expression of related enzymes. The biomodulation of GSH metabolism via agents such as BSO or OTZ, could reverse the growth-promoting effects of GFs and enhance the therapeutic benefit of chemotherapeutic drugs. The use of pro-differentiating agents may also represent a promising anti-tumor strategy to block the pro-tumor effects of GFs. The development of more effective retinoids, used either alone or preferably in combination with other dugs, may also provide more effective anti-tumor benefits. These new types of strategies to neutralize the pro-tumor effects of GFs may well be crucial in the treatment of metastatic disease and the prevention of the recurrence of liver metastases arising from CRC.

9. Acknowledgments

This work was supported by research grants from the University of the Basque Country (Project GIU 10/16) and Gangoiti Barrera Foundation.

10. References

Ahn KS, Sethi G & Aggarwal BB. (2008). Reversal of chemoresistance and enhancement of apoptosis by statins through down-regulation of the NF-kappaB pathway. *Biochem Pharmacol*, Vol.75, No4 (2008 Feb 15), pp 907-13. Epub 2007 Oct 16. ISSN: 0006-2952.

Allendorf J, Ippagunta N & Emond J. (2004). Management of liver metastases: new horizonts for biologically based therapy. *J Surg Res*, Vol.117, No.1 (March 2004), pp.144-153, **ISSN:** 0022-4804.

Bach SP, Williamson SE, Marshman E, Kumar S, O`Dwyer ST, Potten CS & Watson AJ. (2001). The antioxidant N-acetylcysteine increases 5-fluorouracil activity against colorectal cancer xenografts in nude mice. *J Gastrointest Surg*, Vol.5, No.1 (January-February 2001), pp. 91-97, ISSN: 1091-255X.

Bailey HH. (1998). L-S,R-buthionine sulfoximine: historical development and clinical issues. *Chem Biol Interact*, Vol.112, (April 1998), pp.239-254, ISSN: 0009-2797.

Balendiran GK, Dabur R & Fraser D. (2004). The role of glutathione in cancer. *Cell Biochem Funct*, Vol.22, No.6 (November-December 2004), pp.343–352, ISSN: 0263-6484.

Barberá-Guillem E, Alonso-Varona A & Vidal-Vanaclocha F. (1989). Selective implantation and growth in rats and mice of experimental liver metastasis in acinar zone one. *Cancer Res*, Vol.49, No.14 (July 1989), pp.4003-4010, ISSN: 0008-5472.

Bardella C, Dettori D, Olivero M, Coltella N, Mazzone M & Di Renzo MF. (2007). The therapeutic potential of hepatocyte growth factor to sensitize ovarian cancer cells to cisplatin and paclitaxel *in vivo.Clin Cancer Res*, Vol.13, No.7 (April 2007), pp.2191-2198, ISSN: 1078-0432.

Barditch-Crovo P, Noe D, Skowron G, Lederman M, Kalayjian RC, Borum P, Buier R, Rowe WB, Goldberg D & Lietman P. (1998). A phase I/II evaluation of oral L-2-oxothiazolidine-4-carboxylic acid in asymptomatic patients infected with human immunodeficiency virus. *J Clin Pharmacol, Vol.*38, No.4 (April 1998), pp.357-363, ISSN: 0091-2700.

Benvenuti S, Sartore-Bianchi A, Di Nicolantonio F, Zanon C, Moroni M, Veronese S, Siena S & Bardelli A. (2007). Oncogenic activation of the RAS/RAF signaling pathway impairs the response of metastatic colorectal cancers to anti-epidermal growth factor receptor antibody therapies. *Cancer Research,* Vol.67, No.6 (March 2007), pp.2643-2648, ISSN: **0008**-5472.

Bernard O & Balasubramanian KA. (1997). Modulation of glutathione level during butyrate-induced differentiation in human colon derived HT-29 cells. *Mol Cell Biochem,* Vol.170, No.1-2 (May 1997), pp.109-114, ISSN: 0300-8177.

Bilbao P, Del Olmo M, Alonso-Varona A, Castro B, Bilbao J & Palomares T. (2002). L-2-Oxothiazolidine-4-Carboxylate reverses the tumour growth-promoting effect of interleukin-2 and improves the anti-tumour efficacy of biochemotherapy in mice bearing B16 melanoma liver metastases. *Melanoma Res,* Vol.12, No.1 (February 2002), pp.17-26, ISSN: 0960-8931.

Blobe GC & Gordon KJ. (2000). Role of transforming growth factor beta in human disease.*Bioch et Bioph Acta Molec Basis of Disease,* Vol.1782, No.4 (April 2008), pp.1350-1358, ISSN: 0925-4439.

Boubakari, Bracht K, Neumann C, Grunert R & Bednarski PJ. (2004). No correlation between GSH levels in human cancer cell lines and the cell growth inhibitory activities of platinum diamine complexes. *Arch Pharm,* Vol.337, No.12 (December 2004), pp.668-671, ISSN: 0365-6233.

Bours V, Dejardin E, Goujon-Letawe F, Merville MP & Castronovo V. (1994). The NF-kappa B transcription factor and cancer: high expression of NF-kappa B- and I kappa B-related proteins in tumor cell lines. *Biochem Pharmacol,* Vol.47, No.1 (January 1994), pp.145-149, ISSN: 0006-2952.

Brizel DM & Overgaard J (2003). Does amifostine have a role in chemoradiation treatment? *Lancet Oncol.* Vol.4, No.6 (2003 Jun), pp.378-381. ISSN: 1470-2045.

Cadena DL & Gill GN. (1992). Receptor tyrosine kinases. *FASEB J,* Vol.6, No.6 (March 1992), pp.2332-2337, ISSN: 0892-6638.

Cao B, Su Y, Oskarsson M, Zhao P, Kort EJ, Fisher RJ, Wang LM & Vande Woude GF.(2001). Neutralizing monoclonal antibodies to hepatocyte growth factor/scatter factor (HGF/SF) display antitumor activity in animal models. *Proc Natl Acad Sci U S A,* Vol.98, No.13 (June 2001), pp.7443-7448, ISSN: 0027-8424.

Caramés, M, Alonso-Varona A, García-Alonso I & Palomares T. (2010). Glutathione modulators reverse the pro-tumour effect of growth factors enhancing WiDr cell response to chemotherapeutic agents. *Anticancer Res,* Vol.30, No.4 (April 2010), pp.1223-1231, ISSN: 0250-7005.

Carmona-Cuenca I, Herrera B, Ventura JJ, Roncero C, Fernández M & Fabregat I. (2006). EGF blocks NADPH oxidase activation by TGF-beta in fetal rat hepatocytes, impairing oxidative stress, and cell death. *J Cell Physiol,* Vol.207, No.2 (May 2006), pp.322-330, ISSN: 0021-9541.

Castro B, Alonso-Varona A, del Olmo M, Bilbao P & Palomares T. (2002). Role of gamma-glutamyltranspeptidase on the response of poorly and moderately differentieted rhabdomyosarcoma cell lines to buthionine sulfoximine-induced inhibition of glutathione synthesis. *Anti-Cancer Drugs,* Vol.13, No.3 (March 2002), pp.281-291, ISSN: 0959-4973.

Chen JT, Huang CY, Chiang YY, Chen WH, Chiou SH, Chen CY & Chow KC. (2008). HGF increases cisplatin resistance via down-regulation of AIF in lung cancer cells. *Am J Respir Cell Mol Biol.* Vol. 38, No.5 (2008 May), pp.559-65. Epub 2007 Dec 20. ISSN: 1044-1549.

Chen MF, Chen LT & Bouce HW Jr. (1995). 5-Fluorouracil cytotoxicity in human colon HT-29 cells with moderately increased or decreased cellular gluthatione level. *Anticancer Res*, Vol.15, No.1 (January-February 1995), pp.163-167, ISSN: 0250-7005.

Chen X & Batist G. (1998). Sensitization effect of L-2-oxothiazolidine-4-carboxylate on tumor cells to melpahalan and the role of 5-oxo-L-prolinase in glutathione modulation in tumor cells. *Biochem Pharmacol*, Vol.56, No.6 (September 1998), pp.743-749, ISSN: 0006-2952.

Christophi C, Harun N & Fifis T. (2008). Liver regeneration and tumor stimulation-A review of Cytokine and angiogenic factors. *Journal of Gastrointestinal Surgery*, Vol.12, No.5 (May 2008), pp.966-980, ISSN: 1091-255X.

Chung KY, Shia J, Kemeny NE, Shah M, Schwartz GK, Tse A, Hamilton A, Pan D, Schrag D, Schwartz L, Klimstra DS, Fridman D, Kelsen DP & Saltz LB. (2005). Cetuximab shows activity in colorectal cancer patients with tumors that do not express the epidermal growth factor receptor by immunohistochemistry. *Journal of Clinical Oncology*, Vol.23, No.9 (March 2005), pp.1803-1810, ISSN: 0732-183X.

Cudkowicz ME, Sexton PM, Ellis T, Hayden DL, Gwilt PR, Whalen J & Brown RH Jr. (1999). The pharmacokinetics and pharmaco-dynamics of procysteine in amyotrophic lateral sclerosis. *Neurology*, Vol.52, No.7 (April 1999), pp.1492-1494, ISSN: 0028-3878.

Cunningham D, Humblet Y, Siena S, Khayat D, Bleiberg H, Santero A, Bets D, Mueser M, Harstrick A, Verslype C, Chau I & Van Cutsem E. (2004). Cetuximab monotherapy and cetuximab plus irinotecan in irinotecan-refractory metastatic colorectal cancer. *N Engl J Med*, Vol.351, No.4 (July 2004), pp.337-345, ISSN: 0028-4793.

Davis RJ. (1993). The mitogen-activated protein kinase signal transduction pathway. *J Biol Chem*, Vol.268, No.20 (July 1993), pp.14553-14556, ISSN: 0021-9258.

De Jonge HJ, Weidenaar AC, Ter Elst A, Boezen HM, Scherpen FJ, Bouma-Ter Steege JC, Kaspers GJ, Goemans BF, Creutzig U, Zimmermann M, Kamps WA & de Bont ES. (2008). Endogenous vascular endothelial growth factor-C expression is associated with decreased drug responsiveness in childhood acute myeloid leukemia. *Clin Cancer Res*, Vol.14, No.3 (February 2008), pp.924-930, ISSN: 1078-0432.

Del Olmo M, Alonso-Varona A, Castro B, Calle Y, Bilbao P & Palomares T. (2000). Effects of L-2-oxothiazolidine-4-carboxylate on the cytotoxic activity and toxicity of cyclophosphamide in mice bearing B16F10 melanoma liver metastases. *Melanoma Res*, Vol.10, No.2 (April 2000), pp.103-112, ISSN: 0960-8931.

Del Olmo M, Alonso-Varona A, Castro B, Bilbao P, & Palomares T. (2006). Cytomodulation of interleukin-2-effect by L-2-oxothiazolidine-4-carboxylate on human malignant melanoma. *Cancer Immunol Immunother*, Vol.55, No.8 (August 2006), pp.948-957, ISSN: 0340-7004.

Di Renzo MF, Narsimhan RP, Olivero M, Bretti S, Giordano S, Medico E, Gaglia P, Zara P & Comoglio PM. (1991). Expression of the Met/HGF receptor in normal and neoplastic human tissues. *Oncogene*, Vol.6, No.11 (November 1991), pp.1997-2003, ISSN: 0950-9232.

Díaz I, Palomares T, Marín H, Alonso-Varona A, Herrero B & García-Alonso I. (2009). ATRA
      blockage of cancer cells' proliferation *in vitro* depends on the continuous presence
      of the drug. *Br J Surg,* Vol.96, No.S5 (May2009), pp.42, ISSN: 1365-2168.
Dong G, Chen Z, Li ZY, Yeh NT, Bancroft CC & Van Waes C. (2001). Hepatocyte growth
      factor/scatter factor-induced activation of MEK and PI3K signal pathways
      contributes to expression of proangiogenic cytokines interleukin-8 and vascular
      endothelial growth factor in head and neck squamous cell carcinoma. *Cancer Res,*
      Vol.61, No.15 (August 2001), pp.5911-5918, ISSN: 0008-5472.
Duff SE, Jeziorska M, Rosa DD, Kumar S, Haboubi N, Sherlock D, O'Dwyer ST & Jayson GC.
      (2006) Vascular endothelial growth factors and receptors in colorectal cancer:
      implications for anti-angiogenic therapy. *European Journal of Cancer,* Vol.42, No.1
      (January 2006), pp.112-117, ISSN: 0959-8049.
Fan S, Gao M, Meng Q, Laterra JJ, Symons MH, Coniglio S, Pestell RG, Goldberg ID & Rosen
      EM. (2005). Role of NF-kappaB signaling in hepatocyte growth factor/scatter
      factor-mediated cell protection. *Oncogene,* Vol.24, No.10 (March 2005), pp.1749-
      1766, ISSN: 0950-9232.
Ferraro D, Corso S, Fasano E, Panieri E, Santangelo R, Borrello S, Giordano S, Pani G &
      Galeotti T. (2006). Pro-metastatic signaling by c-Met through RAC-1 and reactive
      oxygen species (ROS). *Oncogene,* Vol.25, No.26 (June 2006), pp.3689-3698, ISSN:
      0950-9232.
Garcea G, Sharma RA, Dennison A, Steward WP, Gescher A & Berry DP. (2003).
      Molecular biomarkers of colorectal carcinogenesis and their role in surveillance
      and early intervention. *Eur J Cancer,* Vol.39, No.8 (May 2003), pp.1041–1052,
      ISSN: 0959-8049.
García-Alonso I, Palomares T, Alonso A, Portugal V, Castro B, Caramés J & Méndez J.
      (2003). Effect of hepatic resection on development of liver metastasis. *Rev Esp
      Enferm Dig,* Vol.95, No.11 (November 2003), pp.771-776, ISSN: 1130-0108.
García-Alonso I, Palomares T, Alonso-Varona A, Castro B, Del Olmo M, Portugal V &
      Méndez J (2005). Effects of all-trans retinoic acid on tumor recurrence and
      metastasis. *Rev Esp Enferm Di, Vol.97, No.4* (2005 Apr), pp.240-248, ISSN: 1130-
      0108.
García-Alonso I, Díaz-Sanz I, Palomares T, San Cristóbal J, Martínez-Astorquiza T, Marín H.
      (2008a) Effect of hepatic growth factors on CC-531 adenocarcinoma cancer cells. *Br
      J Surg,* Vol.95, No.S6 (May 2008), pp.19-20, ISSN: 1365-2168.
García-Alonso I, Palomares T, Alonso A, Echenique-Elizondo M, Caramés J, Castro B &
      Méndez J. (2008b). Effect of liver resection on the progression and growth of
      rhabdomyosarcoma metastases in a rat model. *J Surg Res,* Vol.148, No.2 (August
      2008), pp.185-190, ISSN: 0022-4804.
García-Alonso I, Palomares T, Alonso-Varona A, Díaz-Sanz I, Miró B, Méndez J. (2010)
      All-Trans Retinoic Acid blocks the proliferative effect of growth factors on rat
      colocarcinoma cells. *Br J Surg,* Vol.97, No.S4 (June 2010), pp.15, ISSN: 1365-
      2168.
Giantonio BJ, Catalano PJ, Meropol NJ, O'Dwyer PJ, Mitchell EP, Alberts SR, Schawartz MA
      & Benson AB 3rd. (2007). Bevacizumab in combination with oxaliplatin,
      fluorouracil, and leucovorin (FOLFOX4) for previously treated metastatic colorectal

cancer: results from the Eastern Cooperative Oncology Group Study E3200. *J Clin Oncol*, Vol.25, No.12 (April 2007), pp.1539-1544, ISSN: 0732-183X.

Giaccone G & Wang Y. (2011) Strategies for overcoming resistance to EGFR family tyrosine kinase inhibitors. *Cancer treatment reviews*, (February 2011), DOI: 10.1016/j.ctrv.2011.01.003, ISSN: 0305-7372.

Halliwell B. (1991). Reactive oxygen species in living systems: source, biochemistry, and role in human disease. *Am J Med, (suppl. 3C)*, Vol.91, (September 1991), pp.S14-S22, ISSN: 0002-9343.

Hbibi AT, Lagorce C, Wind P, Spano JP, Des Guetz G, Milano G, Benamouzig R, Rixe O, Morere JF, Breau JL, Martin A & Fagard R. (2008). Identification of a functional EGF-R/p60c-src/STAT3 pathway in colorectal carcinoma: analysis of its long-term prognostic value. *Cancer Biomark*, Vol.4, No.2 (June 2008), pp.83-91, ISSN: 1574-0153.

Higuchi Y. (2004). Glutathione depletion-induced chromosomal DNA fragmentation associated with apoptosis and necrosis. *J Cell Mol Med*, Vol.8, No.4 (October-December 2004), pp.455-464, ISSN: 1582-1838.

Hirao S, Yamada Y, Koyama F, Fujimoto H, Takahama Y, Ueno M, Kamada K, Mizuno T, Maemondo M, Nukiwa T, Matsumoto K, Nakamura T & Nakajima Y. (2002). Tumor suppression effect using NK4, a molecule acting as an antagonist of HGF, on human gastric carcinomas. *Cancer Gene Ther*, Vol.9, No.8 (August 2002), pp.700-707, ISSN: 0929-1903.

Hiro J, Inoue Y, Toiyama Y, Miki C & Kusunoki M. (2008). Mechanism of resistance to chemoradiation in p53 mutant human colon cancer. *Int J Oncol*, Vol.32, No.6 (June 2008), pp.1305-1310, ISSN: 1019-6439.

Hurwitz H, Fehrenbacher L, Novotny W, Cartwright T, Hainsworth J, Heim W, Berlin J, Baron A, Griffing S, Holmgren E, Ferrara N, Fyfe G, Rogers B, Ross R & Kabbinavar F. (2004). Bevacizumab plus irinotecan, fluorouracil, and leucovorin for metastatic colorectal cancer. *New England Journal of Medicine*, Vol.350, No.23 (June 2004), pp.2335-2342, ISSN: 0028-4793.

Hwang IT, Chung YM, Kim JJ, Chung JS, Kim BS, Kim HJ. Kim JS & Yoo YD. (2007). Drug resistance to 5-FU linked to reactive oxygen species modulator 1. *Biochem Biophys Res Commun*, Vol.359, No.2 (July 2007), pp.304-310, ISSN: 0006-291X.

Hynes NE & Lane HA. (2005). ERBB receptors and cancer: the complexity of targeted inhibitors. *Nat Rev Cancer*, Vol.5, No.7 (July 2005), pp.341-354, ISSN: 1474-175X.

Ischenko I, Camaj P, Seeliger H, Kleespies A, Guba M, De Toni EN, Schwarz B, Graeb C, Eichhorn ME, Jauch KW & Bruns JC. (2008). Inhibition of Src tyrosine kinase reverts chemoresistance toward 5-fluorouracil in human pancreatic carcinoma cells: an involvement of epidermal growth factor receptor signaling. *Oncogene*, Vol.27, No.57 (December 2008), pp.7212-7222, ISSN: 0950-9232.

Jankowski K, Kucia M, Wyscoczynski M, Reca R, Zhao DL, Trzyna E, Trent J, Peiper S, Zembala M, Ratajczak J, Houghton P, Janowska-Wieczorek A & Ratajczak MZ (2003). Both hepatocyte growth factor (HGF) and stromal-derived factor-1 regulate metastatic behaviour of human rhabdomyosarcoma cells, but only HGF enhances their resistance to radiochemotherapy. *Cancer Res*, Vol.63, No.22 (November 2003), pp.7926-7935, ISSN: 0008-5472.

Jansen BA, Brouwer J & Reedijk J. (2002). Glutathione induces cellular resistance against cationic dinuclear platinum anticancer drugs. *J Inorg Biochem*,Vol.89, No.3-4 (April 2002), pp.197-202, ISSN: 0162-0134.

Jin H, Yang R, Zheng Z, Romero M, Ross J, Bou-Reslan H, Carano RA, Kasman I, Mai E, Young J, Zha J, Zhang Z, Ross S, Schwall R, Colbern G & Merchant M. (2008). MetMAb, the one-armed 5D5 anti-c-Met antibody, inhibits orthotopic pancreatic tumor growth and improves survival. *Cancer Res*, Vol.68, No.11 (June 2008), pp.4360-4368, ISSN: 0008-5472.

Johnson GL & Vaillancourt RR. (1994). Sequential protein kinase reactions controlling cell growth and differentiation. *Curr Opin Cell Biol*, Vol.6, No.2 (April 1994), pp.230-238, ISSN: 0955-0674.

Kalluri R & Zeisberg M. (2006). Fibroblasts in cancer. *Nature Reviews in Cancer*, Vol.6, No.5 (May 2006), pp.392-401, ISSN: 1474-175X.

Kammula US, Kuntz EJ, Francone TD, Zeng Z, Shia J, Landmann RG, Paty PB & Weiser MR. (2007). Molecular co-expression of the c-Met oncogene and hepatocyte growth factor in primary colon cancer predicts tumor stage and clinical outcome. *Cancer Lett*, Vol.248, No.2 (April 2007), pp.219-228, ISSN: 0304-3835.

Kang YJ. (1993). Buthionine sulfoximine spares intracellular glutamate: a possible mechanism for cell growth stimulation. *Cell Mol Biol Res*, Vol.39, No.7 (May 1993), pp.675-684, ISSN: 0968-8773.

Kaur B, Khwaja FW, Severson EA, Matheny SL, Brat DJ & Van Meir EG. (2005). Hypoxia and the hipoxya-inducible factor pathway in glioma growth and angiogenesis. *Neuro-oncol*, Vol.7, No.2 (April 2005), pp.134-153, ISSN: 1522-8517.

Kishida O, Miyazaki Y, Murayama Y, Ogasa M, Miyazaki T, Yamamoto T, Watabe K, Tsutsui S, Kiyohara T, Shimomura I & Shinomura Y. (2005). Gefitinib ("Iressa", ZD1839) inhibits SN-38-triggered EGF signals and IL-8 production in gastric cancer cells. *Cancer Chemother Pharmacol*, Vol.55, No.4 (April 2005), pp.393-403, ISSN: 0344-5704.

Koizumi F, Kanzawa F, Ueda Y, Koh Y, Tsukiyama S, Taguchi F, Tamura T, Saijo N & Nishio K. (2004). Synergistic interaction between the EGFR tyrosine kinase inhibitor gefitinib ("Iressa") and the DNA topoisomerase I inhibitor CPT-11 (irinotecan) in human colorectal cancer cells. *Int J Cancer.*, Vol.108, No.3 (January 2004), pp.464-472, ISSN: 0020-7136.

Kummar S, Gutierrez ME, Maurer BJ, Reynolds CP, Kang M, Singh H, Crandon S, Murgo AJ & Doroshow JH. (2011). Phase I trial of fenretinide lym-x-sorb oral powder in adults with solid tumors and lymphomas. *Anticancer Res*, Vol.31, No.3 (2011 Mar), pp.961-966, ISSN: 0250-7005.

Kuzuya M, Ramos MA, Kanda S, Koike T, Asai T, Maeda K, Shitara K, Shibuya M & Iguchi A. (2001). VEGF protects against oxidized LDL toxicity to endothelial cells by an intracellular glutathione-dependent mechanism through the KDR receptor. *Arterioscler Thromb Vasc Biol*, Vol.21, No.5 (May 2001), pp.765-770, ISSN: 1079-5642.

Lagadec P, Griessinger E, Nawrot MP, Fenouille N, Colosetti P, Imbert V, Mari M, Hofman P, Czerucka D, Rousseau D, Berard E, Dreano M & Peyron JF. (2008). Pharmacological targeting of NF-kappaB potentiates the effect of the topoisomerase inhibitor CPT-11 on colon cancer cells. *Br J Cancer,* Vol.98, No.2 (January 2008), pp.335-344, ISSN: 0007-0920.

Le Bras M, Clément MV, Pervaiz S & Brenner C. (2005). Reactive oxygen species and the mitochondrial signalling pathway of cell death. *Histol Histopathol,* Vol.20, No.1 (January 2005), pp.205-219, ISSN: 0213-3911.

LeGolvan MP & Resnick M. (2010). Pathobiology of colorectal cancer hepatic metastases with an emphasis on prognostic factors. *Journal of Surgical Oncology,* Vol.102, No.8 (December 2010), pp.898-908, ISSN: 0022-4790.

Liu JP, Wei HB, Zheng ZH, Guo WP & Fang JF. (2010). Celecoxib increases retinoid sensitivity in human colon cancer cell lines. *Cell Mol Biol Lett,* Vol.15, No.3 (2010 Sep), pp.440-450, ISSN: 1425-8153.

Lou H & Kaplowitz N (2007). Glutathione depletion down-regulates tumor necrosis factor alpha-induced NF-kappaB activity via IkappaB kinase-dependent and - independent mechanisms. *J Biol Chem,* Vol.282, No.40 (October 2007), pp.29470-29481, ISSN: 0021-9258.

Maellaro E, Dominici S, Del Bello B, Valentini MA, Pieri L, Perego P, Supino R, Zunino F, Lorenzini E, Paolicchi A, Comporti M & Pompella A. (2000). Membrane gamma-glutamyltranspeptidase activity of melanoma cells: effects on cellular H_2O_2 production, cell surface protein thiol oxidation and NF-κB activation status. *J Cell Sci,* Vol.113, No.15 (August 2000), pp.2671-2678, ISSN: 0021-9533.

Markowitz SD & Bertagnolli MM. (2009). Molecular origins of cancer: Molecular basis of colorectal cancer. *New England Journal of Medicine,* Vol.361, No.25 (December 2009), pp.2449-2460, ISSN: 0028-4793.

Martínez-Astorquiza T, Palomares T, San Cristóbal J, Marín H, Quintana A & García-Alonso I. (2008) Effect of all-trans retinoic acid on the development of colon carcinoma liver metastases following partial hepatectomy in rats. *Br J Surg,* Vol.95, No.S6, (May 2008), pp.34, ISSN: 1365-2168.

Meister A & Anderson ME. (1983). Glutathione. *Annu Rev Biochem,* Vol.52, (November 1983), pp.711-760, ISSN: 0066-4154.

Meurette O, Lefeuvre-Orfila L, Rebillard A, Lagadic-Gossmann D & Dimanche-Boitrel MT. (2005). Role of intracellular glutathione in cell sensitivity to the apoptosis induced by tumor necrosis factor {alpha}-related apoptosis-inducing ligand/anticancer drug combinations. *Clin Cancer Res,* Vol.11, No.8 (April 2005), pp.3075-3083, ISSN: 1078-0432.

Mills EM, Takeda K, Yu ZX, Ferrans V, Katagiri Y, Jiang H, Lavigne MC,Leto TL & Guroff G. (1998). Nerve growth factor treatment prevents the increase in superoxide produced by epidermal growth factor in PC12 cells. *J Biol Chem,* Vol.273, No.35 (August 1998), pp.22165-22168, ISSN: 0021-9258.

Moberly JB, Logan J, Borum PR, Story KO, Webb LE, Jassal SV, Mupas L, Rodela H, Alghamdi GA, Moran JE, Wolfson M, Martis L & Oeropoulos DG. (1998). Elevation of whole-blood glutathione in peritoneal dialysis patients by L-2-oxothiazolidine-4-carboxylate, a cysteine prodrug (Procysteine (R)). *J Am Soc Nephrol,* Vol.9, No.6 (June 1998), pp.1093-1099, ISSN: 1046-6673.

Morini M, Cai T, Aluigi MG, Noonan DM, Masiello L, De Flora S, D'Agostini F, Albini A & Fassina G. (1999). The role of the thiol N-acetylcysteine in the prevention of tumor invasion and angiogenesis. *Int. J. Biol. Markers*, Vol.14, No.4 (October-December 1999), pp.268-271, ISSN: 0393-6155.

Morris PE, Papadakos P, Russell JA, Wunderink R, Schuster DP, Truwit JD, Vincent JL & Bernard GR. (2008). A double-blind placebo-controlled study to evaluate the safety and efficacy of L-2-oxothiazolidine-4-carboxylic acid in the treatment of patients with acute respiratory distress syndrome. *Crit Care Med*, Vol.36, No.3 (March 2008), pp.782-788, ISSN: 0090-3493.

Mulder K, Scarfe A, Chua N, Spratlin J. (2011) The role of bevacizumab in colorectal cancer: understanding its benefits and limitations. *Expert Opinion on Biological Therapy*, Vol.11, No.3 (March 2011), pp.405-413, ISSN: 1471-2598.

Murillo MM, Carmona-Cuenca I, Del Castillo G, Ortiz C, Roncero C, Sánchez A, Fernández M & Fabregat I. (2007). Activation of NADPH oxidase by transforming growth factor-beta in hepatocytes mediates up-regulation of epidermal growth factor receptor ligands through a nuclear factor-kappaB-dependent mechanism. *Biochem J*, Vol.405 (part 2), No.? (July 2007), pp.251-259, ISSN: 0264-6021.

Naidu KA, Nasir A, Pinkas H, Kaiser HE, Brady P & Coppola D. (2003). Glutathione-S-transferase pi expression and activity is increased in colonic neoplasia. *In Vivo*, Vol.17, No.5 (September-October 2003), pp.479–482, ISSN: 0258-851X.

Niu G, Wright KL, Huang M, Song LX, Haura E, Turkson J, Zhang SM, Wang TH, Sinibaldi D, Coppola D, Heller R, Ellis LM, Karras J, Bromberg J, Pardoll D, Jove R & Yu H. (2002). Constitutive Stat3 activity up-regulates VEGF expression and tumor angiogenesis. *Oncogene*, Vol.21, No.13 (March 2002), pp.2000-2008, ISSN: 0950-9232.

Odom D, Barber B, Bennett L, Peeters M, Zhao Z, Kaye J, Wolf M, Wiezorek J. (2011) Health-related quality of life and colorectal cancer-specific symptoms in patients with chemotherapy-refractory metastatic disease treated with panitumumab. *Int J Colorectal Dis*, Vol.26, No.2 (February 2011), pp.173-181, ISSN 0179-1958.

Ortiz C, Caja L, Sancho P, Bertran E & Fabregat I. (2008). Inhibition of the EGF receptor blocks autocrine growth and increases the cytotoxic effects of doxorubicin in rat hepatoma cells: role of reactive oxygen species production and glutathione depletion. *Biochem Pharmacol*, Vol.75, No.10 (May 2008), pp.1935-1945, ISSN: 0006-2952.

Palomares T, Alonso-Varona A, Alvarez A, Castro B, Calle Y & Bilbao P. (1997). Interleukin-2 increases intracellular glutathione levels and reverses the growth inhibiting effects of cyclophosphamide on B16 melanoma cells. *Clin Exp Metastasis*, Vol.15, No.3 (May 1997), pp.329-337, ISSN: 0262-0898.

Palomares T, Bilbao P, del Olmo M, Castro B, Calle Y & Alonso-Varona A. (1999). *In vitro* and *in vivo* comparison between the effects of treatment with adenosine triphosphate and treatment with buthionine sulfoximine on chemosensitization and tumour growth of B16 melanoma. *Melanoma Res*, Vol.9, No.3 (June 1999), pp.233-242, ISSN: 0960-8931.

Palomares T, Caramés M, García-Alonso I & Alonso-Varona A. (2009). Glutathione modulation reverses the growth-promoting effect of growth factors, improving the

5-fluorouracil anti-tumour response in WiDr human colon cancer cell line. *Anti-Cancer Res*, Vol.29, No.10 (October 2009), pp.3957-3965, ISSN: 0250-7005.

Qu Z, Van Ginkel S, Roy AM, Westbrook L, Nasrin M, Maxuitenko Y, Frost AR, Carey D, Wang W, Li R, Grizzle WE, Thottassery JV & Kern FG. (2008). Vascular endothelial growth factor reduces tamoxifen efficacy and promotes metastatic colonization and desmoplasia in breast tumors. *Cancer Res*, Vol.68, No.15 (August 2008), pp.6232-6240, ISSN: 0008-5472.

Radominska-Pandya A, Chen G, Czernik PJ, Little JM, Samokyszyn VM, Carter CA, et al. (2000). Direct interaction of all-trans-retinoic acid with protein kinase C (PKC). J Biol Chem, Vol.275, No.29 (July 2000), pp.22324-22330, ISSN: 0021- 9258.

Raffel J, Bhattacharyya AK, Gallegos A, Cui HY, Einspahr JG, Alberts DS & Powis G. (2003). Increased expression of thioredoxin-1 in human colorectal cancer is associated with decreased patient survival. *J Lab Clin Med*, Vol.142, No.1 (July 2003), pp.46–51, ISSN: 0022-2143.

Rao GN. (1996). Hydrogen peroxide induces complex formation of SHC-Grb2-SOS with receptor tyrosine kinase and activates Ras and extracellular signal-regulated protein kinases group of mitogen-activated protein kinases. *Oncogene*, Vol.13, No.4 (August 1996), pp.713-719, ISSN: 0950-9232.

Rhee SG, Bae YS, Lee C, Yang KS, Lee SR & Kwon J. (2000). Hydrogen peroxide in peptide growth factor signaling. Faseb Journal, Vol.14, No.8 (May 2000), pp.A1505-A1505, ISSN: 0892-6638.

Roy S, Khanna S & Sen CK. (2008). Redox regulation of the VEGF signaling path and tissue vascularization: Hydrogen peroxide, the common link between physical exercise and cutaneous wound healing. *Free Radic Biol Medic*, Vol.44, No.2 (January 2008), pp.180-192, ISSN: 0891-5849.

Russo A, DeGraff W, Friedman N & Mitchell JB. (1986). Selective modulation of glutathione levels in human normal versus tumor cells and subsequent differential response to chemotherapy drugs. *Cancer Res*, Vol.46, No.6 (June 1986), pp.2845-2848, ISSN: 0008-5472.

Sadowitz PD, Hubbard BA, Dabrowiak JC, Goodisman J, Tacka KA, Aktas MK, Cunningham MJ, Dubowy RL & Souid AK. (2002). Kinetics of cisplatin binding to cellular DNA and modulations by thiol-blocking agents and thiol drugs. *Drug Metabol Dispos*, Vol.30, No.2 (February 2002), pp.183-190, ISSN: 0090-9556.

Schmid K, Nair J, Winde G, Velic I & Bartcsh H. (2000). Increased levels of DNA adducts in colonic polyps of Fap patients. *Int J Cancer*, Vol.87, No.1 (July 2000), pp.1–4, ISSN: 0020-7136.

Schmidt M & Lichtner RB. (2002). EGF receptor targeting in therapy-resistant human tumors. *Drug Resist Updat*, Vol.5, No.1 (February 2002), pp.11-18, ISSN: 1368-7646.

Schulze-Bergkamen H, Ehrenberg R, Hickmann L, Vick B, Urbanik T, Schimanski CC, Berger MR, Schad A, Weber A, Heeger S, Galle PR & Moehler M. (2008). Bcl-x(L) and Myeloid cell leukaemia-1 contribute to apoptosis resistance of colorectal cancer cells. *World J Gastroenterol*, Vol.14, No.24 (June 2008), pp.3829-3840, ISSN: 1007-9327.

Sen CK, Khanna S, Babior BM, Hunt TK, Ellison EC & Roy S. (2002). Oxidant-induced vascular endothelial growth factor expression in human keratinocytes and cutaneous wound healing. *J Biol Chem*, Vol.277, No.36 (September 2002), pp.33284-33290, ISSN: 0021-9258.

Sethi G, Ahn KS, Chaturvedi MM & Aggarwal BB. (2007). Epidermal growth factor (EGF) activates nuclear factor-kappaB through I kappa B alpha kinase-independent but EGF receptor-kinase dependent tyrosine 42 phosphorylation of I kappa B alpha. *Oncogene*, Vol.26, No.52 (November 2007), pp.7324-7232, ISSN: 0950-9232.

Shen JG, Cheong JH, Noh SH & Wang LB. (2007). Effects of hepatocyte growth factor gene transfection on adriamycin-induced apoptosis of gastric cancer cells *in vitro*. *Zhonghua Zhong Liu Za Zhi*, Vol.29, No.5 (May 2007), pp.338-341, ISSN: 0253-3766.

Shim KS, Kim KH, Han WS & Park EB. (1999). Elevated serum levels of transforming growth factor-beta 1 in patients with colorectal carcinoma: Its association with tumor progression and its significant decrease after curative surgical resection. *Cancer*, Vol.85, No.3 (February 1999), pp.554-561, ISSN: 0008-543X.

Shinomiya N, Gao CF, Xie Q, Gustafson M, Waters DJ, Zhang YW & Woude GF. (2004). RNA interference reveals that ligand-independent met activity is required for tumor cell signaling and survival. *Cancer Res*, Vol.64, No.21 (November 2004), pp.7962-7970, ISSN: 0008-5472.

Sogno I, Venè R, Ferrari N, De Censi A, Imperatori A, Noonan DM, Tosetti F & Albini A. (2010). Angioprevention with fenretinide: targeting angiogenesis in prevention and therapeutic strategies. *Crit Rev Oncol Hematol*, Vol.75, No.1 (July 2010), pp.2-14, ISSN: 1040-8428.

Sreekumar PG, Kannan R, de Silva AT, Burton R, Ryan SJ & Hinton DR. (2006). Thiol regulation of vascular endothelial growth factor-A and its receptors in human retinal pigment epithelial cells. *Biochem Biophys Res Commun*, Vol.346, No.4 (August 2006), pp.1200-1206, ISSN: 0006-291X.

Stabile LP, Lyker JS, Huang L & Siegfried JM. (2004). Inhibition of human non-small cell lung tumors by a c-Met antisense/U6 expression plasmid strategy. *Gene Ther*, Vol.11, No.3 (February 2004), pp.325-335, ISSN: 0969-7128.

Stebbing J, Harrison M, Glynne-Jones R, Bridgewater J & Propper D. (2008). A phase II study to determine the ability of gefitinib to reverse fluoropyrimidine resistance in metastatic colorectal cancer (the INFORM study). *Br J Cancer*, Vol.98, No.4 (February 2008), pp.716-719, ISSN: 0007-0920.

Stoeltzing O, Liu W, Reinmuth N, Parikh A, Ahmad SA, Jung YD, Fan F & Ellis LM. (2003). Angiogenesis and antiangiogenic therapy of colon cancer liver metastasis. *Ann Surg Oncol*, Vol.10, No.7 (August 2003), pp.722-733, ISSN: 1068-9265.

Storz P. (2005). Reactive oxygen species in tumor progression. *Front Biosci*, Vol.10, (May 2005), pp.1881-1896, ISSN: 1093-9946.

Sullivan LA & Brekken RA. (2010). The VEGF family in cancer and antibody-based strategies for their inhibition. *Mabs*, Vol.2, No.2 (March 2010), pp.165-175, ISSN: 19420862.

Sun HC & Tang ZY (2003). Preventive treatments for recurrence after curative resection of hepatocellular carcinoma. A literature review of randomised control trials. *World J Gastroenterol*, Vol.9, No.4 (April 2003), pp.635-640, ISSN: 1007-9327.

Tatebe S, Unate H, Sinicrope FA, Sakatini T, Sugumura K, Makino M, Ito H, Savaraj N, Kaibara N & Kuo MT. (2002). Expression of heavy subunit of gamma-glutamylcysteine synthetase (gamma-GCSh) in human colorectal carcinoma. *Int J Cancer*, Vol.97, No.1 (January 2002), pp.21–27, ISSN: 0020-7136.

Thannickal VJ & Fanburg BL. (2000). Reactive oxygen species in cell signaling. *Am J Physiol Lung Cell Mol Physiol*, Vol.279, No.6 (December 2000), pp.L1005-L1028, ISSN: 1040-0605.

Thrall BD, Raha GA, Springer DL & Meadows GG. (1991). Differential sensitivities of murine melanocytes and melanoma cells to buthionine sulfoximine and anticancer drugs. *Pigment Cell Res*, Vol.4, No.5-6 (December 1991), pp.234-239, ISSN: 0893-5785.

Tol J & Punt CJA. (2010). Monoclonal antibodies in the treatment of metastatic colorectal cancer: a review. *Clinical Therapeutics*, Vol.32, No.3 (March 2010), pp.437-453, ISSN: 0149-2918.

Ushio-Fukai M & Nakamura Y. (2008). Reactive oxygen species and angiogenesis: NADPH oxidase as target for cancer therapy. *Cancer lett*, Vol.266, No.1 (July 2008), pp.37-52, ISSN: 0304-3835.

Vigneron A, Gamelin E & Coqueret O. (2008). The EGFR-STAT3 oncogenic pathway up-regulates the Eme1 endonuclease to reduce DNA damage after topoisomerase I inhibition. *Cancer Res*, Vol.68, No.3 (February 2008), pp.815-825, ISSN: 0008-5472.

Vita JA, Frei B, Holbrook M, Gokce N, Leaf C & Keany JF Jr. (1998). L-2-oxothiazolidine-4-carboxylic acid reverses endothelial dysfunction in patients with coronary artery disease. *J Clin Invest*, Vol.101, No.6 (March 1998), pp.1408-1414, ISSN: 0021-9738.

Voboril R, Hochwald SN, Li J, Brank A, Weberova J, Wessels F, Moldawer LL, Camp ER & MacKay SL. (2004). Inhibition of NF-kappa B augments sensitivity to 5-fluorouracil/folinic acid in colon cancer. *J Surg Res*, Vol.120, No.2 (August 2004), pp.178-188, ISSN: 0022-4804.

Wanebo HJ & Berz D. (2010). The neoadjuvant therapy of colorectal hepatic metastases and the role of biologic sensitizing and resistance factors. *Journal of Surgical Oncology*, Vol.102, No.8 (December 2010), pp.891-897, ISSN: 0022-4790.

Wen JH, Matsumoto K, Taniura N, Tomioka D & Nakamura T. (2007). Inhibition of colon cancer growth and metastasis by NK4 gene repetitive delivery in mice. *Biochem Biophys Res Commun*, Vol.358, No.1 (June 2007), pp.117-123, ISSN: 0006-291X.

Wu YP, Yakar S, Zhao L, Hennighausen L & Le Roith D. (2002). Circulating insulin-like growth factor-I levels regulate colon cancer growth and metastasis. *Cancer Res*, Vol.62, No.4 (February 2002), pp.1030-1035, ISSN: 0008-5472.

Xu JM, Azzariti A, Colucci G & Paradiso A. (2003). The effect of gefitinib (Iressa, ZD1839) in combination with oxaliplatin is schedule-dependent in colon cancer cell lines. *Cancer Chemother Pharmacol*, Vol.52, No.6 (December 2003), pp.442-448, ISSN: 0344-5704.

Yang H, Magilnick N, Xia M & Lu SC. (2008). Effects of hepatocyte growth factor on glutathione synthesis, growth, and apoptosis is cell density-dependent. *Exp Cell Res*, Vol.314, No.2 (January 2008), pp.398-412, ISSN: 0014-4827.

Yoshida A, Takemura H, Inoue H, Miyashita T & Ueda T. (2006). Inhibition of glutathione synthesis overcomes Bcl-2-mediated topoisomerase inhibitor resistance and induces nonapoptotic cell death via mitochondrial-independent pathway. *Cancer Res*, Vol.66, No.11 (June 2006), pp.5772-5780, ISSN: 0008-5472.

Zhang L, Hannay JA, Liu J, Das P, Zhan M, Nguyen T, Hicklin DJ, Yu D, Pollock RE & Lev D. (2006). Vascular endothelial growth factor overexpression by soft tissue sarcoma cells: implications for tumor growth, metastasis, and chemoresistance. *Cancer Res*, Vol.66, No.17 (September 2006), pp.8770-8778, ISSN: 0008-5472.

5

Lipid Peroxidation in Colorectal Carcinogenesis: Bad and Good News

Stefania Pizzimenti, Cristina Toaldo,
Piergiorgio Pettazzoni, Eric Ciamporcero,
Mario Umberto Dianzani and Giuseppina Barrera
University of Turin,
Italy

1. Introduction

During oxidative stress, membrane lipids are one of the major targets of Reactive Oxygen Species (ROS) that are known to elicit oxidative decomposition of polyunsaturated fatty acids (PUFAs) of membrane phospholipids, a process usually referred to lipid peroxidation (Esterbauer et al., 1991). During this process, a number of carbonylic compounds are generated as final products, including acrolein, malondialdehyde (MDA) and 4-hydroxyalkenals (Esterbauer et al., 1991). Among the 4-hydroxyalkenal class, 4-hydroxynonenal (HNE) is the most abundant aldehyde produced (Dianzani et al., 1999). Over the years, HNE has achieved a status as one of the best recognized and most studied of the cytotoxic products of lipid peroxidation (Poli et al., 2008). In addition to studies on its bioactivity, HNE is commonly used as a biomarker for the occurrence and/or the extent of oxidative stress. It appears to be produced specifically by peroxidation of ω-6 PUFAs, such as linoleic acid, arachidonic acid (AA) and γ-linolenic acid (Esterbauer et al., 1982). HNE has three main functional groups: the aldehyde group, the C=C double bond and the hydroxyl group, which can participate, alone or in sequence, in chemical reactions with other molecules (Esterbauer et al., 1991). HNE is a highly electrophilic molecule, which predisposes it to localize in the cell membranes. It can easily react with low molecular weight compounds, such as glutathione, with proteins, with lipids and, at higher concentration, with DNA (Esterbauer et al., 1991; Uchida, 2003). The double bond, the carbonyl group and the hydroxyl group, all contribute to making HNE highly reactive with nucleophiles with the primary reactivity of the molecule lying at the unsaturated bond of the C-3 atom. HNE has been shown to form Michael adducts via the C-3 atom with the sulfhydryl group of Cys residues, the imidazole group of His residues, and the ε-amino group of Lys residues on a large number of proteins (Esterbauer et al., 1991). Recently, it has been proposed that HNE can also modify Arg residues of proteins (Isom et al., 2004). In addition to Michael adduct formation, Lys residues also form Schiff bases and pentylpyrrole adducts with HNE via the C-1 aldehyde group (Sayre et al., 1993; Petersen & Doorn, 2004; Schaur, 2003)

HNE-modified proteins can be removed by the proteasomal system (Siems & Grune, 2003).

Once formed, HNE is rapidly degraded and its metabolism is dependent upon a set of specific enzymes presenting high affinity toward HNE. In particular HNE metabolism can be divided into glutathione-mediated and oxidative/reductive categories (Siems & Grune, 2003). In the first case, HNE binds the thiol group of GSH resulting in the correspondent emiacetal (Balogh & Atkins, 2011). The reaction with GSH can occur in a spontaneous manner, with low efficiency or through the reaction catalyzed by Glutathione S Transferases (GSTs). Moreover, although a number of isoforms of GST manifested HNE conjugating activity, it has been widely reported that the isoform GST A4 presents the highest HNE affinity (Balogh & Atkins , 2011). The oxidative/reductive pathway of HNE involves its NAD/NADP-dependent oxidative conversion to 4-hydroxy-2-nonenoic Acid (HNA) catalyzed by aldheyde dehydrogenases (ALDHs) or the reductive conversion to 1,4-dihydroxy-2-nonene (DHN) catalyzed by alchool dehydrogenase (ADH) or aldhehyde reductase (AR) (Hartley et al., 1995; Vander Jagt et al., 1995). However, the majority of HNE is metabolized through forming GS-HNE (Forman et al., 2003). HNE-GSH is then further metabolized and found in urine, mostly, as the mercapturic acid derivative, HNE-MA (Alary, 1995). Indeed, HNE-GSH adduct is further metabolized by γ-glutamyltranspeptidase (γ-GT) and dipeptidases (DP) to the cysteinyl (CYS)-HNE thioether adduct. The cysteinyl thioether adduct is a substrate for acetyltransferases (AT) that catalyze the acetylation of the cysteinyl adduct to generate the acetylcysteinyl (AcCYS), or mercapturic acid, adduct. HNE metabolites also can be found associated with mercapturic acid, such as DHN-MA, HNE-MA and HNA-lactone (Alary et al., 2003). HNE is also partially excreted first with the bile, then with the faeces, under the form of conjugated metabolites. However, biliary metabolites undergo an enterohepatic cycle that limits the final excretion of faecal metabolites (Alary et al., 2003).

HNE, and in general aldehydes formed during membrane lipid peroxidation, are quite long lived, as compared to reactive free radicals and can widely diffuse and react around the site of origin (Esterbauer 1991). As a consequence, HNE and related aldehydes were proposed as putative ultimate toxic messengers, potentially able to mediate stress-related injury at the molecular level (Uchida, 2003). Indeed, HNE has been detected in vivo in several pathological conditions, which entail increased lipid peroxidation, including inflammation, atherosclerosis, chronic degenerative diseases of the nervous system, and chronic liver diseases, reaching a concentration up to about 10 µM (Parola et al., 1999).

However, under physiological conditions, HNE can be found at low concentrations in human tissues and plasma (0.07-2.8 µM) (Esterbauer et al., 1991, Poli et al., 2008) where it participates in the control of biological processes, such as signal transduction, cell proliferation and differentiation. Indeed, HNE, similarly to ROS, plays an important role in controlling the intracellular signal transduction pathways involved in a number of cell responses (Parola et al., 1999; Dianzani et al., 2003; Leonarduzzi et al., 2004).

The contribution of HNE and lipid peroxidation in carcinogenesis is still controversial. Beside pro-tumoral effects, several authors pointed out their protective role. This "two-faced" role has already emerged for ROS (Halliwell, 2007; Wang & Yi, 2008; Pan et al., 2009; Acharya et al., 2010) and increasing evidence is emerging also for a dual role of lipid peroxidation products (Zhi-Hua et al., 2006; Pizzimenti et al., 2010a).

2. HNE and carcinogenesis

2.1 DNA-adducts, mutagenicity and genotoxicity

2.1.1 DNA-adducts

The most substantial evidence of the genotoxic and mutagenic effect of HNE is the formation of HNE-DNA adducts. ROS and HNE seem to share this feature and this has been proposed as the mechanism of tumor induction (Bartsch & Nair, 2005).

One of the most studied HNE-adducts is the propane-type DNA adduct with deoxyguanosine, the 6-(1-hydroxyhexanyl)-8-hydroxy-1, N2-propano-2'deoxyguanine (HNE-dG) (Winter et al., 1986). AA appears to be a major source of HNE-DNA adducts, producing a total of 20.6 μmol of HNE-dG adducts (Chung et al., 2000), by an in vitro assay using 1 mM AA. HNE-dG is also the main lesion produced upon the addition of HNE to DNA (Chung et al., 2000; Wacker et al., 2001); moreover, an increase of HNE-dG adducts was observed in the liver DNA of rats after treatment with CCl4, a well known inducer of lipid peroxidation (Chung et al., 2000). Taken together, these results generate substantial evidence for the endogenous formation of these adducts, thus it has been proposed that lipid peroxidation is a main endogenous pathway leading to propano adduction in DNA (Chung et al., 1999).

In the presence of peroxides and reactive oxygen species, HNE can be further metabolized to an epoxide intermediate that interacts with DNA, forming etheno-type DNA adducts (Chung et al., 1996). However the etheno-type DNA adducts are produced in significantly lower yield, with respect to the HNE-dG adducts, when a pro-oxidant stimulus, such H_2O_2, or HNE is added to cells. Indeed, in these experimental conditions, HNE-dG represent more than 95% of the overall adducts to DNA, suggesting that HNE-dG may represent the best biomarker of the genotoxic effects of HNE (Douki et al., 2004).

All four bases of DNA are the targets for HNE adduct formation (Chung et al., 1996; De Bont et al., 2004), but with different efficiency: G>C>A>T (Kowalczyk et al., 2004).

HNE-DNA adducts have been identified in tissues of untreated rats and humans (Chung et al., 2000), suggesting that the endogenously produced HNE can form adducts with DNA in the physiological condition also.

Removal of these modified bases from DNA plays an important role in the prevention of mutagenesis and carcinogenesis. Each cell has an efficient defence mechanism to repair these types of damage via DNA repair pathways such as base excision repair (BER), nucleotide excision repair (NER), and mismatch repair (MMR) pathways (Min & Eberel, 2009). In human leukocyte treated with 200 μM HNE, DNA damage was repaired after 12 h and returned to the control level at 24 h (Park & Park, 2011).

It has been demonstrated that NER is a major pathway for repairing HNE-dG adducts, since HNE-dG adducts induce a significantly higher level of genotoxicity and mutagenicity in NER-deficient human and E. coli cells than in NER-proficient cells (Feng et al., 2003). Moreover, other authors suggested that HNE can also contribute to carcinogenesis, by inhibiting the nucleotide excision repair (NER) of DNA damage in cancer cells with concentration higher than 50 μM (Feng et al., 2004). In any case, HNE forms adducts with DNA only at higher concentrations, since it can react quickly with amino and sulphydrylic groups of proteins and, primarly, with the sulphydrylic group of GSH. Indeed, it has been calculated that GSH conjugates were 20000 times more numerous than DNA adducts when HNE was exogenously added to the cultured cells (Falletti & Douki, 2008).

2.1.2 Mutagenicity

In this context, it would be important to know whether the HNE-dG adducts are mutagenic. Several authors suggest this possibility, since HNE has been shown to be mutagenic in mammalian cells (Cajelli et al., 1987). HNE was negative in bacterial mutagenicity tests, however its epoxidized form has been tested positive (Chung et al., 1993). HNE was found to be responsible for recombination, base substitutions and frameshift mutations in M13 phage transfected in E.coli (Kowalczyk et al., 2004).

Moreover it has been reported that 50 µM HNE treatment in human cells induces a high frequency of G.C to T.A mutations at the third base of codon 249 (AGG*) of the p53 gene (Hussain et al., 2000), a mutational hot spot in human cancers, particularly in hepatocellular carcinoma (Hsu et al., 1991). Both eheno and propane type HNE-DNA-adduct at codon 249 can be responsible for such transitions (Feng et al., 2003).

The stereochemistry of HNE-dG adducts seems to play an important role in determining mutations. Indeed, two of the HNE-dG adducts, (6R, 8S, 11R) and (6S, 8R, 11S), were significantly more mutagenic than (6R, 8S, 11S) and (6S, 8R, 11R) HNE-dG adducts. Only one of the HNE stereoisomers was able to form interstrand DNA–DNA cross-links. (Fernandes et al., 2003).

2.1.3 Genotoxicity

The genotoxic property of HNE was demonstrated in different cell types, such as on cultured human lymphocytes (Emerit et al., 1991), in primary hepatocytes (Esterbauer et al., 1991) and cerebral microvascular endothelial cells (Eckl, 2003). In these cell lines an increase of micronuclei (a biomarker of chromosome breakage and/or whole chromosome loss), chromosomal aberrations and sister chromatid exchanges was observed after exposure to HNE at relatively low doses, ranging 0.1-10 µM. However these clastrogenic features of low doses of HNE failed to be confirmed in a recent multicentrum study on DNA of normal peripheral blood lymphocytes (Katic et al., 2010).

Currently, the comet assay has been extensively used to measure DNA strand breaks, since it represents a sensitive and rapid assay to detect the mutagenic and genotoxicity of chemicals and xenobiotics (Tice, et al., 1991).

Unfortunately, most HNE-induced DNA lesions are the stable 1,N2-propano adducts and they are not detected by this technique. By using this assay, the genotoxic property of 5-10 µM HNE in the K562 leukemic cell line has been shown; this feature was highly dependent on cellular GSH/GST/AR system (Yadav et al., 2008). The comet test was also used to demonstrate the genotoxicity of 200 µM HNE in human leukocytes (Park & Park, 2011).

2.2 Results in laboratory animals

To date, in contrast with several in vitro experimental results, tumor bioassays in laboratory animals failed to demonstrate the carcinogenic and mutagenic properties of HNE. HNE, in particular its epoxy derivate, has shown that to be a weak tumor-initiating agent, causing the development of renal preneoplastic tubule lesions in new-born mice (Chung et al., 1993). More interestingly, HNE lacks in vivo genotoxicity in lacI transgenic mice, a model for detecting mutagenicity in target organs, even when lethal doses are applied (Nishikawa et al., 2000).

The big gap between the in vitro and the in vivo data can be partially explained by carefully considering the elevated doses frequently used to demonstrated the carcinogenic properties of HNE in vitro. Indeed, several mutagenic assays with HNE have been performed with high doses of HNE (more than 100 μM). It seems rather unlikely that HNE or other aldehydes can reach overall concentrations in the range of 100 μM in cells and organs (Esterbauer et al., 1991). It is conceivable that such levels may be built up locally, near or within peroxidizing membranes for a short time because of their high lipophilicity. It has been calculated, for example, that the concentration of HNE in the lipid bilayer of isolated peroxidizing microsomes is about 4.5 mM (Koster et al., 1986). Nevertheless, a convincing demonstration that this very high concentration can be reached into the cells has remained elusive. On the other hand, when HNE diffuses out from membranes, its concentration is reduced by the surrounding aqueous phase. Moreover, the cytosolic HNE-metabolizing enzymes destroy HNE produced in excess so that the steady-state HNE concentration into the cells, around 1 μM, is reached quickly (Esterbauer et al., 1991; Dianzani et al., 1999).

2.3 Cellular responses and signal transduction

As previously indicated, the adduct formation between HNE and DNA is only one of the several biological effects determined by this aldehyde. Indeed, HNE is considered as a signalling molecule influencing proliferation, differentiation and apoptosis of cancer cells (Dianzani, 2003; Leonarduzzi et al., 2004; Poli et al., 2008; Pizzimenti et al., 2010b). The majority of experimental evidence indicate an antiproliferative role of HNE, when added at low doses (1-10 μM) to cultured cells. The inhibition of proliferation has been observed in leukemic (HL-60, K562, U937, MEL, ML-1) (Barrera et al., 1991; Barrera et al., 1987, Rinaldi et al., 2000; Pizzimenti et al., 2006), neuroblastoma (SK-N-BE) (Laurora et al. 2005), hepatoma (7777, J42) (Muzio et al., 2001; Canuto et al., 1999), osteosarcoma (SaOS2; HOS) (Calonghi et al., 2002; Sunjic et al., 2005), prostate cancer (PC3) (Pettazzoni et al., 2011) cells. This anti-proliferative effect is sustained by the modulation of key genes involved in cell growth control, such as oncogenes (c-myc, c-myb, fos, AP1, cyclins) and anti-oncogenes (pRB, p53, SUFU-1, Mad-1) (Poli et al., 2008; Pizzimenti et al., 2009).

Interestingly, the effect of HNE in normal cell proliferation is more variable if not opposite to that observed in tumor cells. For example, HNE has no effect on normal myeloid stem cells (Hassane et al., 2008) or on human peripheral blood lymphocytes (Semlitsch et al., 2002), while the respective tumour was sensitive to the anti-proliferative effect of aldehyde. On the contrary, in vascular smooth muscle cells 0.1 μM HNE stimulated cell proliferation (Kakishita et al., 2001).

In several cell lines, the inhibition of proliferation was accompanied by apoptosis. The mechanisms of HNE-induced apoptosis through the extrinsic and intrinsic pathways, its self-regulatory role in this process and its interaction with Fas (CD95), p53, and Daxx has been recently reviewed (Awasti et al., 2008).

HNE is also able to induce differentiation, as observed in HL-60, MEL, K562 and SaOS osteosarcoma cells (Barrera et al., 1991; Rinaldi et al., 2000; Calonghi et al., 2002; Cheng et al., 1999; Fazio et al., 1992). Moreover, HNE was shown to induce features of typical differentiated cells, such as chemotaxis (Curzio et al., 1988), phagocytosis and the ability to induce respiratory burst (Barrera et al., 1991) in myeloid cells. HNE also demonstrated the ability to regulate the replicative potential of cells, by inhibiting the telomerase activity. Indeed, in HNE-treated leukemic cells, the expression of the hTERT gene was down-regulated by modulating the expression of transcription factors belonging to the Myc/Mad/Max network (Pizzimenti et al., 2006).

The anti-tumoral properties of HNE are also sustained by the demonstration of anti-angiogenic properties. Stagos and collaborators demonstrated that 5 and 10 µM HNE were able to inhibit the tube formation of human bone marrow endothelial cells (HBMEC) (Stagos et al., 2009). However, conflicting results have been reported, since it has been demonstrated that 1 µM HNE induces an increase of VEGF expression in human retinal pigment epithelial cells (Ayalasomayajula & Kompella, 2002).

The cellular responses to HNE are sustained by affecting cell signalling at multiple levels. Relevant findings in this area have been extensively reviewed (Poli et al., 2008; Leonarduzzi et al., 2004; Dianzani et al., 1999).

In addition to the above cellular responses presented, HNE activates various cytoprotective, stress response pathways, promoting changes in gene expression that facilitate cell survival and recovery from stress (West & Marnett, 2005). For example, HNE activates the transcription factors Nrf2 (Nuclear factor erythroid-derived 2-like 2) and HSF1 (heat shock factor 1), which mediate the antioxidant and heat shock responses, respectively (Jacobs & Marnett, 2007). Nrf2 acts by binding Antioxidant Responsive Elements (ARE) sequences on promoters of certain genes promoting their expression (Thimmulappa et al., 2002). In regard to HNE metabolism, functional ARE sequences have been found on promoter of GST A4 ALDH and ADH (Reddy et al., 2007; Malhotra et al., 2010). Moreover, Nrf2 promotes de novo GSH synthesis by up-regulating expression of the GSH synthesis pathway (Harvey 2009). Nrf2 is controlled by both translational and post-translational mechanisms, in particular the protein Kelch-like ECH-associated protein 1 (KEAP1) mediates Nrf2 ubiquitinaltion followed by proteasomal destruction (Kaspar et al., 2010). In conditions of oxidative stress or in response to many chemicals KEAP1 undergo conformational changes responsible for loss of Nrf2 binding activity. As a consequence Nrf2 can accumulate, translocate in the nucleus and drive expression of the antioxidant program (Reddy et al., 2007).

The heat shock response mediates the induction of a highly conserved set of heat shock proteins (Hsps) (Mosley, 1997). The inducible expression of Hsps is mediated by heat shock transcription factor 1 (HSF1), which translocates to the nucleus upon activation and enhances the expression of genes to form promoters containing heat shoch elements (HSE), such as Hsp70 (Sarge et al., 1993; Baler et al., 1993). A principal function of Hsps is to chaperone other proteins, binding to nascent polypeptide chains as well as to unfolded and damaged proteins. Their function as protein chaperones aids in the recovery of cells from thermal and chemical-induced damage (Hahn & 1982; Howard, 1993). In addition to acting as protein chaperones, Hsps inhibit cell death by directly inhibiting a variety of pro-apoptotic mediators, such as HNE (Jacobs et al., 2007).

It is very likely that the majority of effects observed on cell signalling and cellular responses can be mediated by the reaction of HNE to proteins and peptides. Quantitatively, proteins and, among peptides, the GSH, represent the most important group of HNE-targeted biomolecules. It was estimated that 1–8% of the HNE formed in cells will modify proteins (Siems & Grune, 2003). Most of the identified targets are enzymes, carriers, receptors, ion channels, transport proteins, cytoskeletal, heat shock proteins and others. The biological significance of the HNE-protein adducts identified have been reviewed by several authors (Uchida, 2003; Poli et al., 2008). Some of the protein-adducts identified can explain the anti-tumoral effect exerced by this aldehyde. For example, it was demonstrated that the inhibition of cell proliferation in the human colorectal carcinoma cell line (RKO) and human lung carcinoma cell line (H1299) by HNE was mediated by the direct reaction of HNE with

IκB kinase (IKK), the key enzyme regulating the NF-κB activation (Ji et al., 2001b). Moreover the HNE adducts with alpha-enolase, at the cellular surface of leukemic cells, suggest a new role for HNE in the control of tumour growth and invasion, since HNE causes a dose- and time-dependent reduction of the plasminogen binding to alpha-enolase. As a consequence, HNE reduces adhesion of HL-60 cells to HUVECs (human umbilical vein endothelial cells) (Gentile et al., 2009).

New perspectives of HNE role in cancer-inducing signaling pathways have recently emerged, by recent findings on microRNA (miRNA) (Pizzimenti et al., 2009), a class of conserved non-coding small RNAs, which regulate gene expression by translation repression of coding mRNAs (Bartel, 2004).

2.4 HNE content in human cancers

Several studies on human cancer tissues have analysed the HNE or HNE-protein adduct content, in order to find a possible correlation between this marker of lipid peroxidation and the progression of cancer.

HNE content has been reported to increase along with the progression of breast cancer (Karihtala et al., 2011) and astrocytoma (Zarkovic et al., 2005). In human renal cell carcinoma, immunohistochemistry for HNE-modified proteins showed positive staining in the cytoplasm of tumor cells, with respect to controls, without correlation to the clinical stage (Okamoto et al., 1994).

However other reports have demonstrated the opposite: a low or undetectable lipid peroxidation, as well as HNE content, such as in hepatomas (Dianzani, 1993).

Several studies have shown elevated lipid peroxidation markers in the sera, plasma or urine of breast carcinoma (Hung et al., 1999; Chandramathi et al., 2009), cervical intraepithelial neoplasia and carcinoma of the cervix (Looi et al., 2008), head and neck squamous cell carcinoma (Gupta et al., 2009) and prostate tumor (Kotrikadze et al., 2008), compared to healthy controls. However, these extratumoral measurement are likely, at least partly, to reflect generalized oxidative stress and / or inflammation in the whole body.

3. HNE and colorectal carcinogenesis

3.1 Sources and fate of HNE in colon

Colon cells can be exposed to HNE derived form different sources (Figure 1). It is possible to find HNE directly in the food (Gasc et al., 2007), since it can derived from lipid peroxidation of PUFAs introduced with diet or from endogenous PUFAs presents in cellular membranes. A small amount of HNE can reach the colon also via bile. Following a single intravenous administration of [3H]-HNE, five metabolites were present in the bile, namely GSH–HNE, GSH–DHN, DHN, and HNA-lactone mercapturic acid conjugates (Laurent et al., 1999). Within 4 hr from injection of the radiolabel 3[H]-HNE, 19.5% of the injected radioactivity was found in the bile, whereas only 3% was found in the feces within 48 hr (Laurent et al., 1999). The existence of an enterohepatic circulation for HNE metabolites has been unequivocally demonstrated (Laurent et al., 1999) using a model linking donor rats (injected intravenously with [4-3H]HNE) and recipient rats (to which the bile from donor rats was delivered intraduodenaly). This enterohepatic circulation, approximately 8% of the total dose, may explain the low amount of radioactivity recovered from faeces when rat were dosed intravenously with [4-3H]HNE.

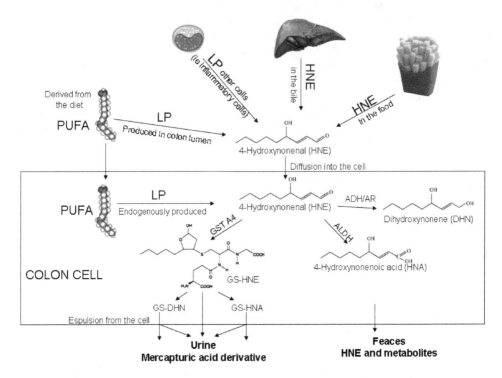

Fig. 1. Sources and fate of HNE in colon

Metabolic transformation of HNE starts in enterocites, where GSH-HNE is the main metabolite produced (Grune et al., 1991). The majority of HNE metabolites are found in the urine. Indeed, following the intravenous administration of [3H]-HNE in rats, 67%, 3%, 0.16%, and 6.5% of the injected radioactive dose was recovered from urine, faeces, liver and remaining tissues, respectively (Alary et al., 2003). The urinary HNE metabolites were separated by HPLC and the resolved peaks were identified as mercapturic acid conjugates of HNA, DHN, HNE and HNA-lactone, where DHN-MA, and to a lesser extent HNA lactone-MA, have been found to be the major urinary metabolites of HNE in rats (Boon et al., 1999). DHN-MA has been confirmed to be the major urinary HNE metabolite also in human urine (Alary et al., 1998).

The microflora of the human intestine can also affect levels of lipid peroxidation, since the antioxidative effect of lactic acid bacteria has been demonstrated (Lin et al., 1999). In particular, the antioxidative activity of Bifidobacterium longum ATCC 15708 and Lactobacillus acidophilus ATCC 4356 was measured based on the inhibition of linoleic acid peroxidation. Both intact cells and intracellular cell-free extracts of B. longum and L. acidophilus demonstrated an antioxidative effect on inhibiting lipid peroxidation. The antioxidative activity ranged from 38 to 48% inhibition of linoleic acid peroxidation. This indicates that B. longum and L. acidophilus have a very strong antioxidative effect on inhibiting lipid peroxidation (Lin et al., 1999).

Low level of HNE and its metabolites can be found also in faecal water (Alary et al., 2003) and numerous studies have emphasized the lipid peroxidation products of faecal water in colon cancer as diet-related factors (Lapre et al., 1992; Glinghammar et al., 1997).

3.2 Pro-tumoral and anti-tumoral role of HNE in colon carcinogenesis

Several authors have reported evidence that sustains the pro-tumoral activity of HNE and other products of lipid peroxidation in colon carcinogenesis. These findings include in vitro (see table 1) and in vivo studies, which demonstrate the genotoxic properties of HNE on coloncarcinoma cell lines, the increase of HNE content along with the progression of colorectal cancer and the increase of HNE-DNA adducts in vivo. However other studies, seem to demonstrate the opposite (see table 1). Consistent with the hypothesis of an anti-tumoral role of HNE are the results showing the inhibition of cell growth, the induction of apoptosis in several colon cancer cell lines, as well as the demonstration that HNE content decreases in biopsies of colon-cancer tissues with respect to normal mucosa. A deeper discussion of these opposite results is here reported.

COLON CANCER CELL LINE	HNE DOSE	OBSERVED EFFECTS	PROTEIN / PATWAY INVOLVED / MAIN RESULTS	REFERENCE
CaCo-2	1 μM	apoptosis, ROS production, enhanced by co-treatement with TGF-β1	HNE activates c-Jun N-terminal kinase (JNK) and Smad4, effects enhanced by co-treatment with TGF-β1	Zanettiet al., 2003; Vizio et al., 2005; Biasi et al., 2006
CaCo-2, HT-29	1 μM	cell growth inhibition, apoptosis	HNE down-regulates telomerase activity and hTERT expression, through modulation of Myc/Mad/Max network	Pizzimenti et al., 2010
CaCo-2	1 μM	cell growth inhibition, apoptosis	HNE induces an increase of c-myc expression and a subsequent down-regulation; HNE increases bax and p-21 expression	Cerbone et al., 2007
RKO	30-75 μM	apoptosis	HNE activates a mitochondrion-dependent pathway, involving cytochrome c release and caspase activation	Ji et al., 2001a
RKO	40 μM	apoptosis	HNE inhibits NF-kB activation by direct interaction with IkB kinase (IKK)	Ji et al., 2001b
RKO	30-60 μM	apoptosis	comparison with other aldehydes producted during lipid peroxidation (HPNE,ONE) and stereoisomers of HNE	West et al., 2004
RKO	5, 20, or 60 μM	5 and 20 μM subcytotoxic, 60 μM apoptosis	by using microarray technology, HNE simultaneously affects multiple stress signaling pathways	West et al., 2005

COLON CANCER CELL LINE	HNE DOSE	OBSERVED EFFECTS	PROTEIN / PATWAY INVOLVED / MAIN RESULTS	REFERENCE
RKO	30-60 µM	apoptosis	beside the activation of pro-apoptotic pathway, HNE activates a protective signal activation through activation of HSF1, Hsp70-1 and Hsp40 and stabilization of Bcl-XL	Jacobs & Marnett, 2007
RKO	45 µM	apoptosis	BAG3, induced by HSF-1, increases cell survival, by stabilizing the level of Bcl-2 family proteins	Jacobs & Marnett, 2009
HCT15	20-80 µM	cell death	AKR1B10-overexpressing cells are resistant to cytotoxicity of HNE	Matsunaga et al., 2011
Apc+/+, Apc+/- colon epithelial cells	10-250 µM	cell death	HNE reduces cellular viability of either Apc+/+ and Apc-/+ cells, with lesser extent in Apc-/+ cells	Pierre et al., 2007
CaCo-2		cell death	HNE increases prostaglandin E2 (PGE2) production and cyclooxygenase (COX)-2 expression; inhibition of AR prevented HNE-induced effects	Tammali et al., 2006
HT-29, HT-29clone19A	100-200 µM	genotoxicity	butyrate reduces DNA damage caused by HNE, through induction of Glutathione S-Transferase	Ebert et al., 2001
primary human colon cells, LT97, HT-29clone19A	100-250 µM	genotoxicity	HNE induces TP53 specific DNA damage	Schaeferhenrich et al., 2003
HT-29	150 µM	genotoxicity	Two fermentation products of wheat bran reduce the genotoxicity of HNE, via up-regulation of the activity of GSTs	Glei et al., 2006
primary human colon cells, LT97	0-250 µM	genotoxicity	HNE induces DNA damage on specific genes (APC,TP53, KRAS)	Glei et al., 2007
HT-29	100-250 µM	genotoxicity	butyrate induces resistance to HNE damage, by inducing GSH syntesis and increasing GSTA4-4 level	Knoll et al., 2005, Scharlau et al., 2009

Table 1. HNE in vitro effects on colon cancer cell lines

3.2.1 HNE-DNA adducts in colon and colon cancer

HNE-dG adducts, were found in normal human colon tissue, as well as DNA adducts with other lipid peroxidation products, such as acrolein and MDA (Chung et al., 2000). The levels of HNE-dG in tissue DNA examined so far are estimated to be in the range of 3-9 adducts per billion bases (3-9 nmol/mol guanine) (Chung et al,. 2000).

The etheno-DNA adducts, inter alia formed from epoxidized HNE, were found at increased level in colonic polyps of familial adenomatous polyposis (FAP) patients. Mean adduct levels in FAP polyps were 65 εdA/109 and 59 εdC/109 parent nucleotides, being 2 to 3 times higher than in unaffected colon tissue (Schmid et al., 2000). Interestingly, the level of etheno-DNA adducts in colon carcinoma tissues were found to be similar to unaffected colon (Schmid et al., 2000), suggesting a possible HNE role in the early events of colon carcinogenesis.

On the contrary, Obtułowicz and collaborators (2010) have found that, in colon cancer patients, the DNA-HNE adducts εdA and εdG, measured both in colon tissues and blood leukocytes, were lower in patients than in controls (Obtułowicz et al., 2010). These authors have measured the two corresponding metabolites also, 1,N6- Ethenoadenine (εAde) and 3,N4-ethenocytosine (εCyt), catalized by BER, the major pathway of etheno adduct elimination from DNA (Obtułowicz et al., 2010). Both excision activities were significantly higher in tumor than in normal colon tissues and this feature could be explained by the increased level of abasic site endonuclease (APE1), belonging to BER system, in coloncancer patients with respect to controls (Obtułowicz et al., 2010).

A possible pro-cancinogenic role of etheno-DNA adducts is also sustained by the finding that in the colon of patients with inflammatory bowel disease εdC, but not εdA, are increased. In particular it has been demonstrated that εdC was 19-fold higher in colonic mucosa of Crohn's disease and 4-fold higher in the colonic mucosa of ulcerative colitis patients, when compared to normal tissues (Nair et al., 2006). Since patients with ulcerative colitis (UC), and Crohn's (CD) have an elevated risk for developing colon cancer (Konner et al., 2003), the authors suggest that the promutagenic etheno-DNA adducts, generated as a consequence of chronic inflammation, can act as a driving force to malignancy in cancer-prone inflammatory diseases (Nair et al., 2006).

HNE can also contribute to induce colon carcinogenesis, by inhibiting the DNA repair mechanism of such adducts. Indeed, Feng and collaborators (2004) demonstrated that 50 μM HNE inhibits NER in the human colon epithelial cell line HCT116. The repair capacity for benzo[a]pyrene diol-epoxide and UV light-induced DNA damage was greatly compromised in cells treated with HNE.

3.2.2 Genotoxicity and mutagenicity of HNE in colon cancer

Comet assay demonstrated that HNE, at concentration higher than 150 μM, displays a genotoxic effect in the colon carcinoma cell line HT-29 (Glei et al., 2006; Ebert et al., 2001; Knoll et al., 2005) and in HT29clone19A, a permanently differentiated sub-clone treated with sodium butyrate (Augeron & Laboisse, 1984). Moreover, such high doses of HNE were able to affect DNA integrity in primary human colon cells (Schaferhenrich et al., 2003; Glei et al., 2007) and in LT97, an established cell line derived from a differentiated microadenoma, representing a model of an early premalignant genotype, carrying adenomatous polyposis coli (APC) and Ki-ras mutated, but normal p53 (Richter et al., 2002), three well-characterized genes involved in coloncancer progression (Fearon et al., 1990).

Genotoxicity of HNE is higly dependent on cellular GSH level. Indeed, GSH depletion leads to and increase of HNE genotoxicity in the HT-29 colon carcinoma cell line (Knoll et al., 2005). Moreover, HNE displayed a higher genotoxicity in LT97 than in HT29clone19A and primary human colon cells. This result can be explained by the lower GST expression found in LT97 compared to HT29clone19A and primary human colon cells (Schaferhenrich et al., 2003).

Recently, by using a refined comet assay (Comet-FISH) (Glei et al., 2009), which combined the classical comet assay with the fluorescence in situ hybridisation, it has been demonstrated that HNE concentrations higher than 150 µM were able to affect DNA integrity on the p53 (Schaferhenrich et al., 2003; Glei et al., 2007), Ki-Ras and APC genes (Glei et al., 2007), in primary human colon cells and the colon adenoma cell LT97. After cell incubation with HNE, the p53 gene, the crucial target gene for the progression of adenoma to carcinoma, migrated more efficiently into the comet tail than the global DNA, indicating a high susceptibility of the p53 gene to HNE (Glei et al., 2007). Moreover, the TP53 gene sensitivity to the DNA damage induced by HNE was significantly higher with respect to APC and KRAS genes. This particular sensitivity is especially apparent in LT97 cells (Glei et al., 2007). This may be due to the fact that LT97 cells normally carry damaged APC and KRAS, but undamaged TP53 (Richter et al., 2002). In normal colonocytes, APC and KRAS were also sensitive to damage (Glei et al., 2007). These findings are highly interesting when considering the sequence of mutational events that occur during human colon carcinogenesis (Vogelstein et al., 1988). APC and KRAS mutations transform normal epithelial (stem) cells into initiated, more rapidly proliferating cells to yield dysplasia and small adenoma. TP53 mutations in adenoma are then crucial alterations leading to further progression and to carcinoma. Based on studies of Glei and collaborators (2007), it is possible to conclude that HNE could potentially contribute to both cancer initiation and progression in the colon, if produced in sufficient amounts. However, as mentioned in the previously chapter, it is unlikely that HNE is reaching such high concentrations (150 µM) in colon in vivo. Moreover it still remains to be studied to what extent the observed genotoxicity of HNE is related to mutagenicity. Consistent with this hypothesis, as previously reported, it has been demonstrated that 50 µM HNE treatment in human TK-6 lymphoblastoid cell line induces a high frequency of G.C to T.A mutations at the third base of codon 249 (AGG*) of the p53 gene (Hussain et al., 2000), a mutational hot spot in human cancers, particularly in hepatocellular carcinoma (Hsu et al., 1991). The adduct of HNE to codon 249 of the p53 gene has been also found by Hu and collaborators (2002). These authors exposed DNA of exons 5, 7 and 8 of human p53 gene, where the large majority of p53 mutations occur, to a very high concentration of HNE (192 mM or more). They identified two main HNE adducts, the first already mentioned at codon 249 (exon 7) and the second at codon 174 (exon 5) (Hu et al., 2002). However, the possible contribution of HNE to p53 mutations, through the formation of DNA adducts remains to demonstrated, since codon 249 and codon 174 of p53 usually are not mutated in colorectal rectal. Indeed, mutations at codon 175, 245, 248, 273, and 282 account for approximately 43% of all p53 mutations in CRC (Soong et al., 2000; Soussi et al., 2000; Soussi & Beroud, 2003).

3.2.3 HNE role in controlling cell proliferation, apoptosis of colon cancer cell

Several findings have been collected through the years related to the anti-proliferative and pro-apoptotic in colon cancer cells. These results, even obtained with very low doses of

HNE, easily reacheable in vivo, cast doubt on the pro-tumoral HNE role. 1 µM HNE is able to inhibit cell proliferation of Caco-2 and HT-29 colon cancer cells (Cerbone et al., 2007; Pizzimenti et al., 2010b; Vizio et al., 2005) and concentrations ranging form 1 to 100 µM are able to induce apoptosis in Caco-2, HT-29, RKO, HCT15 colon cancer cells. (see table I for references). A number of genes or cell signalling pathways have been found to be affected by HNE, and their modulation can explain the biological effects observed.

Results obtained in our laboratories demonstrated that the inhibition of proliferation in Caco-2 and HT-29 colon carcinoma cells by 1 µM HNE is sustained by the down-regulation of telomerase activity and hTERT expression, the catalytic subunit of telomerase (Pizzimenti et al., 2010b). The major mechanism of HNE action seems to be the modulation of expression and activity of transcription factors belonging to the Myc/Mad/Max network (Pizzimenti et al., 2010b).

After HNE treatment, apoptosis of several colon cancer cell lines was investigated by different authors and different pathways were considered to be involved. In Caco-2 human colon adenocarcinoma cell line, 1 µM HNE caused an increase of bax expression (Cerbone et al., 2007) and the apoptosis induction is mediated by JNK activation. Indeed, the HNE-mediated apoptotic cell death was significantly prevented by preincubating the cells with the selective JNK inhibitor SP600125 (Biasi et al., 2006).

Ji and collaborators investigated the mechanism of HNE-induced cell death in human colorectal carcinoma cells and found that HNE-induced apoptosis depends on alteration of mitochondrial function, leading to the release of cytochrome c and subsequent activation of caspase cascade (Ji et al., 2001a). The authors have further demonstrated that HNE inhibited IκB kinase activity by direct interaction with IκB kinase and suggested that HNE is an endogenous inhibitor of NF-κB activation that acts by preventing IκB kinase activation and subsequent IκB degradation (Ji et al., 2001b).

The molecular mechanism of HNE induced apoptosis was investigated in RKO colon cancer cells also. In this cell line, beside the pro-apoptotic stimuli, HNE activates the stress response pathways, that abrogate programmed cell death. Moreover, HNE elicits the nuclear translocation of HSF1 and promotes Hsp40 and Hsp72 expression (Jacobs & Marnett, 2007). The silencing of HSF1 sensitizes the colon cancer cells to HNE-induced apoptosis, through a mechanism involving the control of BCL-XL, BAG3 protein turnover (Jacobs & Marnett, 2007; Jacobs & Marnett, 2009)

3.2.4 HNE content in human colon cancers

Only a few studies have investigated the level of the lipid peroxidation products, in particular HNE, in human colon cancers and results are contradictory. It has been demonstrated that the levels of proteins modified by HNE and MDA in colorectal cancer tissues were significantly increased (Murawaki et al., 2008). By immunohystochemical analysis, Murawaki and collaborators (2008) have demonstrated that the proteins modified by HNE were stained diffusely in the cytoplasm of cancer cells, while they were weakly stained in normal tissues. Similar results have been obtained by Kondo and collaborators (1999). Immunostaining of HNE-histidine adducts was observed in the cytoplasm of colon cancer tissues. Immunoreactivity was also found in the cytosol of infiltrating inflammatory cells. Western blot analysis of HNE-histidine adducts confirmed the results, since larger amounts of modified proteins were detected in carcinomas than in nontumorous epithelial counterparts (Kondo et al., 1999). The authors also demonstrated that HNE content increased along with the progression of colorectal cancer, since tubular adenoma cells revealed a weaker staining, similar to the staining of non-tumorous epithelial cells (Kondo et al., 1999). An increase of HNE content in colon cancer tissues have been found also by Skrzydlewska and collaborators (2005). These authors analyzed the HNE content in homogenates of human colon cancer tissues, by measuring HNE as a fluorimetric derivative. These authors have demonstrated that the level of HNE was significantly increased (P<0.001) in cancer tissue compared to control group, with highest in G3-grade adenocarcinoma and mucinous adenocarcinoma and clinical IV stage of colorectal cancer.

In contrast with these results, other scientists demonstrated a decrease of HNE in colon cancer tissues. Indeed, it was demonstrated that HNE was significantly decreased in cancer specimens, with respect to normal tissues, by measuring the HNE content in tissue biopsies from patients with colon adenocarcinoma of different TNM and G stage (Biasi et al., 2002; Zanetti et al., 2003). This result was confirmed later by the same group (Biasi et al., 2006). Moreover, Chiarpotto and collaborators (1997) have demonstrated that the fluorescent adducts with plasma proteins and HNE were significantly lower in the plasma from cancer patients (all stage G3, pT3pN0) than in controls.

3.2.5 HNE metabolism in colon cancer

In colon cells, the enzymes of HNE metabolism are present. Staining with anti GST A4 specific antibodies revealed a significant expression of GST A4 in columnar and crypt epithelial cells of normal colon mucosae (Desmots et al., 2001), as well as in colon cancer cell lines (Scharmach et al., 2009; Knoll et al., 2005). Moreover, both the oxidative and reductive metabolisms of HNE are well represented in colon cells, since both ALDH or ADH have been found to be significantly expressed in colon mucosae (Seitz et al., 1996; Yin et al., 1994). The expression of AR is also enhanced in various forms of cancer, such as hepatoma (Zeindl-Eberhart et al., 1997) and melanoma cancer (Kawamura et al., 1999).

By affecting HNE metabolism enzymes, it is possibly to modulate the HNE concentration inside cells. This could be critical for cancer growth regulation or DNA genotoxicity. Indeed, butyrate, produced during gut fermentation, has a chemoprotective role toward HNE injury, when added at high concentration, such as 100-200 µM in HT-29 colon cancer cells (Knoll et al., 2005). The chemoprotective effect of butyrate seems to be related to the increasing the expression of glutathione S-transferases GSTP1 (Ebert et al., 2001) and hGSTA4-4 (Knoll et al., 2005) able to catalyze the conjugation of HNE with glutathione. Similar results were obtained in HT-29 cells by using two wheat bran-derived arabinoxylans, fermented under anaerobic conditions in human feces. These two fermentation products inhibited growth and reduced the genotoxicity of HNE (100-200 µM) via up-regulation of the activity of GSTs, in absence of a GSTP1 or hGSTA4-4 increase (Glei et al., 2006).

There is a growing interest in targeting aldose reductase (AR), as a novel therapeutic approach in preventing progression of colon cancer (Tammali et al., 2011). AR besides reducing aldo-sugars efficiently reduces toxic lipid aldehydes and their conjugates with glutathione (Tammali et al., 2006). Indeed, inhibition of AR by sorbinil or by antisense ablation, prevented FGF–induced and PDGF–induced proliferation of Caco-2 cells at S-phase (Tammali et al., 2006). Similar results were also obtained in other colon cancer cell lines, by Ramana and collaborators which show that the inhibition of AR prevents epidermal growth factor (EGF)– and basic fibroblast growth factor (bFGF)–induced HT29, and cell proliferation, by accumulating cells at the G1 phase of the cell cycle, through the AKT/Phosphoinositide 3-Kinase/E2F-1 pathway. Analogous results were obtained in SW480 and HCT-116 colon cancer cells (Ramana et al., 2010).

More interestingly, in vivo studies showed that administration of aldose reductase-small interfering RNA (siRNA), or the AR inhibitor fidarest, to nude mice bearing SW480 human colon adenocarcinoma cells, led to a complete arrest of tumor progression. Such evidence suggests a key role for aldose reductase in growth factor-induced proliferation in colon cancer cells and it points to inhibition of aldose reductase as a novel therapeutic approach in preventing progression of colon cancer (Tammali et al., 2006; Ramana et al., 2010).

Recently, the ATP-depent transporter RLIP76 (Ral binding protein1) has been considered for its role in controlling HNE content inside the cells. Indeed, it has been demonstrated that this transporter with multi-specific transport activity towards glutathione-conjugates and chemotherapeutic agents, is also specific for GSH-HNE (Sharma et al., 2002). The expulsion of GS-HNE from cells represents another critical step in HNE detoxification since it avoids the accumulation of adducted GSH and permits the restoration of GSH/GSSG equilibrium. RLIP76 protein is frequently overexpressed in cancer lesions (Vatsyayan et al., 2010), included colon cancers (Singhal et al., 2007), thus there is a growing interest in considering this protein as target in cancer therapy (Vatsyayan et al., 2010). When RLIP76 is inhibited, a rapid increase in HNE-GSH is observed, both in vitro (Awasthi et al., 2003; Cheng et al., 2001; Yang et al., 2003) and in vivo (Vatsyayan et al., 2010). Recent studies show that the inhibition and/or depletion of RLIP76 by antibodies, siRNA, or antisense can lead to a drastic and sustained regression of lung, kidney, melanoma, prostate, and colon cancer xenografts with no observed recurrence of tumors (Vatsyayan et al., 2010). In particular, it has been shown that xenografts of SW480 human colon cancer cells in nude mice can be completely regressed by anti-RalBP1 immunoglubulin G or by suppression of RalBP1 expression using phosphorothioate antisense against it (Singhal et al., 2007).

The super family of aldo–keto reductase (AKR) enzymes seems to be involved in tumor development, and growing evidence is accumulating, suggesting them as a new class of tumor marker. These enzymes are hydroxysteroid dehydrogenases with a broad substrate specificity for other carbonyl compounds including HNE. The isoform AKR1B10 seems to be particulary involved in the transformation of HNE to the oxidized counterpart 4-oxonon-2-enal (4-ONE) (Martin et al., 2009). AKR1B10 is also up-regulated in many types of solid tumors (Fukumoto et al., 2005; Yoshitake et al., 2007; Breton et al., 2008; Satow et al., 2010), and its gene silencing results in growth inhibition of colorectal cancer cells (Yan et al., 2007), as well as in increasing HNE-elicited cell death (Matsunaga et al., 2011).

Recently, some family members of AKR enzymes have been shown to be overexpressed and linked to resistance against anticancer drugs such as anthracyclines, cisplatin, and methotrexate (Veitch et al., 2009; Cheng al., 2008; Selga et al., 2008). As regarding colon cancer, experimental data suggest that the up-regulation of AKR1B10 was related with acquisition of resistance to the anticancer drug mitomycin-c (MMC) in HT-29 colon cancer cells (Matsunaga et al., 2011). The cytotoxic effects of MMC seems to be mediated by the formation of HNE. Thus, the biological significance of the increasing of AKR1B10 in MCC resistant cancer cells would be an ability to better detoxify cytotoxic aldehydes including HNE. (Matsunaga et al., 2011). In the resistant cells, treatment with an AKR1B10 inhibitor decreased their MMC tolerance (Matsunaga et al., 2011), suggesting its use as adjuvant therapy in drug resistant cells, in which AKR1B10 is over-expressed.

Many dietary cancer chemopreventive compounds, such as cruciferous vegetables, could activate the antioxidant responsive element (ARE), a critical regulatory element in the promoter sequence of genes encoding cellular Phase II detoxifying and antioxidant enzymes. Transcriptional activation of ARE is typically mediated by the transcription Nuclear factor-erythroid 2-related factor 2 (Nrf2). Thus, this transcription factor has emerged as a novel target for the prevention of colon cancer (Saw & Kong, 2011). However, stable RNAi-mediated knockdown of Nrf2 in human colon cancer cells suppressed tumor growth in mouse xenograft settings and colon tumor angiogenesis by inhibiting Hypoxia-Induced Activation of HIF-1a (Kim et al., 2011). Thus, the role of Nfr2 in colon carcinogenesis still has to be explored.

3.2.6 HNE and nutrition

It is well accepted that development and progression of colon cancer is generally associated with lifestyle-dependent risk factors, such as dietary choices (Pearson et al., 2009). HNE can be directly found in food (Gasc et al., 2007) or its production can be enhanced by the presence of some nutrients, i.e. ω-6 PUFAs, or some fermentation products of diet, i.e. butyrate, can modulate the metabolism of this aldehyde, thus modifying its concentration. In this context, it is very interesting to explore the connection between HNE, nutrition and colon carcinogenesis.

HNE has been founded in different foods, correlating with the amount of ω-6 (Surh et al., 2010). UsingGC–MS technology, scientists measured 4-hydroxy-alkenaks content in vegetable oils, fish and shellfish, calculating the HNE dietary intake of the Korean population (Surh et al., 2005). Korean daily exposure to 4-hydroxy- 2-alkenals was found to be of 4.3 mg/day and HNE was found to be more represented (2.7 mg). There was an additional exposure to more than 11.8 mg/day 4-hydroxy-2-alkenal from fried foods. The combined exposure would be, therefore, 16.1 mg/day corresponding to 0.3 mg/kg body weight/day for a 60 kg Korean adult. Additionally, the screening of PUFA-fortified foods including infant formulas and baby foods commercially available on the Korean markets were screened, and it was estimated that 3- month to 1-year-old babies sticking exclusively to these products could be exposed to a maximum 20.2 μg/kg BW/ day of 4-hydroxy-2-alkenals (Surh et al., 2007). However, in spite of the biological toxicity of 4-hydroxy-2-alkenals, the risk for humans cannot be quantified due to the lack of a virtually safe dose of the compound (Surh et al., 2005).

A diet high in red and processed meats can increase colon cancer risk by 12–20%. The mechanism of promotion by haem iron is not known, but may be linked to oxidative stress and subsequent events such as lipid pro-oxidation and HNE production (Sesink et al., 1999; Sawa et al., 1998). Indeed, the dietary haem, in the form of either haemoglobin or meat, promotes precancerous lesions, aberrant crypt foci (ACF) and mucin-depleted foci in the colon of rats (Pierre et al., 2003; Pierre et al., 2004). This haem-induced promotion was associated with increased lipid peroxidation in faecal water and strong cytotoxycity activity of faecal water on the cancerous colonic epithelial cell line (Pierre et al., 2003). Further, Pierre and collaborators (2007), have explored the effect of faecal water components of haem-fed rats, on normal APC +/+ or premalignant APC -/+ cells, demonstrating that the toxic effects observed correlated with the presence of HNE in the faeces. Moreover, the premalignat APC -/+ cells were more resistant to apoptosis with respect to normal APC +/+. The authors suggested, thus, that the premalignant mutation confer to cells the resistance to the inhibitory signal, allowing them to undergo further mutations and follow a tumoural pathway (Pierre et al., 2007).

In a randomized human study, the urinary excretion of DHN-MA, the major metabolite of HNE detectable in urine was compared in volunteers consuming different levels of heme iron. The volunteers fed with a low red meat diet (60 g/day) showed a twofold increase of DHN-MA when supplemented with heme iron as blood sausage (70 g/day). Since colon preneoplastic lesions and DHN-MA excretion in the experimental animal were clearly associated with dietary heme iron, urinary DHN-MA was suggested as a promising biomarker of colon carcinogenesis (Pierre et al., 2006).

The role of fat present in the diet in coloncarcinogenesis has been explored by several authors and comprehensive reviews have been published. In particular, diets rich in ω-6 PUFAs, contained in vegetable oils, seem to enhance the development of colon tumors, whereas ω-3 PUFA-containing diets, such as fish oil, reduce colon cancer incidence (Reddy, 2002; Kim & Milner, 2007). Thus, it is possible to suggest a putative HNE role in colon carcinogenesis, since HNE is derived from peroxidation of ω-6. However, the complexity of the issue forces us to be more cautious. Indeed, Eder and collaborators investigated the impact of different fatty-acids composition in the diet on cancer development, measuring the formation of the promutagenic HNE-dG in the mucosa of several organs, such as colon. The correlation between adduct levels and the different fatty acids assumption was not uniform for all organs and they didn't find a clear relationship between fatty acids and adduct levels in the colon (Eder et al., 2008). Moreover, beside lipid peroxidation products it is necessary to consider the eicosanoids, also derived from PUFAs. Indeed, eicosanoids have different properties in cancer cell growth, invasion and angiogenesis when derived from ω-6 or ω-3 fatty acids (Berquim et al., 2008), thus suggesting a role in carcinogenesis.

Epidemiological studies show a reduction in risk for individuals and populations consuming high amounts of vegetables. The protective effect of vegetables may be due to their content of complex carbohydrates such as dietary fiber and starch (Scheppach et al., 1999). A substantial amount of starch escapes digestion in the small intestine (Englyst et al., 1992) and this fraction is called enzyme-resistant starch (RS). Starch and dietary fiber together are the principal substrates controlling the pattern of fermentation in the colon and, thus, the metabolism of compounds, like bile acids, nitrate and enzyme activityes (bacterial and antioxidant enzymes), which have been implicated in carcinogenesis. The effect of enzyme-resistant starch (RS) on the development of colon cancer was reported to include both chemopreventive and tumorigenic activity in humans. Indeed, an inverse association between starch consumption and large bowel cancer incidence has been found in an international comparison in 12 populations worldwide (Cassidy et al., 1994). However, an increased cancer risk with high-starch intake has been also reported (Franceschi et al., 1998; Favero et al., 1999). Wacker and collaborators (2002) have studied the number of 1,N2-propanodeoxyguanosine-30- monophosphate (HNE-dGp) adducts in the colonic mucosa of volunteers fed with starchy foods enriched with a highly resistant amylomaize starch (Hylon VII) and they found an increase of the HNE-dGp adduct, whereas there was no evidence for an increased cell proliferation in the upper crypt.

Finally, as already mentioned, nutrients can modulate the HNE level in the colon, by affecting its metabolism. This is the case of fermented products of diet, such as butyrate (Knoll et al., 2005; Glei et al., 2006) and wheat bran-derived arabinoxylans, that can affect the HNE levels, by upregulating GSTs activities.

4. Conclusion

Lipid peroxidation is a physiological and pathological process that elicits a number of electrophilic compounds able to modulate several cellular processes. Among these, HNE is the most studied aldehyde, due to its high biological activity. Since HNE is a normal constituent of the diet or can be produced in the gut, colon cells can be exposed to this aldehyde.

Low doses of HNE are able to inhibit cell proliferation and induce differentiation of colon cancer cells. Conversely, a high concentration of HNE exhibits genotoxic and mutagenic activity. We believe that the concentration of HNE and other lipid peroxidation products in the colon, represent a steady state level between production and catabolism. The alteration of this equilibrium elicits a stress condition for colon cells and, possibly, could be involved in colon carcinogenesis, although there is no scientific consensus in supporting its pro-tumoral action.

Results on HNE content in human biopsies of coloncancer tissues are contradictory, and the positive correlation between HNE content and cancer progression doesn't allow an assumption whether the HNE increase during the progression of colon cancer may represent a cause or a consequence of this process. However, in colon cancer cells, HNE induces apoptosis and telomerase inhibition. Thus, we can hypothesize that HNE, produced during radiotherapy or chemotherapy, can participate to the control of tumor growth and tumor cell death.

5. References

Acharya, A., Das, I., Chandhok, D. & Saha, T. (2010). Redox regulation in cancer: a double-edged sword with therapeutic potential. Oxidative Medicine and Cellular Longevity, Vol.3, No.1, (January 2010), pp. 23-34, ISSN 1942-0900

Alary, J., Debrauwer, L., Fernandez, Y., Cravedi, J.P., Rao D. & Bories, G. (1998). 1,4-Dihydroxynonene mercapturic acid, the major end metabolite of exogenous 4-hydroxy-2-nonenal, is a physiological component of rat and human urine. Chemical Research in Toxicology, Vol. 11, No.2, (February 1998), pp. 130–135, ISSN 0893-228X

Alary, J., Gueraud, F. & Cravedi, J.P. (2003). Fate of 4-hydroxynonenal in vivo: Disposition and metabolic pathways. Molecular Aspects in Medicine, Vol.24, No.4-5, (August-October 2003), pp. 177–187, ISSN 0098-2997

Augeron, C. & Laboisse C.L. (1984). Emergence of permanently differentiated cell clones in a human colonic cancer cell line in culture after treatment with sodium butyrate. Cancer Research, Vol.44, No.9, (September 1984), pp. 3961–3969, ISSN 0008-5472

Awasthi, S., Singhal, S.S., Singhal, J., Yang, Y., Zimniak, P. & Awasthi, Y.C. (2003). Role of RLIP76 in lung cancer doxorubicin resistance: III. Anti-RLIP76 antibodies trigger apoptosis in lung cancer cells and synergistically increase doxorubicin cytotoxicity. International Journal of Oncology, Vol.22, No.4, (April 2003), pp. 721–732, ISSN 1019-6439

Awasthi, Y.C., Sharma, R., Sharma, A., Yadav, S., Singhal, S.S., Chaudhary, P. & Awasthi, S. (2008). Self-regulatory role of 4-hydroxynonenal in signaling for stress-induced programmed cell death. Free Radical Biology & Medicine, Vol.45, No.2, (July 2008), pp. 111-118, ISSN 0891-5849

Ayalasomayajula, S.P. & Kompella, U.B. (2002), Induction of vascular endothelial growth factor by 4-hydroxynonenal and its prevention by glutathione precursors in retinal pigment epithelial cells. European Journal of Pharmacology, Vol.449, No.3, (August 2002), pp. 213-220, ISSN 0014-2999

Baler, R., Dahl, G., & Voellmy, R. (1993). Activation of human heat shock genes is accompanied by oligomerization, modification, and rapid translocation of heat shock transcription factor HSF. Molecular and Cellular Biology, Vol.13, No.4, (April 1993), pp. 2486-2496, ISSN 0270-7306

Balogh, L.M. & Atkins, W.M. (2011). Interactions of glutathione transferases with 4-hydroxynonenal. Drug Metabolism Review, Vol.43, No.2, (May 2011), pp.165-178, ISSN 0360-2532

Barrera, G., Martinotti, S., Fazio, V., Manzari, V., Paradisi, L., Parola, M., Frati, L. & Dianzani, M.U. (1987). Effect of 4-hydroxynonenal on c-myc expression. Toxicologic Pathology, Vol.15, No.2, (1987), pp. 238-240, ISSN 0192-6233

Barrera, G., Di Mauro, C., Muraca, R., Ferrero, D., Cavalli, G., Fazio, V.M., Paradisi, L. & Dianzani, M.U. (1991). Induction of differentiation in human HL-60 cells by 4-hydroxynonenal.; a product of lipid peroxidation. Experimental Cell Research, Vol.197, No.2, (December 1991), pp. 148-152, ISSN 0014-4827

Bartel, D.P. (2004). MicroRNAs: genomics, biogenesis, mechanism, and function. Cell, Vol.116, No.2, (January 2004), pp. 281-297, ISSN 0092-8674

Bartsch, H. & Nair, J. (2005). Accumulation of lipid peroxidation-derived DNA lesions: potential lead markers for chemoprevention of inflammation-driven malignancies. Mutation Research, Vol.591, No.1-2, (December 2005), pp. 34-44, ISSN 0027-5107

Berquin, I.M., Edwards, I.J. & Chen, Y.Q. (2008). Multi-targeted therapy of cancer by omega-3 fatty acids. Cancer Letters, Vol.269, No.2, (October 2008), pp.363-377, ISSN 0304-3835

Biasi, F., Tessitore, L., Zanetti, D., Cutrin, J.C., Zingaro, B., Chiarpotto, E., Zarkovic, N., Serviddio, G. & Poli G. (2002). Associated changes of lipid peroxidation and transforming growth factor beta1 levels in human colon cancer during tumour progression. Gut, Vol.50, No.3, (March 2002), pp.361-367, ISSN 0017-5749

Biasi, F., Vizio, B., Mascia, C., Gaia, E., Zarkovic, N., Chiarpotto, E., Leonarduzzi, G. & Poli G. (2006). c-Jun N-terminal kinase upregulation as a key event in the proapoptotic interaction between transforming growth factor-beta1 and 4-hydroxynonenal in colon mucosa. Free Radical Biology & Medicine, Vol.41, No.3, (August. 2006), pp.443-54, ISSN 0891-5849

Boon, P.J., Marinho, H.S., Oosting, R. & Mulder, G.J. (1999). Glutathione conjugation of 4-hydroxytrans-2,3-nonenal in the rat in vivo, the isolated perfused liver and erythrocytes. Toxicology and Applied Pharmacology, Vol.159, No.3, (September 1999), pp.214-223, ISSN 0041-008X

Breton, J., Gage, M.C., Hay, A.W., Keen, J.N., Wild, C.P., Donnellan C, Findlay, J.B. & Hardie, L.J. (2008). Proteomic screening of a cell line model of esophageal carcinogenesis identifies cathepsin D and aldo-keto reductase 1C2 and 1B10 dysregulation in Barrett's esophagus and esophageal adenocarcinoma. Journal of Proteome Research, Vol.7, No.5 (May 2008), pp.1953-1962, ISSN 1535-3893

Cajelli, E., Ferraris, A. & Brambilla, G. (1987). Mutagenicity of 4-hydroxynonenal in V79 Chinese hamster cells. Mutation Research, Vol.190, No.2, (February 1987), pp.169-171, ISSN 0027-5107

Calonghi, N., Boga, C., Cappadone, C., Pagnotta, E., Bertucci, C., Fiori, J. & Masotti, L. (2002). Cytotoxic and cytostatic effects induced by 4-hydroxynonenal in human osteosarcoma cells. Biochemical Biophysical Research Communcations, Vol.293, No.5, (May 2002), pp.1502-1507, ISSN 0006-291X

Canuto, R.A., Muzio, G., Ferro, M., Maggiora, M., Federa, R., Bassi, A.M., Lindahl, R. & Dianzani, M.U. (1999). Inhibition of class-3 aldehyde dehydrogenase and cell growth by restored lipid peroxidation in hepatoma cell lines. Free Radical Biology & Medicine, Vol.26, No.3-4, (February 1999), pp. 333-340, ISSN 0891-5849

Cassidy, A., Bingham, S. & Cummings, J. (1994). Starch intake and colorectal cancer risk: an international comparison. British Journal of Cancer, Vol.69, No.5, (May 1994), pp. 937-942, ISSN 0007-0920

Cerbone, A., Toaldo, C., Laurora, S., Briatore, F., Pizzimenti, S., Dianzani, M.U., Ferretti, C. & Barrera G. (2007). 4-Hydroxynonenal and PPARgamma ligands affect proliferation, differentiation, and apoptosis in colon cancer cells. Free Radical Biology & Medicine, Vol. 42, No.11, (June 2007), pp.1661-1670, ISSN 0891-5849

Chandramathi, S., Suresh, K., Anita, Z.B. & Kuppusamy, U.R. (2009). Comparative assessment of urinary oxidative indices in breast and colorectal cancer patients. Journal of Cancer Research and Clinical Oncology, Vol.135, No.2, (February 2009), pp.319–323, ISSN 0171-5216

Chen, J., Adikari, M., Pallai, R., Parekh, H.K. & Simpkins, H. (2008). Dihydrodiol dehydrogenases regulate the generation of reactive oxygen species and the development of cisplatin resistance in human ovarian carcinoma cells. Cancer Chemotherapy and Pharmacology, Vol.61, No.6, (May 2008), pp.979–987, ISSN 0344-5704

Cheng, J.Z., Singhal, S.S., Saini, M., Singhal, J., Piper, J.T., Van Kuijk, F.J., Zimniak, P., Awasthi, Y.C. & Awasthi, S. (1999). Effects of mGST A4 transfection on 4-hydroxynonenal-mediated apoptosis and differentiation of K562 human erythroleukemia cells. Archives of Biochemistry and Biophysics, Vol.372, No.1, (December 1999), pp. 29-36, ISSN 0003-9861

Cheng, J.Z., Sharma, R., Yang, Y., Singhal, S.S., Sharma, A., Saini, M.K., Singh, S.V., Zimniak, P., Awasthi, S. & Awasthi, Y,C. (2001). Accelerated metabolism and exclusion of 4-hydroxy-nonenal through induction of RLIP76 and hGST5.8 is an early adaptive response of cells to heat and oxidative stress. The Journal of Biological Chemistry, Vol.276, No.44, (November 2001), pp.41213–41223, ISSN 0021-9258

Chiarpotto, E., Scavazza, A., Leonarduzzi, G., Camandola, S., Biasi, F., Teggia, P.M., Garavoglia, M., Robecchi, A., Roncari, A. & Poli, G. (1997). Oxidative damage and transforming growth factor beta 1 expression in pretumoral and tumoral lesions of human intestine. Free Radical Biology & Medicine, Vol.22, No.5, (1997), pp.889-894, ISSN 0891-5849

Chung, F.L., Chen, H.J., Guttenplan, J.B., Nishikawa, A. & Hard, G.C. (1993). 2,3-epoxy-4-hydroxynonanal as a potential tumor-initiating agent of lipid peroxidation. Carcinogenesis, Vol.14, No.10, (October 1993), pp. 2073-2077, ISSN 0143-3334

Chung, F.L., Nath, R.G., Nagao, M., Nishikawa, A., Zhou, G.D. & Randerath, K. (1999). Endogenous formation and significance of 1,N2-propanodeoxyguanosine adducts. Mutation Research, Vol. 424, No.1-2, (March 1999), pp.71-78, ISSN 0027-5107

Chung, F.L., Nath, R.G., Ocando, J., Nishikawa, A. & Zhang, L. (2000). Deoxyguanosine adducts of t-4-hydroxy-2-nonenal are endogenous DNA lesions in rodents and humans: detection and potential sources. Cancer Research, Vol.60, No.6, (March 2000), pp.1507-1511, ISSN 0008-5472

Chung, F.L., Chen, H.J. & Nath, R.G. (1996). Lipid peroxidation as a potential endogenous source for the formation of exocyclic DNA adducts. Carcinogenesis, Vol.17, No.10, (October 1996), pp.:2105-2111, ISSN 0143-3334

Curzio M. (1988). Interaction between neutrophils and 4-hydroxyalkenals and consequences on neutrophil motility. Free Radical Research Communications, Vol.5, No.2, (1988), pp.55-66, ISSN 8755-0199

De Bont, R. & van Larebeke, N. (2004). Endogenous DNA damage in humans: a review of quantitative data. Mutagenesis, Vol.19, No.3, (May 2004), pp.169-185, ISSN 0267-8357

Desmots, F., Rissel, M., Loyer, P., Turlin, B. & Guillouzo, A. (2001). Immunohistological analysis of glutathione transferase A4 distribution in several human tissues using a specific polyclonal antibody. Journal of Histochemistry and Cytochemistry, Vol.49, No.12, (December 2001), pp.1573-1580, ISSN 0022-1554

Dianzani, M.U. (1993). Lipid peroxidation and cancer. Critical Reviews in Oncology/Hematology, Vol.15, No.2, (October 1993), pp.125-147, ISSN 1040-8428

Dianzani, M.U., Barrera, G. & Parola, M. (1999). 4-Hydroxy-2,3-nonenal as a signal for cell function and differentiation. Acta Biochimica Polonica, Vol.46, No.1, (1999), pp.61-75, ISSN 0001-527X

Dianzani, M.U. (2003). 4-hydroxynonenal from pathology to physiology. Molecular Aspects in Medicine, Vol.24, No.4-5, (August-October 2003), pp.263-272, ISSN 0098-2997

Douki, T., Odin, F., Caillat, S., Favier, A. & Cadet, J. (2004). Predominance of the 1,N2-propano 20-deoxyguanosine adduct among 4-hydroxy-2-nonenal-induced DNA lesions. Free Radical Biology & Medicine, Vol. 37, No.1, (July 2004), pp.62-70, ISSN 0891-5849

Ebert, M.N., Beyer-Sehlmeyer, G., Liegibel, U.M., Kautenburger, T., Becker, T.W. & Pool-Zobel B.L. (2001). Butyrate induces glutathione S-transferase in human colon cells and protects from genetic damage by 4-hydroxy-2-nonenal. Nutrition and Cancer, Vol.41, No.1-2, (2001), pp.156-164, ISSN 0163-5581

Eckl, P.M. (2003). Genotoxicity of HNE. Molecular Aspects in Medicine, Vol.24, No.4-5, (August-October 2003), pp.161-165, ISSN 0098-2997

Eder, E., Wacker, M., Lutz, U., Nair, J., Fang, X., Bartsch, H., Beland, F.A., Schlatter, J. & Lutz, W.K. (2006). Oxidative stress related DNA adducts in the liver of female rats fed with sunflower-, rapeseed-, olive- or coconut oil supplemented diets. Chemico-Biological Interactions, Vol.159, No.2, (February 2006), pp. 81-89, ISSN 0009-2797

Emerit, I., Khan, S.H. & Esterbauer H. (1991). Hydroxynonenal, a component of clastogenic factors? Free Radical Biology & Medicine, Vol.10, No.6, (1991), pp.371-377. ISSN 0891-5849

Englyst, H.N., Kingman, S.M. & Cummings, J.H. (1992). Classification and measurement of nutritionally important starch fractions. European Journal of Clinical Nutrition, Vol. Suppl 2:S, (October 1992), pp.33-50, ISSN 0954-3007

Esterbauer, H., Cheeseman, K.H., Dianzani, M.U., Poli, G. & Slater, T.F. (1982). Separation and characterization of the aldehydic products of lipid peroxidation stimulated by ADP-Fe2+ in rat liver microsomes. Biochemical Journal, Vol.208, No.1, (October 1982), pp.129-140, ISSN 0264-6021

Esterbauer, H., Schaur, R.J. & Zollner, H. (1991). Chemistry and biochemistry of 4-hydroxynonenal, malonaldehyde and related aldehydes. Free Radical Biology & Medicine, Vol.11, No.1, (1991), pp. 81-128, ISSN 0891-5849

Falletti, O. & Douki, T. (2008). Low glutathione level favors formation of DNA adducts to 4-hydroxy-2(E)-nonenal, a major lipid peroxidation product. Chemical Research in Toxicology, Vol.21, No.11, (November 2008), pp.2097-2105, ISSN 0893-228X

Favero, A., Parpinel, M. & Montella, M. (1999). Energy sources and risk of cancer of the breast and colon-rectum in Italy. Advances in Experimental Medicine and Biology, Vol.472, (1999), pp. 51-55, ISSN 0065-2598

Fazio, V.M., Barrera, G., Martinotti, S., Farace, M.G., Giglioni, B., Frati, L., Manzari, V. & Dianzani, M.U. (1992). 4-Hydroxynonenal, a product of cellular lipid peroxidation, which modulates c-myc and globin gene expression in K562 erythroleukemic cells. Cancer Research, Vol.52, No.18, (September 1992), pp.4866-4871. ISSN 0008-5472

Fearon, E.R. & Vogelstein, B. (1990). A genetic model for colorectal tumorigenesis. Cell, Vol.61, No.5, (June 1990), pp.759-767, ISSN 0092-8674

Feng, Z.H., Hu, W.W., Amin, S. & Tang, M.S. (2003). Mutational spectrum and genotoxicity of the major lipid peroxidation product, trans-4-hydroxy-2-nonenal, induced DNA adducts in nucleotide excision repairproficient and -deficient human cells. Biochemistry, Vol.42, No.25, (July 2003), pp.7848-7854, ISSN 0006-2960

Feng, Z., Hu, W. & Tang, M.S. (2004). Trans-4-hydroxy-2-nonenal inhibits nucleotide excision repair in human cells: a possible mechanism for lipid peroxidation-induced carcinogenesis. Proceedings of the National Academy of Sciences of the United States of America, Vol.101, No.23, (June 2004), pp.8598-8602, ISSN 0027-8424

Fernandes, P.H., Wang, H., Rizzo, C.J. & Lloyd, R.S. (2003). Site-specific mutagenicity of stereochemically defined 1,N-2-deoxyguanosine adducts of trans-4-hydroxynonenal in mammalian cells. Environmental and Molecular Mutagenesis, Vol.42, No.2, (2003), pp.68-74, ISSN 0893-6692

Forman, H.J., Fukuto, J.M., Miller, T., Zhang, H., Rinna, A. & Levy, S. (2008).The chemistry of cell signaling by reactive oxygen and nitrogen species and 4-hydroxynonenal. Archives of Biochemistry and Biophysics, Vol.477, No,2, (September 2008), pp.183-195, ISSN 0003-9861

Franceschi, S., La Vecchia, C., Russo, A., Favero, A., Negri, E., Conti, E., Montella, M., Filiberti, R., Amadori, D. & Decarli, A. (1998). Macronutrient intake and risk of colorectal cancer in Italy. International Journal of Cancer, Vol.76, No.3, (May 1998), pp.321-324, ISSN 0020-7136

Fukumoto, S., Yamauchi, N., Moriguchi, H., Hippo, Y., Watanabe, A., Shibahara, J., Taniguchi, H., Ishikawa, S., Ito, H., Yamamoto, S., Iwanari, H., Hironaka, M.,

Ishikawa, Y., Niki, T., Sohara, Y., Kodama, T., Nishimura, M., Fukayama, M., Dosaka-Akita, H. & Aburatani, H. (2005).

Overexpression of the aldo-keto reductase family protein AKR1B10 is highly correlated with smokers' non-small cell lung carcinomas. Clinical Cancer Research, Vol.11, No.5, (March 2005), pp.1776-1785, ISSN 1078-0432

Gasc, N., Taché, S., Rathahao, E., Bertrand-Michel, J., Roques, V. & Guéraud, F. (2007). 4-hydroxynonenal in foodstuffs: heme concentration, fatty acid composition and freeze-drying are determining factors. Redox Report, Vol.12, No.1, (2007), pp.40-44, ISSN 1351-0002

Gentile, F., Pizzimenti, S., Arcaro, A., Pettazzoni, P., Minelli, R., D'Angelo, D., Mamone, G., Ferranti, P., Toaldo, C., Cetrangolo, G., Formisano, S., Dianzani, M.U., Uchida, K., Dianzani, C. & Barrera, G. (2009). Exposure of HL-60 human leukaemic cells to 4-hydroxynonenal promotes the formation of adduct(s) with alpha-enolase devoid of plasminogen binding activity. Biochemical Journal, Vol.422, No.2, (August 2009), pp.285-294, ISSN 0264-6021

Glei, M., Hofmann, T., Küster, K., Hollmann, J., Lindhauer, M.G. & Pool-Zobel B.L. (2006) Both wheat (Triticum aestivum) bran arabinoxylans and gut flora-mediated fermentation products protect human colon cells from genotoxic activities of 4-hydroxynonenal and hydrogen peroxide. Journal of Agricultural and Food Chemistry, Vol.54, No.6, (March 2006), pp.2088-2095, ISSN 0021-8561

Glei, M., Schaeferhenrich, A., Claussen, U., Kuechler, A., Liehr, T., Weise, A., Marian, B., Sendt, W. & Pool-Zobel B.L. (2007). Comet fluorescence in situ hybridization analysis for oxidative stress-induced DNA damage in colon cancer relevant genes. Toxicological Sciences, Vol.96, No.2 (April 2007), pp. 279-284, ISSN 1096-6080

Glei, M., Hovhannisyan, G. & Pool-Zobel, B.L. (2009) Use of Comet-FISH in the study of DNA damage and repair: review. Mutation Research, Vol.681, No.1, (January-February 2009), pp.33-43, ISSN 0027-5107

Glinghammar, B., Venturi, M., Rowland, I.R. & Rafter, J.J. (1997). Shift from a dairy product-rich to a dairy product-free diet: influence on cytotoxicity and genotoxicity of fecal water — potential risk factors for colon cancer. American Journal of Clinical Nutrition, Vol.66, No.5, (November 1997), pp. 1277-1282, ISSN 0002-9165

Grune, T., Siems, W., Kowalewski, J., Zollner, H. & Esterbauer H. (1991). Identification of metabolic pathways of the lipid peroxidation product 4-hydroxynonenal by enterocytes of rat small intestine. Biochemical International, Vol.25, No.5, (December 1991), pp.963-971, ISSN 0158-5231

Gupta, A., Bhatt, M.L. & Misra, M.K. (2009). Lipid peroxidation and antioxidant status in head and neck squamous cell carcinoma patients. Oxidative Medicine and Cellular Longevity, Vol.2 , No.2, (April-June 2009), pp.68-72, ISSN 1942-0900

Hahn, G.M. & Li, G.C. (1982). Thermotolerance and heat shock proteins in mammalian cells. Radiation Research, Vol.92, No.3, (December 1982), pp.452-457, ISSN 0033-7587

Halliwell, B. (2007). Oxidative stress and cancer: have we moved forward? Biochemical Journal, Vol.401, No.1, (January 2007), pp.1-11, ISSN 0264-6021

Hartley, D.P, Ruth, J.A. & Petersen, D.R. (1995). The hepatocellular metabolism of 4-hydroxynonenal by alcohol dehydrogenase, aldehyde dehydrogenase, and glutathione S-transferas,. Archives of Biochemistry and Biophysics, Vol.316, No.1, (January 1995), pp.197-205, ISSN 0003-9861

Harvey, C.J., Thimmulappa, R.K., Singh, A., Blake, D.J., Ling, G., Wakabayashi, N., Fujii, J., Myers, A. & Biswal, S. (2009). Nrf2-regulated glutathione recycling independent of biosynthesis is critical for cell survival during oxidative stress. Free Radical Biology and Medicine, Vol.46, No.4, (Febraury 2009), pp.443-453, ISSN 0891-5849

Hassane, D.C., Guzman, M.L., Corbett, C., Li, X., Abboud, R., Young, F., Liesveld, J.L.,Carroll, M. & Jordan, C.T. (2008). Discovery of agents that eradicate leukemia stem cells using an in silico screen of public gene expression data. Blood, Vol.111, No.12, (June 2008), pp.5654-5662, ISSN 0006-4971

Howard, M.K., Burke, L.C., Mailhos, C., Pizzey, A., Gilbert, C.S., Lawson, W.D., Collins, M.K., Thomas, N.S. & Latchman, D.S. (1993). Cell cycle arrest of proliferating neuronal cells by serum deprivation can result in either apoptosis or differentiation. Journal of Neurochemistry, Vol.60, No.5, (May 1993), pp.1783-1791, ISSN 0022-3042

Hsu, I.C., Metcalf, R.A., Sun, T., Welsh, J.A., Wang, N.J. & Harris, C.C. (1991). Mutational hotspot in the p53 gene in human hepatocellular carcinomas. Nature, Vol.350, No.6317, (April 1991), pp.427-428, ISSN 0028-0836

Hu, W., Feng, Z., Eveleigh, J., Lyer, G., Pan, J., Amin, S., Chung, F.T. & Tang, M.S. (2002). The major lipid peroxidation product, trans-4-hydroxy-2-nonenal, preferentially forms DNA adducts at codon 249 of human p53 gene, a unique mutational hotspot in hepatocellular carcinoma. Carcinogenesis, Vol.23, No.11, (November 2008), pp.1781-1789, ISSN 0143-3334

Huang, Y.L., Sheu, J.Y. & Lin, T.H. (1999). Association between oxidative stress and changes of trace elements in patients with breast cancer. Clinical Biochemistry, Vol.32, No.2, (March 1999), pp.131-136, ISSN 0009-9120

Hussain, S.P., Raja, K., Amstad, P.A., Sawyer, M., Trudel, L.J., Wogan, G.N., Hofseth, L.J., Shields, P.G., Billiar, T.R., Trautwein, C., Hohler, T., Galle, P.R., Phillips, D.H., Markin, R., Marrogi, A.J. & Harris, C.C. (2000). Increased p53 mutation load in nontumorous human liver of wilson disease and hemochromatosis: oxyradical overload diseases. Proceedings of the National Academy of Sciences of the United States of America, Vol.97, No.23, (November 2000), pp.12770-12775, ISSN 0027-8424

Isom, A.L., Barnes, S., Wilson, L., Kirk, M., Coward, L. & Darley-Usmar, V. (2004). Modification of Cytochrome c by 4-hydroxy- 2-nonenal: evidence for histidine, lysine, and arginine-aldehyde adducts. Journal of The American Society for Mass Spectrometry, Vol.15, No.8, (August 2004), pp.1136-1147, ISSN 1044-0305

Jacobs, A.T. & Marnett, L.J. (2007). Heat shock factor 1 attenuates 4-Hydroxynonenal-mediated apoptosis: critical role for heat shock protein 70 induction and stabilization of Bcl-XL. The Journal of Biological Chemistry, Vol.282, No.46, (November 2007), pp.33412-33420, ISSN 0021-9258

Jacobs, A.T. & Marnett, L.J. (2009). HSF1-mediated BAG3 expression attenuates apoptosis in 4-hydroxynonenal-treated colon cancer cells via stabilization of anti-apoptotic Bcl-2 proteins. The Journal of Biological Chemistry, Vol.284, No.14, (April 2009), pp.9176-9183, ISSN 0021-9258

Ji, C., Amarnath, V., Pietenpol, J.A. & Marnett, L.J. (2001a). 4-hydroxynonenal induces apoptosis via caspase-3 activation and cytochrome c release. Chemical Research in Toxicology, Vol.14, No.8, (August 2001), pp.1090-1096, ISSN 0893-228X

Ji, C., Kozak, K.R. & Marnett, L.J. (2001b). IkappaB kinase, a molecular target for inhibition by 4-hydroxy-2-nonenal. The Journal of Biological Chemistry, Vol.276, No.21, (May 2001), pp.18223-18228, ISSN 0021-9258

Kakishita, H. & Hattori, Y. (2001).Vascular smooth muscle cell activation and growth by 4-hydroxynonenal. Life Sciences, Vol.69, No.6, (June 2001), pp.689-97, ISSN 0024-3205

Karihtala, P., Kauppila, S., Puistola, U. & Jukkola-Vuorinen, A. (2011). Divergent behaviour of oxidative stress markers 8-hydroxydeoxyguanosine (8-OHdG) and 4-hydroxy-2-nonenal (HNE) in breast carcinogenesis. Histopathology, Vol.58, No.6, (May 2011), pp.854-862, ISSN 1365-2559

Kaspar, J.W. & Jaiswal, A.K. (2010).An autoregulatory loop between Nrf2 and Cul3-Rbx1 controlstheir cellular abundance. The Journal of Biological Chemistry, Vol.285, No.28, (July 2010), pp.21349-21358, ISSN 0021-9258

Katic, J., Cemeli, E., Baumgartner, A., Laubenthal, J., Bassano, I., Stølevik, S.B., Granum, B., Namork, E., Nygaard, U.C., Løvik, M., van Leeuwen, D., Vande Loock, K., Anderson, D., Fucić, A. & Decordier, I. (2010). Evaluation of the genotoxicity of 10 selected dietary/environmental compounds with the in vitro micronucleus cytokinesis-block assay in an interlaboratory comparison. Food and Chemical Toxicology, Vol.48, No.10, (June 2010), pp.2612-2623, ISSN 0278-6915

Kawamura, I., Lacey, E., Inami, M., Nishigaki, F., Naoe, Y., Tsujimoto, S., Manda, T. & Goto, T. (1999). Ponalrestat, an aldose reductase inhibitor, inhibits cachexia syndrome in nude mice bearing human melanomas G361 and SEKI. Anticancer Research, Vol.19, No.5B, (September-October 1999), pp.4091-4097, ISSN 0250-7005

Kim, Y.S. & Milner, J.A. (2007). Dietary modulation of colon cancer risk. Journal of Nutrition, Vol.137, No.11 Suppl, (November 2007), pp.2576S-2579S, ISSN 0022-3166

Kim, T.H., Hur, E.G., Kang, S.J., Kim, J.A., Thapa, D., Lee, Y.M., Ku, S.K., Jung, Y. & Kwak, M.K. (2011). NRF2 blockade suppresses colon tumor angiogenesis by inhibiting hypoxia-induced activation of HIF-1α. Cancer Research, Vol.71, No.6, (March 2011), pp.2260-2275, ISSN 0008-5472

Knoll, N., Ruhe, C., Veeriah, S., Sauer, J., Glei, M., Gallagher, E.P. & Pool-Zobel, B.L. (2005). Genotoxicity of 4-hydroxy-2-nonenal in human colon tumor cells is associated with cellular levels of glutathione and the modulation of glutathione S-transferase A4 expression by butyrate. Toxicological Sciences, Vol.86, No.1, (July 2005), pp.27-35, ISSN 1096-6080

Kondo, S., Toyokuni, S., Iwasa, Y., Tanaka, T., Onodera, H., Hiai, H. & Imamura, M. (1999). Persistent oxidative stress in human colorectal carcinoma, but not in adenoma. Free Radical Biology and Medicine, Vol.27, No.3-4, (August 1999), pp.401-410, ISSN 0891-5849

Konner, J., O'Reilly, E. (2002). Pancreatic cancer; epidemiology, genetics, and approaches to screening. Oncology (Williston Park, N.Y.), Vol.16, No.12, (December 2002), pp.1631-1638, ISSN 0890-9091

Koster, J.F., Slee, R.G., Montfoort, A., Lang, J. & Esterbauer, H. (1986). Comparison of the inactivation of microsomal glucose-6-phosphatase by in situ lipid peroxidation-derived 4-hydroxynonenal and exogenous 4-hydroxynonenal. Free radical research communications, Vol.1, No.4, (1986), pp.273-287, ISSN 8755-0199

Kotrikadze, N., Alibegashvili, M., Zibzibadze, M., Abashidze, N., Chigogidze, T., Managadze, L. & Artsivadze, K. (2008). Activity and content of antioxidant enzymes in prostate tumors. Experimental Oncology, Vol.30, No.3, (September 2008), pp.244-247, ISSN 1812-9269

Kowalczyk, P., Ciesla, J.M., Komisarski, M., Kusmierek, J.T. & Tudek, B. (2004). Long-chain adducts of trans-4-hydroxy-2-nonenal to DNA bases cause recombination, base substitutions and frameshift mutations in M13 phage. Mutation Research, Vol.550, No.1-2, (June 2004), pp.33-48, ISSN 1383-5718

Lapre, J.A. & Vandermeer, R. (1992) Diet-induced increase of colonic bile acids stimulates lytic activity of fecal water and proliferation of colonic cells. Carcinogenesis, Vol.13, No.1, (January 1992), pp.41-44, ISSN 0143-3334

Laurent, A., Alary, J., Debrauwer, L. & Cravedi, J.P. (1999). Analysis in the rat of 4-hydroxynonenal metabolites excreted in bile: Evidence of enterohepatic circulation of these byproducts of lipid peroxidation. Chemical Research in Toxicology, Vol.12, No.10, (October 1999), pp.887-894, ISSN 0893-228X

Laurora, S., Tamagno, E., Briatore, F., Bardini, P., Pizzimenti, S., Toaldo, C., Reffo, P., Costelli, P., Dianzani, M.U., Danni, O. & Barrera, G. (2005). 4-Hydroxynonenal modulation of p53 family gene expression in the SK-N-BE neuroblastoma cell line. Free Radical Biology and Medicine, Vol.38, No.2, (January 2005), pp.215-25, ISSN 0891-5849

Leonarduzzi, G., Robbesyn, F. & Poli, G. Signaling kinases modulated by 4-hydroxynonenal. (2004). Free Radical Biology and Medicine, Vol.37, No.11, (December 2004), pp.1694-1702, ISSN 0891-5849

Lin, M.Y. & Yen, C.L. (1999). Antioxidative ability of lactic acid Bacteria. Journal of Agricultural and Food Chemistry, Vol.47, No.4, (April 1999), pp.1460-1466, ISSN 0021-8561

Looi, M.L., Mohd Dali, A.Z., Md Ali, S.A., Wan Ngah, W.Z. & Mohd Yusof, Y.A. (2008). Oxidative damage and antioxidant status in patients with cervical intraepithelial neoplasia and carcinoma of the cervix. European Journal of Cancer Prevention, Vol.17, No.6, (November 2008), pp.555-560, ISSN 0959-8278

Malhotra, D., Portales-Casamar, E., Singh, A., Srivastava, S., Arenillas, D., Happel, C., Shyr, C., Wakabayashi, N., Kensler, T.W., Wasserman, W.W. & Biswal, S. (2010). Global mapping of 22 binding sites for Nrf2 identifies novel targets in cell survival response through ChIP-Seq profiling and network analysis. Nucleic Acids Research, Vol.38, No.17, (September 2010), pp.5718-5734, ISSN 0305-1048

Martin, H.J. & Maser, E. (2009). Role of human aldo-keto-reductase AKR1B10 in the protection against toxic aldehydes. Chemico-Biological Interactions, Vol.178, No.1-3, (March 2009), pp.145-150, ISSN 0009-2797

Matsunaga, T., Yamane, Y., Iida, K., Endo, S., Banno, Y., El-Kabbani, O. & Hara, A. (2011). Involvement of the aldo-keto reductase, AKR1B10, in mitomycin-c resistance through reactive oxygen species-dependent mechanisms. Anti-Cancer Drugs, Vol.22, No.5, (June 2011), pp.402-408, ISSN 1473-5741

Min, K. & Ebeler, S.E. (2009).Quercetin inhibits hydrogen peroxide-induced DNA damage and enhances DNA repair in Caco-2 cells. Food and Chemical Toxicology. Vol.47, No.11, (November 2009), pp.2716-2722, ISSN 0278-6915

Moseley, P.L. (1997). Heat shock proteins and heat adaptation of the whole organism. Journal of Applied Physiology, Vol.83, No.5, (November 1997), pp.1413-1417, ISSN 8750-7587

Murawaki, Y., Tsuchiya, H., Kanbe, T., Harada, K., Yashima, K., Nozaka, K., Tanida, O., Kohno, M., Mukoyama, T., Nishimuki, E., Kojo, H., Matsura, T., Takahashi, K., Osaki, M., Ito, H., Yodoi, J., Murawaki, Y. & Shiota, G. (2008). Aberrant expression of selenoproteins in the progression of colorectal cancer. Cancer Letters, Vol.259, No.2, (Febraury 2008), pp.218-230, ISSN 0304-3835

Muzio, G., Canuto, R.A., Trombetta, A. & Maggiora, M. (2001). Inhibition of cytosolic class 3 aldehyde dehydrogenase by antisense oligonucleotides in rat hepatoma cells. Chemico-Biological Interactions, Vol.130-132, No.1-3, (January 2001), pp.219-225, ISSN 0009-2797

Nair, J., Gansauge, F., Beger, H., Dolara, P., Winde, G. & Bartsch, H. (2006). Increased etheno-DNA adducts in affected tissues of patients suffering from Crohn's disease, ulcerative colitis, and chronic pancreatitis. Antioxidants & Redox Signaling, Vol.8, No.5-6, (May-June 2006), pp.1003-1010, ISSN 1523-0864

Nishikawa, A., Furukawa, F., Kasahara, K., Ikezaki, S., Itoh, T., Suzuki, T., Uchida, K., Kurihara, M., Hayashi, M., Miyata, N. & Hirose, M. (2000). Trans-4-hydroxy-2-nonenal, an aldehydic lipid peroxidation product, lacks genotoxicity in lacI transgenic mice. Cancer Letters, Vol.148, No.1, (January 2000), pp.81-86, ISSN 0304-3835

Obtułowicz, T., Winczura, A., Speina, E., Swoboda, M., Janik, J., Janowska, B., Cieśla, J.M., Kowalczyk, P., Jawien, A., Gackowski, D., Banaszkiewicz, Z., Krasnodebski, I., Chaber, A., Olinski, R., Nair, J., Bartsch, H., Douki, T., Cadet, J. & Tudek, B. (2010). Aberrant repair of etheno-DNA adducts in leukocytes and colon tissue of colon cancer patients. Free Radical Biology and Medicine, Vol.49, No.6, (September 2010), pp.1064-1071, ISSN 0891-5849

Okamoto, K., Toyokuni, S., Uchida, K., Ogawa, O., Takenawa, J., Kakehi, Y., Kinoshita, H., Hattori-Nakakuki, Y., Hiai, H. & Yoshida, O. (1994). Formation of 8-hydroxy-2'-deoxyguanosine and 4-hydroxy-2-nonenal-modified proteins in human renal-cell carcinoma. International Journal of Cancer, Vol.58, No.6, (September 1994), pp.825-829, ISSN 1097-0215

Pan, J.S., Hong, M.Z. & Ren, J.L. (2009). Reactive oxygen species: a double-edged sword in oncogenesis. World Journal of Gastroenterology, Vol.15, No.14, (April 2009), pp.1702-1707, ISSN 1007-9327

Park, J.H. & Park, E. (2011). Influence of iron-overload on DNA damage and its repair in human leukocytes in vitro. Mutation Research, Vol.718, No.1-2, (January 2011), pp.56-61, ISSN 1383-5718

Parola, M., Bellomo, G., Robino, G., Barrera, G. & Dianzani, M.U. (1999). 4-Hydroxynonenal as a biological signal: molecular basis and pathophysiological implications.

Antioxidants & Redox Signaling, Vol.3, No.1, (Fall 1999), pp.255-284, ISSN 1523-0864

Pearson, J.R., Gill, C.I. & Rowland, I.R. (2004). Diet, fecal water, and colon cancer--development of a biomarker. Nutrition Reviews, Vol.67, No.9, (September 2009), pp.509-526, ISSN 0029-6643

Petersen, D.R. & Doorn, J.A. (2004). Reactions of 4-hydroxynonenal with proteins and cellular targets. Free Radical Biology and Medicine, Vol.37, No.7, (October 2004), pp.937-945, ISSN 0891-5849

Pettazzoni, P., Pizzimenti, S., Toaldo, C., Sotomayor, P., Tagliavacca, L., Liu, S., Wang, D., Minelli, R., Ellis, L., Atadja, P., Ciamporcero, E., Dianzani, M.U., Barrera, G. & Pili, R. (2011). Induction of cell cycle arrest and DNA damage by the HDAC inhibitor panobinostat (LBH589) and the lipid peroxidation end product 4-hydroxynonenal in prostate cancer cells. Free Radical Biology and Medicine, Vol.50, No.2, (January 2011), pp.313-322, ISSN 0891-5849

Pierre, F., Tache, S., Petit, C.R., Van der Meer, R. & Corpet, D.E. (2003) Meat and cancer: haemoglobin and haemin in a low-calcium diet promote colorectal carcinogenesis at the aberrant crypt stage in rats. Carcinogenesis, Vol.24, No.10, (October 2003), pp.1683-1690, ISSN 0143-3334

Pierre, F., Freeman, A., Tache, S., Van der Meer, R. & Corpet, D.E. (2004). Beef meat and blood sausage promote the formation of azoxymethaneinduced mucin-depleted foci and aberrant crypt foci in rat colons. Journal of Nutrition, Vol.134, No.10, (October 2004), pp.2711-2716, ISSN 0022-3166

Pierre, F., Peiro, G., Tache, S., Cross, A.J., Bingham, S.A., Gasc, N., Gottardi, G., Corpet, D.E. & Guéraud, F. (2006). Newmarker of colon cancer risk associated with heme intake: 1,4-dihydroxynonane mercapturic acid. Cancer Epidemiology, Biomarkers & Prevention, Vol.15, No.11, (November 2006), pp.2274-2279, ISSN 1538-7755

Pierre, F., Tache, S., Guéraud, F., Rerole, A.L., Jourdan, M.L. & Petit, C. (2007). Apc mutation induces resistance of colonic cells to lipoperoxide-triggered apoptosis induced by faecal water from haem-fed rats. Carcinogenesis, Vol.28, No.2, (February 2007), pp.321-327, ISSN 0143-3334

Pizzimenti, S., Briatore, F., Laurora, S., Toaldo, C., Maggio, M., De Grandi, M., Meaglia, L., Menegatti, E., Giglioni, B., Dianzani, M.U. & Barrera, G. (2006). 4-Hydroxynonenal inhibits telomerase activity and hTERT expression in human leukemic cell lines. Free Radical Biology and Medicine, Vol.40, No.9, (May 2006), pp.1578-1591, ISSN 0891-5849

Pizzimenti, S., Ferracin, M., Sabbioni, S., Toaldo, C., Pettazzoni, P., Dianzani, M.U., Negrini, M. & Barrera, G. (2009). MicroRNA expression changes during human leukemic HL-60 cell differentiation induced by 4-hydroxynonenal, a product of lipid peroxidation. Free Radical Biology and Medicine, Vol.46, No.2, (January 2009), pp.282-288, ISSN 0891-5849

Pizzimenti, S., Toaldo, C., Pettazzoni, P., Dianzani, M.U. & Barrera, G. (2010a). The "Two-Faced" Effects of Reactive Oxygen Species and the Lipid Peroxidation Product 4-Hydroxynonenal in the Hallmarks of Cancer. Cancers, Vol.2, No.2, (March 2010), pp.338-363, ISSN 1097-0142

Pizzimenti, S., Menegatti, E., Berardi, D., Toaldo, C., Pettazzoni, P., Minelli, R., Giglioni, B., Cerbone, A., Dianzani, M.U., Ferretti, C. & Barrera, G. (2010b). 4-hydroxynonenal, a lipid peroxidation product of dietary polyunsaturated fatty acids, has anticarcinogenic properties in colon carcinoma cell lines through the inhibition of telomerase activity. The Journal of Nutritional Biochemistry, Vol.21, No.9, (September 2010), pp.818-826, ISSN 0955-2863

Poli, G., Schaur, R.J., Siems, W.G. & Leonarduzzi, G. (2008). 4-hydroxynonenal: a membrane lipid oxidation product of medicinal interest. Medicinal Research Reviews, Vol.28, No.4, (July 2008), pp.569-631, ISSN 0198-6325

Poljak-Blazi, M., Kralj, M., Hadzija, M.P., Zarković, N., Zarković, K. & Waeg, G. (2000). Involvement of lipid peroxidation, oncogene expression and induction of apoptosis in the antitumorous activity of ferric-sorbitol-citrate. Cancer Biotherapy and Radiopharmaceuticals, Vol.15, No.3, (June 2000), pp.285-293, ISSN 1084-9785

Ramana, K.V., Tammali, R. & Srivastava, S.K. (2010). Inhibition of aldose reductase prevents growth factor-induced G1-S phase transition through the AKT/phosphoinositide 3-kinase/E2F-1 pathway in human colon cancer cells. Molecular Cancer Therapeutics, Vol.9, No.4, (April 2010), pp.813-824, ISSN 1535-7163

Reddy, B.S. (2002). Types and amount of dietary fat and colon cancer risk: Prevention by omega-3 fatty acid-rich diets. Environmental Health and Preventive Medicine, Vol.7, No.3, (July 2002), pp.95-102, ISSN 1342-078X

Reddy, N.M., Kleeberger, S.R., Yamamoto, M., Kensler, T.W., Scollick, C., Biswal, S. & Reddy, S.P. (2007). Genetic dissection of the Nrf2-dependent redox signaling-regulated transcriptional programs of cell proliferation and cytoprotection. Physiological Genomics, Vol.32, No.1, (December 2007), pp. 74-81, ISSN 1094-8341

Richter, M., Jurek, D., Wrba, F., Kaserer, K., Wurzer, G., Karner-Hanusch, J. & Marian B. (2002). Cells obtained from colorectal microadenomas mirror early premalignant growth patterns in vitro. European Journal of Cancer, Vol.38, No.14, (September 2002), pp. 1937-1945. ISSN 0959-8049

Rinaldi, M., Barrera, G., Aquino, A., Spinsanti, P., Pizzimenti, S., Farace, M.G., Dianzani, M.U. & Fazio, V.M. (2000). 4-Hydroxynonenal-induced MEL cell differentiation involves PKC activity translocation. Biochemical and Biophysical Research Communications, Vol.272, No.1, (May 2000), pp. 75-80, ISSN 0006-291X

Sarge, K.D., Murphy, S.P., & Morimoto, R.I. (1993). Activation of heat shock gene transcription by heat shock factor 1 involves oligomerization, acquisition of DNA-binding activity, and nuclear localization and can occur in the absence of stress. Molecular and Cellular Biology, Vol.13, No.3, (March 1993), pp. 1392-1407, ISSN 0270-7306

Satow, R., Shitashige, M., Kanai, Y., Takeshita, F., Ojima, H., Jigami, T., Honda, K., Kosuge, T., Ochiya, T., Hirohashi, S. & Yamada T. (2010). Combined functional genome survey of therapeutic targets for hepatocellular carcinoma. Clinical Cancer Research, Vol.16, No.9, (May 2010), pp. 2518-2528, ISSN 1078-0432

Saw, C.L. & Kong, A.N. (2011). Nuclear factor-erythroid 2-related factor 2 as a chemopreventive target in colorectal cancer. Expert Opinion on Therapeutic Targets, Vol.15, No.3, (March 2011), pp. 281-295, ISSN 1472-8222

Sawa,T., Akaike,T., Kida, K., Fukushima,Y., Takagi, K., & Maeda, H. (1998). Lipid peroxyl radicals from oxidized oils and heme-iron: implication of a high-fat diet in colon carcinogenesis. Cancer Epidemiology, Biomarkers & Prevention, Vol.7, No.11, (November 1998), pp. 1007–1012, ISSN 1055-9965

Sayre, L.M., Arora, P.K., Iyer, R.S. & Salomon, R.G. (1993). Pyrrole formation from 4-hydroxynonenal and primary amines. Chemical Research in Toxicology , Vol.6, No.1, (January-February 1993), pp. 19-22, ISSN 0893-228X

Schaeferhenrich, A., Beyer-Sehlmeyer, G., Festag, G., Kuechler, A., Haag, N., Weise, A., Liehr, T., Claussen, U., Marian, B., Sendt, W., Scheele, J. & Pool-Zobel B.L. (2003). Human adenoma cells are highly susceptible to the genotoxic action of 4-hydroxy-2-nonenal. Mutation Research - Fundamental and Molecular Mechanisms of Mutagenesis, Vol.526, No.1-2, (May 2003), pp. 19-32, ISSN: 0027-5107

Scharlau, D., Borowicki, A., Habermann, N., Hofmann, T., Klenow, S., Miene, C., Munjal, U., Stein, K. & Glei M. (2009). Mechanisms of primary cancer prevention by butyrate and other products formed during gut flora-mediated fermentation of dietary fibre. Mutatation Research - Reviews, Vol.682, No.1, (July-August 2009), pp. 39-53, ISSN 1383-5742

Scharmach, E., Hessel, S., Niemann, B. & Lampen, A. (2009). Glutathione S-transferase expression and isoenzyme composition during cell differentiation of Caco-2 cells. Toxicology, Vol.265, No.3, (November 2009), pp. 122-126, ISSN 0300-483X

Schaur, R.J. (2003). Basic aspects of the biochemical reactivity of 4-hydroxynonenal. Molecular Aspects of Medicine, Vol.24, No. 4-5, (August-October 2003), pp. 149-59, ISSN: 0098-2997

Scheppach, W., Bingham, S., Boutron-Ruault, M., Verdier, M. G. D., Moreno, V., Nagengast, F., Reifen, R., Riboli, E., Seitz, H. &Wahrendorf, J. (1999). WHO consensus statement on the role of nutrition in colorectal cancer. European Journal of Cancer Prevention, Vol.8, No.1, (February 1999), pp. 57–62, ISSN 0959-8278

Schmid, K., Nair, J., Winde, G., Velic, I., & Bartsch, H. (2000). Increased levels of promutagenic etheno-DNA adducts in colonic polyps of FAP patients. International Journal of Cancer , Vol.87, No.1, (July 2000), pp. 1-4, ISSN 0020-7136

Seitz, H.K., Egerer, G., Oneta, C., Krämer, S., Sieg, A., Klee, F. & Simanowski, U.A. (1996). Alcohol dehydrogenase in the human colon and rectum. Digestion, Vol.57, No.2, pp. 105-108, ISSN 0012-2823

Selga, E., Noé, V., & Ciudad, C.J. (2008). Transcriptional regulation of aldo-keto reductase 1C1 in HT29 human colon cancer cells resistant to methotrexate: role in the cell cycle and apoptosis. Biochemical Pharmacology,. Vol.75, No.2, (January 2008), pp. 414–426, ISSN 0006-2952

Semlitsch, T., Tillian, H.M., Zarkovic, N., Borovic, S., Purtscher, M., Hohenwarter, O., & Schaur, R.J. (2002). Differential influence of the lipid peroxidation product 4-hydroxynonenal on the growth of human lymphatic leukaemia cells and human peripheral blood lymphocytes. Anticancer Research, Vol.22, No.3, (May-June 2002), pp. 1689-1697, ISSN 0250-7005

Sesink, A.L.A., Termont, D.S.M.L., Kleibeuker, J.H. & Vandermeer, R. (1999). Red meat and colon cancer: the cytotoxic and hyperproliferative effects of dietary heme. Cancer Research, Vol.59, No.22, (November 1999), pp. 5704–5709, ISSN 0008-5472

Sharma, R., Sharma, A., Yang, Y., Awasthi, S., Singhal, S.S., Zimniak, P. & Awasthi, Y.C. (2002). Functional reconstitution of Ral-binding GTPase activating protein, RLIP76, in proteoliposomes catalyzing ATP-dependent transport of glutathione conjugate of 4-hydroxynonenal. Acta Biochimica Polonica, Vol.49, No.3, pp. 693-701, ISSN 0001-527X

Siems, W. & Grune, T. (2003). Intracellular metabolism of 4-hydroxynonenal. Molecular Aspects of Medicine, Vol.24, No.4-5, (August-October 2003), pp. 167- 175, ISSN: 0098-2997

Singhal, S.S., Singhal, J., Yadav, S., Dwivedi, S., Boor, P.J., Awasthi, Y.C., & Awasthi, S. (2007). Regression of lung and colon cancer xenografts by depleting or inhibiting RLIP76 (Ral-binding protein 1). Cancer Research, Vol.67, No. 9, (May 2007), pp. 4382-4389, ISSN 0008-5472

Skrzydlewska, E., Sulkowski, S., Koda, M., Zalewski, B., Kanczuga-Koda, L. & Sulkowska, M. (2005). Lipid peroxidation and antioxidant status in colorectal cancer. World Journal of Gastroenterology, Vol.11, No.3, pp. 403-406, ISSN 1007-9327

Soong, R., Powell, B., Elsaleh, H., Gnanasampanthan, G., Smith, D.R., Goh, H.S., Joseph, D. & Iacopetta, B. (2000). Prognostic significance of TP53 gene mutation in 995 cases of colorectal carcinoma. Influence of tumour site, stage, adjuvant chemotherapy and type of mutation. European Journal of Cancer, Vol. 36, No.16, (October 2000), pp. 2053-2060, ISSN 0959-8049

Soussi, T., Dehouche, K. & Beroud, C. (2000). p53 website and analysis of p53 gene mutations in human cancer: forging a link between epidemiology and carcinogenesis. Human Mutation, Vol.15, No.1, pp. 105-113, ISSN: 1059-7794

Soussi, T. & Beroud, C. (2003). Significance of p53 mutations in human cancer: a critical analysis of mutations at CpG dinucleotides. Human Mutation, Vol.21, No3, pp. 192-200, ISSN: 1059-7794

Stagos, D., Zhou, H., Ross, D. & Vasiliou, V. (2009). 4-HNE inhibits tube formation and up-regulates chondromodulin-I in human endothelial cells. Biochemical and Biophysical Research Communications, Vol.379, No.3, (February 2009), pp. 654-658, ISSN 0006-291X

Sunjic, S.B., Cipak, A., Rabuzin, F., Wildburger, R. & Zarkovic, N. (2005). The influence of 4-hydroxy-2-nonenal on proliferation, differentiation and apoptosis of human osteosarcoma cells. Biofactors, Vol. 24, No.1-4, pp. 141-148, ISSN 1872-8081

Surh, J., & Kwon, H. (2005). Estimation of daily exposure to 4-hydroxy-2-alkenals in Korean foods containing n-3 and n-6 polyunsaturated fatty acids. Food Additives & Contaminants., Vol.22, No.8, (August 2005), pp. 701-708, ISSN 1944-0049

Surh, J., Lee, S. & Kwon, H. (2007). 4-Hydroxy-2-alkenals in polyunsaturated fatty acids-fortified infant formulas and other commercial food products. Food Additives & Contaminants, Vol. 24, No.11, (November 2007), pp. 1209-1218, ISSN 1944-0049

Surh, J., Lee, B.Y. & Kwon, H. (2010). Influence of Fatty Acids Compositions and Manufacturing Type on the Formation of 4-Hydroxy-2-alkenals in Food Lipids. Food Science and Biotechnology, Vol.19, No.2, (April 2010), pp.297-303, ISSN 1226-7708

Tammali, R., Ramana, K.V., Singhal, S.S., Awasthi, S., & Srivastava, S.K. (2006). Aldose reductase regulates growth factor-induced cyclooxygenase-2 expression and prostaglandin E2 production in human colon cancer cells. Cancer Research, Vol.66, No.19, (October 2006), pp. 9705-9713, ISSN 0008-5472

Tammali, R., Srivastava, S.K. & Ramana, K.V. (2011). Targeting aldose reductase for the treatment of cancer. Current Cancer Drug Targets, Vol.11, No.5, (June 2011), pp. 560-571, ISSN 1568-0096

Thimmulappa, R.K., Mai, K.H., Srisuma, S., Kensler, T.W., Yamamoto, M. & Biswal, S. (2002). Identification of Nrf2-regulated genes induced by the chemopreventive agent sulforaphane by oligonucleotide microarray. Cancer Research, Vol.62, No.18, (September 2002), pp. 5196-5203, ISSN 0008-5472

Tice, R.P., Andrews, P.W., Hirai, O. & Singh, N.P. (1991). The single cell gel (SCG) assay: an electrophoretic technique for the detection of DNA damage in individual cells. Advances in Experimental Medicine and Biology, Vol. 283, pp. 157-164, ISSN 0065-2598

Uchida, K. (2003). 4-Hydroxy-2-nonenal: a product and mediator of oxidative stress. Progress in lipid research, Vol.42, No.4, (July 2003), pp. 318-343, ISSN 0163-7827

Vander Jagt, D.L., Kolb, N.S., Vander Jagt, T.J., Chino, J., Martinez, F.J., Hunsaker, L.A. & Royer, R.E. (1995). Substrate specificity of human aldose reductase: Identification of 4-hydroxynonenal as an endogenous substrate. Biochimica et Biophysica Acta, Vol.1249, No.2, (June 1995), pp. 117-126, ISSN 0006-3002

Vatsyayan, R., Lelsani, P.C., Awasthi, S., & Singhal, S.S. (2010). RLIP76: a versatile transporter and an emerging target for cancer therapy. Biochemical Pharmacology, Vol.79, No.12, (June 2010), pp. 1699-1705, ISSN 0006-2952

Veitch, Z.W., Guo, B., Hembruff, S.L., Bewick, A.J., Heibein, A.D., Eng, J., Cull, S., Maclean, D.A., & Parissenti, A.M. (2009). Induction of 1C aldoketoreductases and other drug dose-dependent genes upon acquisition of anthracycline resistance. Pharmacogenetics and Genomics, Vol.19, No.6, (June 2009), pp. 477-488, ISSN 1744-6872

Vizio, B., Poli, G., Chiarpotto, E. & Biasi, F. (2005). 4-hydroxynonenal and TGF-beta1 concur in inducing antiproliferative effects on the CaCo-2 human colon adenocarcinoma cell line. Biofactors., Vol.24, No.1-4, pp. 237-246, ISSN 1872-8081

Vogelstein, B., Fearon, E.R., Hamilton, S.R., Kern, S.E., Preisinger, A.C., Leppert, M., Nakamura, Y., White, R., Smits, A.M. & Bos, J.L. (1988). Genetic alterations during colorectal tumor development. The New England Journal of Medicine, Vol.319, No.9, (September 1988), pp. 525-532, ISSN 0028-4793

Wacker, M., Wanek, P., Eder, E., Hylla, S., Gostner, A. & Scheppach, W. (2002). Effect of enzyme-resistant starch on formation of 1,N(2)-propanodeoxyguanosine adducts of trans-4-hydroxy-2-nonenal and cell proliferation in the colonic mucosa of healthy volunteers. Cancer Epidemiology, Biomarkers & Prevention, Vol.11, No.9, (September 2002), pp. 915-920, ISSN 1055-9965

Wacker, M., Wanek, P. & Eder, E. (2001). Detection of 1,N2-propanodeoxyguanosine adducts of trans-4-hydroxy-2-nonenal after gavage of trans-4-hydroxy-2-nonenal or induction of lipid peroxidation with carbon tetrachloride in F344 rats. Chemico-Biological Interactions, Vol.137, No.3, (September 2001), pp. 269-283, ISSN 0009-2797

Wang, J. & Yi, J. (2008). Cancer cell killing via ROS: to increase or decrease, that is the question. Cancer Biology and Therapy, Vol.7, No.12, (December 2008), pp. 1875-1884, ISSN 1538-4047

West, J.D., Ji, C., Duncan, S.T., Amarnath, V., Schneider, C., Rizzo, C.J., Brash, A.R. & Marnett L.J. (2004). Induction of apoptosis in colorectal carcinoma cells treated with 4-hydroxy-2-nonenal and structurally related aldehydic products of lipid peroxidation. Chemical Research in Toxicology, Vol. 17, No. 4, (April 2004), pp. 453-462, ISSN 0893-228X

West, J.D. & Marnett, L.J. (2005). Alterations in gene expression induced by the lipid peroxidation product, 4-hydroxy-2-nonenal. Chemical Research in Toxicology, Vol.18, No.11, (November 2001), pp. 1642-1653, ISSN 0893-228X

Winter, C.K., Segall. H.J. & Haddon.W.F. (1986). Formation of cyclic adducts of deoxyguanosine with the aldehydes trans-4-hydroxy-2-hexenal and trans-4-hydroxy-2-nonenal in vitro. Cancer Research, Vol.46, No.11, (November 1986), pp. 5682-5686, ISSN 0008-5472

Yadav, U.C., Ramana, K.V., Awasthi, Y.C. & Srivastava, S.K. (2008). Glutathione level regulates HNE-induced genotoxicity in human erythroleukemia cells. Toxicology and Applied Pharmacology, Vol.227, No.2, (March 2008), pp. 257-264, ISSN 0041-008X

Yan, R., Zu, X., Ma, J., Liu, Z., Adeyanju, M. & Cao, D. (2007). Aldo-keto reductase family 1B10 gene silencing results in growth inhibition of colorectal cancer cells: implication for cancer intervention. International Journal of Cancer, Vol.121, No.10, (November 2007), pp. 2301–2306, ISSN 0020-7136

Yang, Y., Sharma, A., Sharma, R., Patrick, B., Singhal, S.S., Zimniak, P., Awasthi, S. & Awasthi, Y.C. (2003). Cells preconditioned with mild, transient UVA irradiation acquire resistance to oxidative stress and UVA-induced apoptosis: role of 4-hydroxynonenal in UVA mediated signalling for apoptosis. The Journal of Biological Chemistry, Vol.278, No.42, (October 2003), pp. 41380–41388, ISSN 0021-9258

Yin, S.J., Liao, C.S., Lee, Y.C., Wu, C.W. & Jao, S.W. (1994).Genetic polymorphism and activities of human colon alcohol and aldehyde dehydrogenases: no gender and age differences. Alcoholism, clinical and experimental research, Vol.18, No.5, (October1994), pp. 1256-1260, ISSN 1530-0277

Yoshitake, H., Takahashi, M., Ishikawa, H., Nojima, M., Iwanari, H., Watanabe, A., Aburatani, H., Yoshida, K., Ishi, K., Takamori, K., Ogawa, H., Hamakubo, T., Kodama, T. & Araki, Y. (2007). Aldo-keto reductase family 1, member B10 in uterine carcinomas: a potential risk factor of recurrence after surgical therapy in cervical cancer. International Journal of Gynecological Cancer. Vol.17, No.6, (November-December 2007), pp. 1300–1306, ISSN 1048-891X

Zanetti, D., Poli, G., Vizio, B., Zingaro, B., Chiarpotto, E. & Biasi, F. (2003). 4-hydroxynonenal and transforming growth factor-beta1 expression in colon cancer. Molecular Aspects of Medicine, Vol.24, No.4-5, (August-October 2003), pp. 273-280, ISSN 0098-2997

Zarkovic, K., Juric, G., Waeg, G., Kolenc, D. & Zarkovic, N. (2005). Immunohistochemical
    appearance of HNE-protein conjugates in human astrocytomas. Biofactors, Vol.24,
    No.1-4, pp. 33-40, ISSN 1872-8081

Zeindl-Eberhart, E., Jungblut, P.R., Otto, A., Kerler, R., Rabes, H.M. (1997). Further
    characterization of a rat hepatomaderived aldose-reductase-like protein-organ
    distribution and modulation in vitro. European Journal of Biochemistry, Vol.247,
    No.3, (August 1997), pp. 792–800, ISSN 0014-2956

Zhi-Hua, C. & Etsuo, N. (2006). 4-Hydroxynonenal (4-HNE) has been widely accepted as an
    inducer of oxidative stress. Is this the whole truth about it or can 4-HNE also exert
    protective effects? IUBMB Life, Vol.58, No.5-6, (May-june 2006), pp. 372–373, ISSN
    1521-6543

6

Human Tip60 (NuA4) Complex and Cancer

Hiroshi Y. Yamada
University of Oklahoma Health Sciences Center (OUHSC),
USA

1. Introduction

Recent publications implicate human Tip60 (NuA4) complex in colorectal and other cancers. Our lab and others discovered deregulations in the components of human Tip60 (NuA4) complex in advanced colon cancers, and the functional significance and the potential as a therapeutic target, has been investigated. Human Tip60 (NuA4) complex likely represents a fusion form of yeast NuA4 and SWR1 complexes, and the functions seem to be evolutionarily preserved. This notion has greatly contributed in understanding functions of human Tip60 (NuA4) complex. The Tip60 (NuA4) complex is a multiprotein complex with at least 16 subunits. It is thought to function in at least two ways; (a) as a chromatin remodeling factor, it controls chromatin structure and transcription through its Histone Acetyl Transferase (HAT) activity, and (b) it controls activities of other non-histone proteins, such as metabolic enzymes, through protein acetylation. Through the enzymatic activity and other interactions, Tip60 (NuA4) complex is involved in wide variety of cellular functions, including transcriptional activation, DNA repair, cell cycle progression, chromosome stability, stem cell maintenance and differentiation, and cell migration and invasion. This review will discuss functions of Tip60 (NuA4) complex, consequences of the defect in the subunit, its connection to human cancer, and its potential as a therapeutic target in clinic.

2. A chromatin remodeling factor with Histone Acetyl Transferase (HAT) activity, Tip60 (NuA4) complex

Readout of genomic information is regulated through multiple mechanisms. A major part of the regulatory role is played by chromatin remodeling factors; enzyme complexes that modify DNA or chromatin proteins. The modifications change local chromatin structure, thus change accessibility of transcription factors and availability of genomic information (Kouzarides 2007). In the case of Histones and major chromatin proteins, protein modifications occur in a variety of ways, including phosphorylation, acetylation, methylation, ubiquitylation, and ADP-ribosylation. These different types of modifications may functionally influence each other, creating possibilities of multiple layers of regulations, which have been referred as the "Histone code". Although the possibility has been pointed out, the multiple layers of regulations (the "Histone code") have not fully been deciphered yet.

Among the modifications, acetylation has a defined role: To change surface charge distribution of the target protein and change accessibility to DNA and/or to other proteins.

The histones are acetylated and deacetylated on lysine residues in the N-terminal tail. These acetylation/deacetylation reactions are catalyzed by two groups of enzymes, Histone Acetyl Transferase (HAT) and Histone DeACetylase (HDAC), respectively. Histones are not the only target for these enzymes. HATs and HDACs can acetylate/deacetylate non-histone proteins as well.

In this review, we will focus on a human multisubunit and multifunctional HAT complex, Tip60 (NuA4) (Nucleosomal Acetyltransferase of H4) complex. We will describe the complex and known functions from the standpoint of each subunit and discuss new insights relevant to cancer, especially in colon cancer. We will also discuss the possibility of targeting Tip60 (NuA4) subunits for therapeutic purposes.

3. Human Tip60 (NuA4) complex; Its components and functions

Human Tip60 (NuA4) complex is a multiprotein complex with at least 16 subunits, and it has HAT activity (Cai et al., 2003, Doyon et al., 2004). The subunit composition suggests that Human Tip60 (NuA4) complex is a fusion form of two yeast HAT complexes, NuA4 and SWR (Allard et al, 1999) (Table 1). As seen in Table1, these two yeast HAT complexes share four components (Eaf2, Arp4, Act1 and Yaf9), together they correspond to all human subunits. Supporting the fusion theory, the expression of a chimeric Eaf1-Swr1 protein provides a scaffold for the complex assembly and recreates a single human-like complex in yeast cells (Auger et al, 2008).

Historically speaking, yeast has been a superior model system to investigate functions of molecular and cellular machineries with its genetical tractability, its ease of experimental manipulations, feasibility for biochemistry and its short life cycle and time span for experiments. Several cellular functions of NuA4 and SWR complex were identified directly with yeast studies and later confirmed in human cultured cells. The known acetylation targets of yeast NuA4 in vivo are histone H4 (Mitchell et al., 2008) and the histone H2A variant Htz1 (Babiarz et al., 2006, Keogh et al., 2006, Mizuguchi et al., 2004). Yeast NuA4 complex also targets non-histone proteins, which are equally important to evaluate cellular functions of NuA4 complex. With yeast protein array, Lin et al. (2009) screened the target proteins. Among 5800 proteins screened for in vitro acetylation with NuA4 complex, 91 candidates were identified, 20 were selected for validation, and 13 were validated. The functions of validated proteins encompass metabolism, transcription, cell cycle, RNA processing, and stress response. The authors focused on Pck1, a key metabolic enzyme that regulates gluconeogenesis, and showed that Pck1 activity and glucose secretion is regulated through NuA4-mediated acetylation in yeast and in human hepatocellular carcinoma cells HepG2. Thus NuA4 is implicated in metabolism and energy generation through its non-histone targets.

The human TIP60 complex has at least three interrelated enzymatic activities: histone H4/H2A acetyltransferase, ATP-dependent H2AZ-H2B histone dimer exchange, and DNA helicase (Auger et al., 2008). Only a limited number of non-histone targets, including human Pck1, has been identified so far (Liu et al., 2009).

Knockdown and/or mutational studies have been performed to identify functions of the subunits of human Tip60 (NuA4) complex. The studies implicate following biological events to Tip60 (NuA4) complex, directly or indirectly.

- DNA repair
- Transcriptional regulation
- Chromatin structure alteration
- Interaction and/or regulation with factors relevant to tumorigenesis (e.g. c-myc, E1A, E2F1, p53, STAT3, NF-kappaB)
- Cell migration and invasion
- Mitosis
- Genomic instability
- Stem cell maintenance and differentiation

In addition, RNAi-based screening with nematode *C. elegans* implicated Tip60 (NuA4) complex in attenuation of *ras*-signaling involving development of vulva in the model. The *C. elegans* MLL (Mixed Lineage Leukaemia (MLL)) complex-like complex cooperates with the TIP60 (NuA4) complex to regulate the expression of a novel *ras*-signaling attenuator, AJM-1 (Fischer et al., 2010).

4. Functions of each subunit

In the following section we will discuss each of the subunits.

4.1 TRRAP/Tra1/*

(human protein/yeast protein in NuA4 complex/ yeast protein in Swr complex. Asterisk * if not applicable)

Human TRRAP (transformation/transcription domain-associated protein) has a FATC (FRAP, ATM, TRRAP C-terminal) domain and a kinase domain, and belongs to ATM/PI3K family. However, TRRAP does not appear to possess kinase activity, because the kinase domain in TRRAP lacks the conserved amino acids required for ATP binding and catalytic activity for phosphate transfer. For that reason, it is speculated that TRRAP has evolved as a specialized PIKK member to serve as an adaptor/scaffold for protein–protein interaction and multiprotein assemblies or as a platform for recruitment of different regulatory factors and complexes to chromatin (Murr et al 2007). The FATC domain in the C-terminus likely affects the protein stability in an oxidation/redox-dependent manner (Dames et al., 2005). TRRAP is a common component of many HAT complexes (e.g. SAGA, PCAF and Tip60 (NuA4) complex). As such, targeting TRRAP will influence a broader range of biological events and pathways than targeting more specialized components in Tip60 (NuA4) complex.

TRRAP is one of the frequently mutated genes in melanoma. TRRAP harbored a recurrent mutation that clustered in one position (p. Ser722Phe) in 6 out of 167 affected individuals (~4%), although the effects of the mutation on the protein function is unclear (Wei et al., 2011). Expression profiling revealed that TRRAP is frequently both amplified and overexpressed in Pancreatic Ductal AdenoCarcinoma (PDAC), and the overexpression is associated with poor prognosis (Bashyam et al., 2005, Loukopoulos et al,2007). In brain tumor-initiating cell, knockdown of TRRAP significantly increased differentiation and decreased cell cycle progression, leading to overall inhibition of tumor formation. The result indicates a critical role for TRRAP in maintaining a tumorigenic, stem cell-like state (Wurdak et al., 2010). TRRAP is shown to regulate a major player in colon cancer, beta-catenin. TRRAP interacts with Skp1/SCF and mediates its recruitment to beta-catenin target promoter in chromatin. TRRAP deletion leads to a reduced level of beta-catenin

Human Tip60 (NuA4) complex subunits	Yeast NuA4 complex subunits	Yeast SWR1 complex subunits	Protein domain(s)	Yeast null phenotype	Inhibition (e.g. siRNA) in cultured cells	Knockout in mouse	Relationship to cancer (See text)
TRRAP (transformation/transcription domain-associated protein)	Tra1		ATM/PI3K family kinase, FATC domain	inviable	Mitotic defect with Mad1 and Mad2 misregulation	Embryonic lethal	High expression in mouse leukemogenic cell lines; co-factor for c-myc oncogenic transformation
hDomino p400/EP400	Eaf1 (HAS/SANT)	Swr1 (HAS/SWI2)	SWI2/SNF2 related, ATPase, Trico Peptide Repeat (TPR) domain	Viable; decreased growth, genome instability		Embryonic lethal	
Brd8 (Bromodomain 8)		Bdf1	Bromodomain	Viable; decreased growth, multidrug sensitivity, enhanced salt sensitivity by mitochondrial dysfunction	Enhanced spindle poison sensitivity	ND	Protein accumulated in rat colon cancer and human colon cancer cell lines
EPC1/EPC-like (Enhancer of Polycomb homolog)	Epl1			inviable			Locates in chromosomal breaking point in ATLL
Tip60 (TAT interactive protein)	Esa1			inviable		Embryonic lethal	Prostate cancer promotion; tumor suppressor candidate/ expression reduced in cancers
DMAP1 (DNA methyltransferase 1-associated protein 1)	Eaf2/swc4	Eaf2/swc4	a SWI3-ADA2-N-CoR-TF IIIB (SANT) domain	Inviable; G2/M arrest		lethal during preimplantation	Binds to DNA methyltransferase 1 (DNMT1), which is progressively upregulated in colon adenoma-carcinoma sequence
ING3 (Inhibitor of Growth Protein 3)	Yng2		PHD finger	Viable			Tumor suppressor candidate; Overexpression inhibits cell growth and promote apoptosis; allelic loss detected in head and neck cancers
YL-1 (Vacuolar protein sorting-associated protein 72 homolog)		Vps72		Viable; decreased fitness			
RuvBL1		Rvb1/Tip49A		inviable			Binds to beta-catenin
RuvBL2		Rvb2/Tip49B		inviable			
BAF53a	Arp4	Arp4	Actin-related	inviable			
Actin	Act1	Act1	actin	inviable			
MRG15	Eaf3			Viable; increased lifespan			
GAS41	Yaf9	Yaf9		Viable; Enhanced spindle poison sensitivity, multidrug sensitivity, decreased chromosome maintenance			
?	Eaf5			Viable			
MRGBP	Eaf7			Viable; decreased fitness			Overexpressed in human colon cancer
hEaf6	Eaf6			Viable			

Table 1. Subunits of Human Tip60 (NuA4); (columns from left) subunits of the yeast counterpart complexes NuA4 and SWR1; notable protein domains; yeast mutant phenotypes that implicate functions; inhibition in cultured cells and mice; and information relevant to cancer. ND: Not Determined. The order listed is following the size of the protein. Larger subunit is shown on top.

ubiquitination, lower degradation rate and accumulation of beta-catenin protein. Furthermore, recruitment of Skp1 to chromatin and ubiquitination of chromatin-bound beta-catenin are abolished upon TRRAP knock-down, leading to an abnormal retention of beta-catenin at the chromatin and concomitant hyperactivation of the canonical Wnt pathway (Finkbeiner et al., 2008). TRRAP is also involved in DNA damage repair. TRRAP depletion impairs both DNA-damage-induced histone H4 hyperacetylation and accumulation of repair molecules at sites of Double Strand Breaks (DSBs), resulting in defective homologous recombination (HR) repair, albeit with the presence of a functional ATM-dependent DNA-damage signaling cascade (Murr et al., 2006). TRRAP regulates expressions of many cancer-relevant genes, including mitotic checkpoint proteins Mad1 and Mad2 (Li et al., 2004) and mdm2 (Ard et al., 2002).

Consistent with the loss of mitotic checkpoint proteins essential for cellular survival, null mutation of Trrap (mouse homolog of human TRRAP) results in peri-implantation lethality due to a blocked proliferation of blastocysts. Loss of Trrap blocks cell proliferation because of an aberrant mitotic exit accompanied by cytokinesis failure and endoreduplication. Trrap-deficient cells failed to sustain mitotic arrest despite chromosome missegregation and disrupted spindles, and display compromised cdk1 activity. Thus, Trrap is essential for early development and required for the mitotic checkpoint, presumably through expression control of mad1 and mad2, and normal cell cycle progression (Herceg et al., 2001).

In yeast, deletion of TRRAP homolog Tra1 is also lethal. Tra1 is identified as a component of multiple yeast transcription regulator complexes, Ada-Spt, SAGA and NuA4 (Saleh et al., 1998; Grant et al., 1998; Allard et al., 1999). Tra1 directly interacts with the acidic transcriptional activators Gcn4, Hap4, and Gal4 (Brown et al., 2001). Tra1 is required for both the acetylation of Histone H4 surrounding the promoters and the transcription of Gcn4-dependent genes, suggesting that Tra1 may mediate the recruitment of NuA4 to certain promoters.

4.2 hDomino p400/Eaf1/Swr1

hDomino (also known as p400, EP400, E1A binding protein p400) is a DEXH-box class of RNA-dependent ATPase subunit in Tip60 (NuA4) complex, and can destabilize histone-DNA interactions in reconstituted nucleosomes in an ATP-dependent manner. hDomino also contains a highly conserved SANT (SWI3–ADA2–NcoR–TFIIIB) domain, a histone tail-binding module (Boyer et al. 2004). The protein is related to yeast Swi2/Snf2 (SWItch 2/Sucrose NonFermentable 2) and to Domino in fruit fly Drosophila. Drosophila Domino was isolated in search of immune system mutants devoid of circulating larval hemocytes from P-element insertion-based mutant library. Because of the very striking lymph gland phenotype that results in mutant larvae with two black dots visible on the anterior half, the authors named the mutation domino (Braun et al., 1997).

Through the Swi2/Snf2 domain, hDomino binds to adenovirus oncoprotein E1A. Mutational loss of E1A binding results in the loss of transformation, indicating that the binding plays a critical role in cellular transformation. hDomino also binds to c-myc with different protein components (Fuchs et al., 2001). In most human colorectal carcinoma, the ratio between Tip60 and p400 mRNAs is affected. Reversing the p400/Tip60 imbalance by Tip60 overexpression or the use of siRNAs resulted in increased apoptosis and decreased proliferation of colon-cancer-derived cells, suggesting that this ratio defect is important for cancer progression (Mattera et al., 2009).

In mice, p400 knockout results in embryonic lethality. Homozygous knockout mice died on embryonic day 11.5 (E11.5), and displayed an anemic appearance and slight deformity of the neural tube. Their results suggest that p400/mDomino plays a critical role in embryonic hematopoiesis by regulating the expression of developmentally essential genes such as those in the Hox gene cluster (Ueda et al., 2007). Tip60-p400 is necessary to maintain characteristic features of Embryonic Stem Cells (ESCs) (Fazzio et al., 2008). Through an RNAi screen in mouse ESCs of 1008 loci encoding chromatin protein, the authors identified 68 proteins that exhibit diverse phenotypes upon knockdown, including seven subunits of the Tip60-p400 complex, Trrap, Tip60, p400, DMAP1, RuvBL1, RuvBL2 and GAS41. Phenotypic analyses revealed that p400 localization to the promoters of both silent and active genes is dependent upon histone H3 lysine 4 trimethylation (H3K4me3). The Tip60-p400 knockdown gene expression profile is enriched for developmental regulators and significantly overlaps with that of the transcription factor Nanog. Depletion of Nanog reduces p400 binding to target promoters without affecting H3K4me3 levels. Together, these data indicate that Tip60-p400 integrates signals from Nanog and H3K4me3 to regulate gene expression in ESCs (Fazzio et al., 2008).

Yeast p400 homolog Eaf1 (Esa1-associated Factor 1, VID21) is the only subunit exclusively found in the NuA4 complex in biochemical preparation. Eaf1 is the platform on which four different functional modules of the other subunits are assembled into the native complex (Auger et al., 2008). Although eaf1 deletion strain is viable, the cells show genome instability and high incidences of sporulation defects and aneuploidy. The mutant is also highly sensitive to DNA damage-inducing stress such as X-ray (Auger et al., 2008; Hughes et al., 2000; Krogan et al., 2004).

4.3 Brd8/*/Bdf1

Human Brd8 was functionally identified as a Thyroid hormone receptor coactivator p120 (Monden et al., 1997; Yuan et al., 1998). Later, its role as a transcriptional coactivator with RXR/PPAR-gamma was also reported, establishing the role as a nuclear receptor coactivator (Monden et al., 1999). Human Brd8 has one or two Bromodomain(s), depending on the isoform. The Bromodomain is a domain that can bind to acetylated lysine, typically observed in histones, suggesting its role in regulating protein-protein interactions in histone-directed chromatin remodeling and gene transcription. (Zeng and Zhou, 2002; Mujtaba et al., 2007).

Brd8 was isolated through a HeLa cell-based expression cloning for genes that influence sensitivity to a microtubule inhibitor (Yamada and Gorbsky, 2006). Ectopic expression of Brd8 provides partial resistance to microtubule inhibitors and proteasome inhibitor, and knockdown sensitized cells to the drugs, suggesting Brd8 influences sensitivity to microtubule inhibitors and proteasome inhibitor (Yamada and Rao, 2008). Human Brd8 protein is overexpressed in human metastatic colorectal cancer cell lines. Brd8 is also overexpressed in advanced colon adenocarcinoma in rats induced with Dextran sulfate and azoxymethane (an inflammatory colon cancer model system). SiRNA-mediated Brd8 knockdown resulted in cell death in HCT116 and growth delay in DLD1, both are colorectal cancer cells (Yamada and Rao, 2008). With shRNA, an independent lab showed that inhibition of Brd8 resulted in growth inhibition (Yamaguchi et al., 2010), thus Brd8 is suspected to provide survival fitness and growth advantage. In our lab, transcriptome analysis showed little difference in the amount of Brd8 transcripts in colonic normal-looking epithelial and cancer cells, yet the protein accumulates in cancer cells. The protein accumulation is enhanced with an addition of proteasome inhibitor in cultured human colon cancer cells, suggesting that a post translational, proteasome-dependent pathway is involved in the regulation (unpublished results).

Yeast homolog Bdf1p (Bromo Domain Factor 1) contains two bromodomains and is thought to correspond to a missing piece of TFIID (Matangkasombut et al., 2000). Bdf1 deletion in yeast is viable, but affects general transcription including small nuclear RNA, sporulation, mitochondrial function and stress-induced cell death (Lygerou et al., 1994; Liu et al, 2009). Overexpression of Bdf1 can suppress phenotypes and defects of yaf9 (human GAS41 homolog) deletion, indicating functional overlap between Bdf1 and Yaf9 (Bianchi et al., 2004).

4.4 Epc1/Epl1/*

In *Drosophila*, EPC1 (Enhancer of PolyComb 1) mutation was isolated as a mutation that enhances the effect of homeotic proteins Polycomb. Although homozygotic mutations of Epc1 in *Drosophila* are lethal in the embryo, heterozygous mutations do not by themselves result in a zygotic homeotic phenotype (Stankunas et al, 1998). Epc1 protein is a chromatin protein with no known enzymatic activity by itself.

EPC1 deregulation is observed in Adult T-cell leukemia/lymphoma (ATLL), a malignant tumor caused by latent human T-lymphotropic virus 1 (HTLV-1) infection. In acute-type ATLL, there is a common breakpoint cluster region at 10p11.2. The chromosomal breakpoints are localized within the enhancer of polycomb 1 (EPC1) gene locus (Nakahata et al., 2009).

In mice development, Epc1 is involved in skeletal muscle differentiation. The expression of *Epc1* mRNA is gradually decreased with aging from embryonic day 11.5 to postnatal week 8. Epc1 is highly expressed in skeletal muscles and heart ventricle in week 8 mice (Kee et al., 2007). Epc1 knockdown caused a decrease in the acetylation of histones associated with serum response element (SRE) of the skeletal alpha-actin promoter. The Epc1.SRF (Serum Response Factor) complex bound to the SRE, and the knockdown of Epc1 resulted in a decrease in SRF binding to the skeletal alpha-actin promoter. Epc1 recruited histone acetyltransferase activity, which was potentiated by cotransfection with p300 but abolished by siRNA-mediated p300 inhibition. Epc1 directly bound to p300 in myoblast cells. Epc1 heterozygous mice showed distortion of skeletal alpha-actin, and the isolated myoblasts from the mice had impaired muscle differentiation. These results suggest that Epc1 is required for skeletal muscle differentiation by recruiting both SRF and p300 to the SRE of muscle-specific gene promoters (Kim et al., 2009).

Deletion of Yeast homolog Epl1 (Enhancer of Polycomb Like 1) is inviable, causes cells to accumulate in G2/M and global loss of acetylated histones H4 and H2A (Boudreault et al., 2003).

4.5 Tip60/Esa1/*

TIP60 in humans and Esa1 in yeast are the catalytic (acetyltransferase) subunit of the NuA4 complex (Ikura et al., 2000; Smith et al., 1998) and play a central role in Tip60 (NuA4) complex function. MYC associates with TIP60 and recruits it to chromatin *in vivo* with four other components of the TIP60 complex: TRRAP, p400, RuvBL1 and RuvBL2 (Frank et al., 2003)

The Tip60 histone acetyltransferase has been recently shown to be underexpressed in many human cancers from various origins (Lleonart et al., 2006; Gorrini et al., 2007). Moreover, in a model of tumor induction mice, it has been shown to function as a haploinsufficient tumor suppressor, providing a causal link between Tip60 underexpression and tumorigenesis (Gorrini et al., 2007).

A down-regulation of the TIP60 gene was observed in 28 out of 46 (61%) specimens of primary gastric cancer (Sakuraba et al, 2011). As mentioned in p400, in colon cancer expression ratio of Tip60-p400 is altered, and it may be involved in tumor growth (Mattera et al., 2009).

In yeast the catalytic subunit Esa1 is the only HAT protein essential for viability and is responsible for the bulk of histone H4 and H2A acetylation in vivo (Doyon and Cote, 2004). *esa1* temperature sensitive (ts) mutants provoke a *RAD9*-dependent G2/M delay (Megee et al., 1995; Clarke et al., 1999). Yeast Esa1 mutation is inviable, and *esa1* conditional mutation serve to dissolve whole complex (Allard et al., 1999).

4.6 DMAP1/Eaf2/Eaf2

Human DMAP1 and its yeast homolog Eaf2 contain a highly conserved SANT (SWI3–ADA2–NcoR–TFIIIB) domain, a histone tail-binding module (Boyer et al. 2004). DMAP1 (DNA methyltransferase (DNMT)-1 associated protein 1) is a subunit of the TIP60-p400 complex that maintains embryonic stem (ES) cell pluripotency (Fazzio et al., 2008) and also a subunit of a complex containing the somatic form of DNA methyltransferase 1 (DNMT1s). The lack of DNMT1 in the purified TIP60-p400 complex indicates that DMAP1 interacts with DNMT1 in a distinct complex, thus DMAP1 functions in two distinct manner, as a Tip60 (NuA4) complex and with DNMT1 (Cai et al. 2003, Doyon et al., 2004). The non-catalytic amino terminus of DNMT1 binds to HDAC2 and can mediate transcriptional repression (Rountree et al, 2000). DNMT1 is essential for epidermal progenitor cell function and replenishing the tissue (Sen et al., 2010).

DMAP1 associated proteins (DNMT1,3A and 3B) were progressively upregulated in colorectal adenoma-carcinoma sequence (Schmidt et al., 2007). Since counteracting demethylase MBD2 amount remained unchanged, the authors suggested that epigenetic regulation in the adenoma-carcinoma sequence may be driven by increased methylating activity by DNMTs rather than suppressed demethylation.

In mice, DMAP1 homozygous knockout resulted in lethality during preimplantation (Mohan et al., 2010). Reduction of the expression of DMAP1 caused a loss of characteristic ES cell morphology and activation of genes associated with cell differentiation (Fazzio et al., 2008), and it is a likely cause of the embryonic lethal phenotype. Dmap1 knockdown in mouse embryonic fibroblasts (MEFs) lead to spontaneous double-strand breaks (DSBs), resulting in growth arrest because of p53-dependent cell cycle checkpoint activation (Negishi et al., 2009).

Yeast homolog Eaf2 (also known as SWC4) is a shared component of NuA4 and SWR1 complexes. Mutant yeasts are highly sensitive to DNA breaks induced by DNA-damaging agents, suggesting an essential role for these two proteins in DNA repair (Auger et al., 2008).

4.7 Ing3/Yng2/*

Human ING1 (Inhibitor of Growth 1) was identified as a tumor suppressor candidate, and subsequently the "Ing family" proteins (ING1-ING5) were investigated. Human Ing3 is a

47kd protein with a C-terminal plant homeodomain (PHD)-finger motif, common in proteins involved in chromatin remodeling and is a sequence-specific histone recognition protein module (Gunduz et al., 2002; Nagashima et al., 2003; Sanchez and Zhou, 2011). p47ING3 activates p53-transactivated promoters, including promoters of p21/waf1 and bax. Thus p47ING3 modulates p53-mediated transcription, cell cycle control, and apoptosis. Later, ING family proteins are identified as components of chromatin remodeling complexes; ING1 in mSin3A HDAC, ING2 in an HDAC complex similar to ING1, ING3 in Tip60 (NuA4) HAT complex, ING4 in HBO1 HAT, and ING5 fractionates with two distinct complexes containing HBO1 or nucleosomal H3-specific MOZ/MORF HATs. (Doyon et al., 2006).

Consistent with the proposed function as a tumor suppressor, a decrease of ING3 expression or LOH are observed in tumors. Decreased or no expression of ING3 mRNA was observed in 50% of primary head and neck squamous cell carcinomas (HNSCC) as compared with that of matched normal samples. About 63% of tongue and larynx tumors showed the decrease, and a tendency of higher mortality was observed in cases with decreased ING3 expression. It suggests that the ING3 gene functions as a tumor suppressor in a subset of HNSCC (Gunduz et al., 2002). Expression of ING3 is correlated with poor prognosis in HNSCC (Gunduz et al., 2008). Distorted ING3 expression has been found in several lymphoma-derived cell lines (Fadlelmola et al., 2008). Nuclear ING3 expression was reduced in melanomas in a Skp2-ubiquitin/proteasome pathway-dependent manner (Chen et al., 2010). This reduction was correlated with a poorer patient survival (Wang et al., 2007). Decreased ING3 expression is associated with melanoma progression and poor prognosis.

The yeast Saccharomyces cerevisiae has three homologs of ING family proteins. Homolog of human ING3 is Yng2 (Loewith et al., 2000). Yng2 is a plant homeodomain (PHD)-finger protein and a NuA4 complex subunit. Deletion of YNG2 results in several phenotypes, including an abnormal multibudded morphology, an inability to utilize nonfermentable carbon sources, heat shock sensitivity, slow growth, temperature sensitivity, and sensitivity to caffeine (Loeweth et al., 2000). Also notable was its requirement for normal progression through mitosis and meiosis. Some of the phenotypes were suppressed by HDAC inhibitor Tricostatin A, demonstrating that the phenotypes are based on defects in acetylation cycle (Choy et al., 2001). Yng2p is stabilized by the proteasome inhibitor MG-132, and is likely regulated through an ubiquitin-proteasome pathway (Lin et al., 2008).

4.8 YL-1/*/Vps72

Human YL-1 is a nuclear protein with an acidic region and a proline-rich region (Horikawa et al., 1995), and was identified as a component of Tip60 (NuA4) complex with biochemical purification and mass spectrometry. YL-1 is also a part of human counterpart of yeast SWR1 complex (Cai et al., 2005). Notably, mammalian SRCAP and Drosophila Tip60 complexes are associated with histone H2AZ or its fly counterpart H2AvD. These similarities suggest that YL-1 may serve as a binding module for histone H2AZ in metazoans, as does Swc2 in yeast (Wu et al., 2005).

In the Kirsten sarcoma virus–transformed NIH3T3 cells highly expressing the exogenous human YL-1 protein, the anchorage-independent growth (colony-forming ability in soft agar medium) was markedly suppressed. However, in contrast to the suppression of anchorage-independent growth, the forced expression of YL-1 did not affect the transformed phenotypes in adherent culture and tumorigenicity in nude mice. The data suggest that YL-

1 is involved in the transformation process, and once cells are transformed, additional YL-1 expression does not play additional role in tumor growth (Horikawa et al., 1995).

Yeast homolog VPS72 (Vascular Protein Sorting 72, also known as SWC2) is a histone variant H2AZ (Htz1p)-binding component of the SWR1 complex, which exchanges Htz1p for chromatin-bound histone H2A (Wu et al., 2005).

4.9 RuvBL1/*/Rvb1(Tip49A) and
4.10 RuvBL2/*/Rvb2(Tip49B)

RuvBL1 and RuvBL2 belong to the family of AAA+ ATPases (ATPases Associated with various cellular Activities). Ruvbl1 is also called Pontin, NMP238, ECP54, TAP54α, TIH1 or Tip49, while Ruvbl2 is also called Reptin, ECP51, TAP54α, TIH2 or Tip48. RuvBL1 and RuvBL2 bind each other and function as a hexameric helicase (Ikura et al., 2000; Shen et al., 2000). The names come from their homology with the bacterial RuvB helicase, which is involved in DNA recombination and repair. In bacteria, the ruvA-ruvB complex in the presence of ATP renatures cruciform structure in supercoiled DNA with palindromic sequence, indicating that it may promote strand exchange reactions in homologous recombination. RuvAB is a helicase that mediates the Holliday junction migration by localized denaturation and reannealing.

Human RuvBL1 and RuvBL2 are components of multiple multiprotein complexes, INO80, SRCAP, URI-1, R2TP and Tip60 (NuA4) complex. RuvBL1 and RuvBL2 were co-immunoprecipitated or affinity-purified with at least 48 proteins (Grigoletto et al., 2011).

Human RuvBL1 and RuvBL2 are overexpressed in a variety of cancers inculding colorectal (Carlson et al., 2003). Regulation of COX-2 transcription in a colon cancer cell line by Pontin52/TIP49a, (Lauscher et al.; 2007; Ki et al., 2007), gastric (Li et al., 2010), bladder (Sanchez-Carbayo et al., 2006), mesothelioma (Zhan et al., 2007), non-small cell lung cancer (Dehan et al., 2007), as well as in several types of acute (Andersson et al., 2007) or chronic leukemias (Haslinger et al., 2004), in multiple myeloma (Zhan et al., 2007) and high-grade lymphoma (Nishiu et al., 2002). In ovarian cancer cell lines, microcell-mediated chromosome transfer and expression microarray analysis identified nine genes associated with functional suppression of tumorogenicity; AIFM2, AKTIP, AXIN2, CASP5, FILIP1L, RBBP8, RGC32, RUVBL1 and STAG3. Two SNPs in RUVBL1 were associated with increased risk of serous ovarian cancer (Notaridou et al., 2011). The expression of an ATPase-deficient mutant form of RuvBL1/TIP49 substantially inhibited β-catenin-mediated neoplastic transformation of immortalized rat epithelial cells and anchorage-independent growth of human colon cancer cells with deregulated β-catenin (Feng et al., 2003).

Disruption of the yeast RuvBL1 (Kanemaki et al., 1999; Lim et al., 2000) or RuvBL2 genes (Lim et al., 2000) is lethal.

4.11 BAF53a (ACTL6a)/Arp4/Arp4

Human BAF53a (BRG1-associated factor 53a) is also known as ACTL6a (Actin-like 6a). As the name implies, the protein has a 36% identity and 50% similarity with the human beta-actin. BAF53 is a part of Tip60 (NuA4) complex (Cai et al., 2003, Doyon et al., 2004, 2006). In addition, BAF53a is also a part of other multiple multiprotein complexes, including INO80, SWI/SNF, and myc-containing nuclear cofactor complex (Park et al., 2002; Sung et al., 2001). For SWI/SNF-like protein complex, beta-actin and BAF53 are required for maximal ATPase activity of BRG1 and are also required with BRG1 for association of the complex with chromatin/matrix (Zhao et al., 1998). Baf53 protein was also identified as a major binding target for HIV Tat protein through affinity chromatography coupled with mass spectrometry. The result suggests that Baf53 and Tip60 (NuA4) complex is a major target for HIV-1 proviral gene silencing and activation (Gautier et al., 2009).

In yeast, Arp4/Act3 was identified as a component of NuA4 complex with affinity-purification followed by mass spectrometry (Galarneau et al., 2000). *ARP4* gene is essential for growth in yeast (Harata et al., 1994). In temperature-sensitive *arp4* mutants, NuA4 complex disintegrated and lost its activity in restrictive temperature, demonstrating the critical role of Arp4 in the NuA4 complex (Galarneau et al., 2000). Upon DNA damage, Arp4 recognizes and interacts with histone H2A phosphorylated at serine 129. This action recruits NuA4 to regions of DNA double-strand breaks where histone H4 acetylation is required for DNA double-strand break repair (Bird et al., 2002; Downs et al., 2004).

4.12 Actin/Act1/Act1

A major cytoskeletal protein beta-actin is also a subunit of Tip60 (NuA4) complex (Cai et al., 2003; Doyon et al., 2004, 2006). As in BAF53a, Actin is also a subunit of other multiprotein complex. Inhibition of Actin with the Actin monomer sequestering natural product Latrunculin B blocks chromatin-dependent ATPase activation of the BAF complex, indicating that Actin is a functionally critical component of SWI/SNF complex (Zhao et al., 1998). As a major cytoskeletal component, beta-actin (Actb) gene is an essential gene, and its hypomorph is embryonic lethal in mice (Tondeleir et al., 2009).

In yeast, in addition to cytoskeletal roles, Act1 is shown to be a component of distinctive chromatin remodeling complexes including INO80, SWR and NuA4 (Shen et al., 2000; Krogan et al., 2003; Galarneau et al., 2000). Act1 deletion is lethal.

4.13 MRG15/Eaf3/*

MRG 15 (Morf-related genes (Mrg) on chromosomes 15 (Mrg15)) belongs to Morf family proteins. From cellular senescent study to identify single chromosomes from normal human cells that can inhibit growth of immortal human cells, an intronless transcription factor-like protein, mortality factor on chromosome 4 (*MORF4*) was identified. From structural homology, other family proteins including MRG15 and MRGX were identified and investigated. MRG15 has helix-loop-helix and leucine zipper domains, which are typically found in transcriptional regulators, and a chromodomain thought to be involved in protein-protein interaction in chromatin remodeling factors. MRG15 and -MRGX are expressed ubiquitously in all cells and tissues. Currently, MRG proteins, which have pro-growth activity, are hypothesized to antagonize growth inhibition activity by Morf4.

Mrg15 knockout mice are embryonic lethal, and mouse embryonic fibroblasts derived from Mrg15 null embryos proliferate poorly, enter senescence rapidly, and have impaired DNA repair compared to wild type mice (Tominaga et al., 2005). Mrg15 null embryonic neural stem and progenitor cells also have a decreased capacity for proliferation and differentiation (Garcia et al., 2007). Expression of the cyclin-dependent kinase inhibitor p21 is specifically up-regulated in Mrg15 deficient neural stem/progenitor cells (NSCs). Mrg15 deficient NSCs exhibit severe defects in DNA damage response following ionizing radiation (Chen et al., 2011).

So far, cancer association of Mrg15 has been poorly shown. No alterations or mutations were identified for MRG15/MORF4L1 in unclassified FA patients and Breast Cancer (BrCa) familial cases. No significant associations between common MORF4L1 variants and BrCa risk for BRCA1 or BRCA2 mutation carriers were identified (Martrat et al., 2011).

Yeast Eaf3 is a shared component of the NuA4 complex and Rpd3 histone deacetylase complex. The loss of Eaf3 greatly alters the genomic profile of histone acetylation (Reid et al., 2004).

4.14 GAS41/Yaf9/Yaf9

GAS41 (Glioma Amplified Sequence 41) is a nuclear protein containing a C-terminal alpha-acidic activation domain and an N-terminal YEATS domain (Fischer et al., 1997). The YEATS domain family of proteins is well conserved from yeast to human, and functions as transcriptional regulators as a part of multiprotein complexes. GAS41 is associated with TFIIF via its YEATS domain. GAS41 is also a subunit of the human TIP60 and SCRAP complexes (Doyon et al., 2004; Cai et al., 2005). In addition, GAS41 physically interacts with transforming acidic coiled-coil 1(TACC1) protein, microtubule-associated colonic and hepatic tumor overexpressed (ch-TOG) protein and nuclear matrix (NuMA) protein (Lauffart et al., 2002; Harborth et al., 2000).

Yeast homolog Yaf9 encodes a protein of 226 residues, containing an N-terminal YEATS domain and a C-terminal predicted coiled-coil sequence (Le Masson et al., 2003). Deletion of Yaf9 shows pleiotropic effect, including sensitivity to a variety of drugs such as cadmium, cecium chrolide, cycloheximide, and microtubule inhibitor benomyl. The phenotype is associated with a change in transcriptome. The transcriptomic change can be suppressed by Bdf1 multicopy expression, suggesting functional overlapping between these two components (Bianchi et al., 2004). Since human Brd8 (Bdf1) was isolated from a screen that influenced sensitivity to microtubule inhibitors, it is tempting to speculate that Brd8-GAS41 (Bdf1-yaf9) may be an interface module to genes involved in sensitivity to microtubule inhibitors.

4.15 */Eaf5/*

Yeast Eaf5 (Esa1p-associated factor 5) is a component of yeast NuA4 complex (Nourani et al., 2001). Its direct human counterpart is unclear. Eaf5 protein forms subcomplex with Eaf7, and Eaf5 interacts with NuA4 complex (Mitchell et al., 2008). Eaf5 deletion strain is viable, and shows resistance to chemicals such as acetic acid and lactic acid (Kawahata et al., 2006).

Deletion strains of eaf5 and eaf7 display similarity in microarray transcriptional profiles (Krogan et al., 2006).

4.16 MRGBP/Eaf7/*

MRGBP (MRG Binding Protein) was identified as a NuA4 component with biochemical purification (Cai et al., 2003). MRGBP is also a component of the human INO80 complex (Jin et al., 2005). Crystal structure determination of the MRG domain indicated that MRGBP has structural similarity to DNA binding domains of the tyrosine site-specific recombinases XerD, lambda integrase, and Cre (Bowman et al., 2006).

In human colon cancer, MRGBP was upregulated in the majority of the cancers. Inhibition of MRGBP with shRNA in vitro resulted in an inhibition of cell growth (Yamaguchi et al., 2010). High levels of MRGBP expression were observed more frequently in human colonic carcinomas (45%) than adenomas (5%), linking its role to malignant properties of colorectal tumors (Yamaguchi et al., 2011).

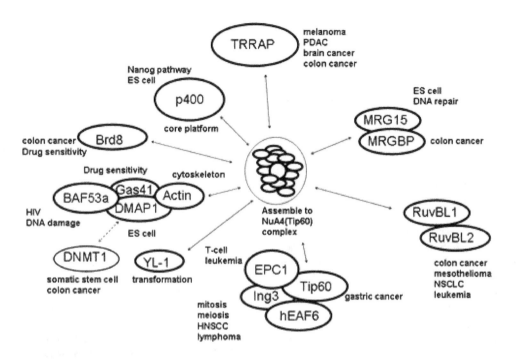

Fig. 1. Tip60 (NuA4) complex is assembled by combining subcomplexes and subunits. Each subunit of Tip60 (NuA4) complex is linked to different biological events, presumably because each subunit represents an interface to the proteins involved in the particular events. Inhibition of a subunit results in different phenotypes, which may provide intervention opportunities for cancer prevention and/or therapeutic purpose. Abbreviations: PDAC (Pancreatic Ductal Adeno Carcinoma); ES cell (Embryonic Stem cell); NSCLC (Non Small Cell Lung Cancer); HNSCC (Head and Neck Small Cell Carcinoma).

4.17 hEaf6/Eaf6/*

Human Eaf6 was isolated as a component of Tip60 (NuA4) complex (Doyon et al., 2004). hEaf6 is also a component of HBO and/or MOZ/MORF HAT complex (Ullah et al., 2008; Saksouk et al., 2009).

5. Relevance to colon cancer

Among multiple subunits, Brd8, MRGBP, RuvBL1 and RuvBL2 show particularly strong connections to colon cancer. These subunits are overexpressed in colon cancer (Yamada and Rao, 2009; Yamaguchi et al.,2010, 2011; Carlson et al., 2003; Lauscher et al., 2007; Graudens et al., 2006; Ki et al., 2007). Brd8 plays a role in survival and/or drug resistance of cultured colon cancer cells. MRGBP also plays a role in survival of cultured colon cancer cells. RuvBL1 is an important cofactor in beta-catenin/TCF gene regulation, and expression of its dominant-negative form inhibited β-catenin-mediated neoplastic transformation of immortalized rat epithelial cells and anchorage-independent growth of human colon cancer cells with deregulated β-catenin (Feng et al., 2003).

In addition, DMAP1 associated proteins (DNMT1,3A and 3B) were progressively upregulated in colorectal adenoma-carcinoma sequence (Schmidt et al., 2007). DNMT1 may play a role in colon cancer progression directly or indirectly.

6. Subunit-specific targeting strategy

As in above, deregulations in subunits of human Tip60 (NuA4) complex are common in various cancers, and the complex is gaining attention as a potential target for cancer therapy. However, concerns for targeting whole Tip60 (NuA4) complex are raised because the complex plays essential roles for cellular survival and targeting the core components of the complex would impair the essential functions, which may lead to general toxicity to both normal and cancer cells. Although many successful drugs in existence do target essential and ubiquitous cellular components (e.g. Taxol for microtubule, Velcade for proteasome), the concern needs to be addressed.

As a rebuttal, targeting of each component has been proposed. Although the Tip60 (NuA4) complex is thought to function as a complex, targeting each subunit does not necessarily show the same biological effect and phenotype empirically, suggesting unique roles of each subunit. This fact may be exploited for developing therapeutic strategy. Further investigation of the unique roles of each subunit would allow us to develop subunit-specific targeting strategies for therapeutic purpose.

Extrapolating from yeast and mice results, the following subunits of Tip60 (NuA4) complex are essential for cellular survival; TRRAP, p400, EPC1, Tip60, DMAP1, RuvBL1, RuvBL2, BAF53a and Actin. Inhibiting these subunits may require caution. Components whose inhibition may not directly or immediately kill cells are; Brd8, ING3, YL-1, MRG15, GAS41, MRGBP and hEaf6. Inhibition of these components may prove valuable as an adjuvant approach to improve other therapies such as chemo- and radio-therapies.

In some subunits and associating factors (Brd8, MRGBP, DNMT1), overexpression is correlated to stage advancement of colon cancer, thus drug-mediated inhibition seems intuitively appropriate. GAS41 and Brd8 may have a more prominent effect on cellular sensitivity to anti-microtubule drugs. It is possible that chemoresistance of colon cancer is at least in part provided by deregulation of these subunits, and drug-mediated inhibition of these subunits results in enhancement of the effect of these drugs.

7. Conclusion

Accumulating evidence supports that the Tip60 (NuA4) complex plays a role in various cancers including that in colon, and possibly in drug sensitivity/resistance of cells. Targeting the components may prove successful in preventing cancer and/or in killing or chemosensitizing cancer cells. Since the major hindrance to a colon cancer cure is its chemoresistance, chemosensitizing through modulation of the Tip60 (NuA4) complex component seems to be a novel and attractive strategy. However, thus far validation of Tip60 (NuA4) complex, or the subunit(s), as a therapeutic target is yet to be performed. Continuing investigation is required to translate current knowledge to clinical or translational studies. Strategies for targeting (e.g. siRNA, small molecule) should be explored.

8. Acknowledgements

Dr. Chinthalapally V. Rao (OUHSC) for support. Dr. Kiyoshi Yamaguchi for sharing manuscript prior to publication. A part of this work is supported by Kerley-Cade chair Research endowment (OUHSC).

9. References

Allard, S.; Utley, R.T.; Savard, J.; Clarke, A.; Grant, P.; Brandl, C. J.; Pillus, L.; Workman, J.L.; Côté, J. (1999). NuA4, an essential transcription adaptor/histone H4 acetyltransferase complex containing Esa1p and the ATM-related cofactor Tra1p. *EMBO J* Vol. 18(18), pp. 5108-5119.

Andersson, A.; Ritz, C.; Lindgren, D.; Eden, P.; Lassen, C.; Heldrup, J.; et al. (2007). Microarray-based classification of a consecutive series of 121 childhood acute leukemias: prediction of leukemic and genetic subtype as well as of minimal residual disease status. *Leukemia* Vol. 21, pp. 1198–1203.

Ard, P.G.; Chatterjee, C.; Kunjibettu, S.; Adside, L.R.; Gralinski, L.E.; McMahon, S.B. (2002). Transcriptional regulation of the mdm2 oncogene by p53 requires TRRAP acetyltransferase complexes. *Mol Cell Biol* Vol. 22(16), pp.5650-5661.

Auger, A.; Galarneau, L.; Altaf, M.; Nourani, A.; Doyon, Y.; Utley, R. T.; Cronier, D.; Allard, S.; Côté, J.(2008). Eaf1 is the platform for NuA4 molecular assembly that evolutionarily links chromatin acetylation to ATP-dependent exchange of histone H2A variants. *Mol Cell Biol* Vol. 28 (7), pp.2257-2270.

Babiarz, J. E.; Halley, J. E. ; Rine, J. (2006). Telomeric heterochromatin boundaries require NuA4-dependent acetylation of histone variant H2A.Z in Saccharomyces cerevisiae. Genes Dev Vol. 20, pp. 700-710.

Basso, K.; Margolin, A.A.; Stolovitzky, G.; Klein, U.; Dalla-Favera, R.; Califano, A. (2005). Reverse engineering of regulatory networks in human B cells. *Nat. Genet* Vol. 37, pp. 382–390.

Bianchi, M.M.; Costanzo, G.; Chelstowska, A.; Grabowska, D.; Mazzoni, C.; Piccinni, E.; Cavalli, A.; Ciceroni, F.; Rytka, J.; Slonimski, P.P.; Frontali, L.; Negri, R. (2004). The bromodomain-containing protein Bdf1p acts as a phenotypic and transcriptional multicopy suppressor of YAF9 deletion in yeast. *Mol Microbiol* Vol. 53(3), pp. 953-968.

Bird, A. W.; Yu, D. Y.; Pray-Grant, M. G.; Qiu, Q.; Harmon, K. E.; Megee, P. C.; Grant, P. A.; Smith, M. M.; Christman, M. F. (2002). Acetylation of histone H4 by Esa1 is required for DNA double-strand break repair. *Nature* Vol. 419, pp. 411-415

Boudreault, A.A.; Cronier, D.; Selleck, W.; Lacoste, N.; Utley, R.T.; Allard, S.; Savard, J.; Lane, W.S.; Tan, S.; Côté, J. (2003). Yeast enhancer of polycomb defines global Esa1-dependent acetylation of chromatin. *Genes Dev* Vol. 17(11), pp. 1415-1428.

Bowman, B.R.; Moure, C.M.; Kirtane, B.M.; Welschhans, R.L.; Tominaga, K.; Pereira-Smith, O.M.; Quiocho, F.A. (2006). Multipurpose MRG domain involved in cell senescence and proliferation exhibits structural homology to a DNA-interacting domain. *Structure* Vol.14(1), pp.151-158.

Boyer, L.A.; Latek, R.R.; Peterson, C.L. (2004) The SANT domain: a unique histone-tail-binding module? Nat. Rev. *Mol Cell Biol* Vol. 5, pp. 158–163.

Braun, A.; Lemaitre, B.; Lanot, R.; Zachary, D.; Meister, M. (1997) Drosophila immunity: analysis of larval hemocytes by P-element-mediated enhancer trap. *Genetics* Vol. 147 (2), pp. 623-634.

Brown, C. E.; L. Howe; K. Sousa, S. C.; Alley, M. J.; Carrozza, S.; Tan, and J. L. Workman. (2001). Recruitment of HAT complexes by direct activator interactions with the ATM-related Tra1 subunit. *Science* Vol. 292, pp. 2333-2337.

Cai, Y.; Jin, J.; Tomomori-Sato, C.; Sato, S.; Sorokina, I.; Parmely, T. J.; Conaway, R. C.; Conaway, J. W. (2003) Identification of new subunits of the multiprotein mammalian TRRAP/TIP60-containing histone acetyltransferase complex. *J Biol Chem* Vol. 278 (44), pp. 42733-42736.

Cai, Y.; Jin, J.; Florens, L.; Swanson, S.K.; Kusch, T.; Li, B.; Workman, J.L.; Washburn, M.P.; Conaway, R.C.; Conaway, J.W. (2005). The mammalian YL1 protein is a shared subunit of the TRRAP/TIP60 histone acetyltransferase and SRCAP complexes. *J Biol Chem* Vol. 280(14), pp. 13665-13670.

Carlson, M.L.; Wilson, E.T.; Prescott, S.M. (2003). Regulation of COX-2 transcription in a colon cancer cell line by Pontin52/TIP49a. *Mol Cancer* Vol. 2, pp. 42.

Chen, M.; Pereira-Smith, O.M.; Tominaga, K. (2011). Loss of the chromatin regulator MRG15 limits neural stem/progenitor cell proliferation via increased expression of the p21 Cdk inhibitor. *Stem Cell Res* Vol. 7(1), pp. 75-88.

Choy, J.S.; Tobe, B.T.; Huh, J.H.; Kron, S.J. (2001). Yng2p-dependent NuA4 histone H4 acetylation activity is required for mitotic and meiotic progression. *J Biol Chem* Vol. 276(47), pp. 43653-43662.

Chua, P.; Roeder, G.S. (1995). Bdf1, a yeast chromosomal protein required for sporulation. *Mol Cell Biol* Vol. 15(7), pp. 3685-3696.

Couture, J.F.; Trievel, R.C. (2006). Histone-modifying enzymes: encrypting an enigmatic epigenetic code. *Curr Opin Struct Biol* Vol. 16(6), pp.753-760.

Dames, S.A.; Mulet, J.M.; Rathgeb-Szabo, K.; Hall, M.N.; Grzesiek, S. (2005).The solution structure of the FATC domain of the protein kinase target of rapamycin suggests a role for redox-dependent structural and cellular stability. *J Biol Chem* Vol. 280 (21), pp. 20558-20564.

Dehan, E.; Ben-Dor, A.; Liao, W.; Lipson, D.; Frimer, H.; Rienstein, S.; Simansky, D.; Krupsky, M.; Yaron, P.; Friedman, E.; Rechavi, G.; Perlman, M, et al. (2007). Chromosomal aberrations and gene expression profiles in non-small cell lung cancer. *Lung Cancer* Vol. 56, pp. 175–184.

Downs, J. A.; Allard, S.; Jobin-Robitaille, A.; Javaheri, A.; Auger, N.; Bouchard, S.; Kron, S. J.; Jackson, S. P.; Cote, J. (2004). Binding of chromatin-modifying activities to phosphorylated histone H2A at DNA damage sites. *Mol Cell* Vol. 16, pp.979-990.

Doyon, Y.; Selleck, W.; Lane, W. S.; Tan, S.; Côté, J. (2004) Structural and functional conservation of the NuA4 histone acetyltransferase complex from yeast to humans. *Mol cell biol* Vol. 5, pp.1884-1896.

Doyon, Y.; Cayrou, C.; Ullah, M.; Landry, A.J.; Côté, V.; Selleck, W.; Lane, W.S.; Tan, S.; Yang, X.J.; Côté, J. (2006). ING tumor suppressor proteins are critical regulators of chromatin acetylation required for genome expression and perpetuation. *Mol Cell* Vol. 21(1), pp. 51-64.

Fadlelmola, F.M.; Zhou, M.; de Leeuw, R.J.; Dosanjh, N. S.; Harmer, K.; Huntsman, D. et al. (2008). Sub-megabase resolution tiling (SMRT) array-based comparative genomic hybridization profiling reveals novel gains and losses of chromosomal regions in Hodgkin lymphoma and anaplastic large cell lymphoma cell lines. *Mol Cancer* Vol. 7, pp. 2.

Fazzio, T.G.; Huff, J.T.; Panning, B. (2008). An RNAi screen of chromatin proteins identifies Tip60-p400 as a regulator of embryonic stem cell identity. *Cell* Vol. 134(1), pp. 162-174.

Feng, Y.; Lee, N.; Fearon, E.R. (2003) .TIP49 regulates beta-catenin-mediated neoplastic transformation and T-cell factor target gene induction via effects on chromatin remodeling. *Cancer Res* Vol. 63(24), pp.8726-8734.

Fischer, U.; Heckel, D.; Michel, A.; Janka, M.; Hulsebos, T.; Meese, E. (1997). Cloning of a novel transcription factor-like gene amplified in human glioma including astrocytoma grade I. *Hum Mol Genet* Vol. 6, pp. 1817-1822.

Fuchs, M.; Gerber, J.; Drapkin, R.; Sif, S.; Ikura, T.; Ogryzko, V.; Lane, W.S.; Nakatani, Y.; Livingston, D.M. (2001). The p400 complex is an essential E1A transformation target. *Cell* Vol. 106(3), pp. 297-307.

Galarneau, L.; Nourani, A.; Boudreault, A.A.; Zhang, Y.; Héliot, L.; Allard, S.; Savard, J.; Lane, W.S.; Stillman ,D.J.; Côté, J. (2000). Multiple links between the NuA4 histone acetyltransferase complex and epigenetic control of transcription. *Mol Cell* Vol. 5(6), pp. 927-937.

Garcia, S.N.; Kirtane, B.M.; Podlutsky, A.J.; Pereira-Smith, O.M.; Tominaga, K. (2007). Mrg15 null and heterozygous mouse embryonic fibroblasts exhibit DNA-repair defects post exposure to gamma ionizing radiation. *FEBS Lett* Vol. 581(27), pp. 5275-5281.

Gautier, V.W.; Gu, L.; O'Donoghue, N.; Pennington, S.; Sheehy, N.; Hall, W.W. (2009). In vitro nuclear interactome of the HIV-1 Tat protein. *Retrovirology* Vol. 6, pp. 47.

Grant, P.A.; Schieltz, D.; Pray-Grant, M.G.; Yates, J.R. 3rd.; Workman, J.L.(1998). The ATM-related cofactor Tra1 is a component of the purified SAGA complex. *Mol Cell* Vol. 2(6), pp. 863-867.

Grigoletto, A.; Lestienne, P.; Rosenbaum, J. (2011). The multifaceted proteins Reptin and Pontin as major players in cancer. *Biochim Biophys Acta* Vol. 1815(2), pp. 147-157.

Gunduz, M.; Ouchida, M.; Fukushima, K.; Ito, S.; Jitsumori, Y.; Nakashima, T.; Nagai, N.; Nishizaki, K.; Shimizu, K. (2002). Allelic loss and reduced expression of the ING3, a candidate tumor suppressor gene at 7q31, in human head and neck cancers. *Oncogene* Vol. 21(28), pp. 4462-4470.

Gunduz, M.; Beder, L.B.; Gunduz, E.; Nagatsuka, H.; Fukushima, K.; Pehlivan, D.; Cetin, E.; Yamanaka, N.; Nishizaki, K.; Shimizu K.; Nagai, N. (2008). Downregulation of

ING3 mRNA expression predicts poor prognosis in head and neck cancer. *Cancer Sci* Vol. 99(3), pp. 531-538.

Harata, M.; Karwan, A.; Wintersberger, U. (1994). An essential gene of Saccharomyces cerevisiae coding for an actin-related protein. *Proc. Natl. Acad. Sci. USA* Vol. 91, pp. 8258-8262.

Harborth, J.; Weber, K.; Osborn, M. (2000). GAS41, a highly conserved protein in eukaryotic nuclei, binds to NuMA. *J Biol Chem* Vol. 275(41), pp.31979-31985.

Haslinger, C.; Schweifer, N.; Stilgenbauer, S.; Dohner, H.; Lichter, P.; Kraut, N.; Stratowa, C.; Abseher, R. (2004). Microarray gene expression profiling of B-cell chronic lymphocytic leukemia subgroups defined by genomic aberrations and VH mutation status. *J Clin Oncol* Vol. 22, pp. 3937-3949.

Herceg, Z.; Hulla, W.; Gell, D.; Cuenin, C.; Lleonart, M.; Jackson, S.; Wang, Z. Q. (2001). Disruption of Trrap causes early embryonic lethality and defects in cell cycle progression. *Nat Genet* Vol. 29(2), pp. 206-211.

Horikawa, I.; Tanaka, H.; Yuasa, Y.; Suzuki, M.; Oshimura, M. (1995a). Molecular cloning of a novel human cDNA on chromosome 1q21 and its mouse homolog encoding a nuclear protein with DNA-binding ability. *Biochem Biophys Res Commun* Vol. 208(3), pp. 999-1007.

Horikawa, I.; Tanaka, H.; Yuasa, Y.; Suzuki, M.; Shimizu, M.; Oshimura, M. (1995b). Forced expression of YL-1 protein suppresses the anchorage-independent growth of Kirsten sarcoma virus-transformed NIH3T3 cells. *Exp Cell Res* Vol. 220(1), pp. 11-17.

Hughes, T. R.; C. J. Roberts, H.; Dai, A. R.; Jones, M. R.; Meyer, D.; Slade, J.; Burchard, S.; Dow, T. R.; Ward, M. J.; Kidd, et al. (2000). Widespread aneuploidy revealed by DNA microarray expression profiling. *Nat Genet* Vol. 25, pp. 333-337.

Ikura, T.; Ogryzko, V.V.; Grigoriev, M.; Groisman, R.; Wang, J.; Horikoshi, M.; Scully, R.; Qin, J.; Nakatani Y. (2000). Involvement of the TIP60 histone acetylase complex in DNA repair and apoptosis. *Cell* Vol.102(4), pp.463-473.

Imbeaud, S. (2006). Deciphering cellular states of innate tumor drug responses. *Genome Biol* Vol. 7, pp. R19.

Jin, J.; Cai, Y.; Yao, T.; Gottschalk, A.J.; Florens, L.; Swanson, S.K.; Gutiérrez, J.L.; Coleman, M.K.; Workman, J.L.; Mushegian, A.; Washburn, M.P.; Conaway, R.C.; Conaway, J.W. (2005) A mammalian chromatin remodeling complex with similarities to the yeast INO80 complex. *J Biol Chem* Vol. 280(50), pp. 41207-41212.

Kanemaki, M.; Kurokawa, Y.; Matsu-ura, T.; Makino, Y. Masani, A.; Okazaki, K.; Morishita, T.; Tamura, T.A. (1999). TIP49b, a new RuvB-like DNA helicase, is included in a complex together with another RuvB-like DNA helicase, TIP49a, *J Biol Chem* Vol, 274 , pp. 22437-22444.

Kawahata, M. Masaki, K.; Fujii, T.; Iefuji, H. (2006). Yeast genes involved in response to lactic acid and acetic acid: acidic conditions caused by the organic acids in Saccharomyces cerevisiae cultures induce expression of intracellular metal metabolism genes regulated by Aft1p. *FEMS Yeast Res* Vol. 6(6), pp. 924-936.

Keogh, M. C.; Mennella, T. A.; Sawa, C.; Berthelet, S.; Krogan, N. J.; Wolek, A.; Podolny, V.; Carpenter, L. R.; Greenblatt, J. F.; Baetz, K.; Buratowski, S. (2006). The

Saccharomyces cerevisiae histone H2A variant Htz1 is acetylated by NuA4. *Genes Dev* Vol. 20, pp. 660-665.

Ki, D.H.; Jeung, H.C.; Park, C.H.; Kang, S.H.; Lee, G.Y.; Lee, W.S.; Kim, N.K.; Chung, H.C.; Rha, S.Y. (2007). Whole genome analysis for liver metastasis gene signatures in colorectal cancer. *Int J Cancer* Vol. 121, pp. 2005-2012.

Kim, J.R.; Kee, H.J.; Kim, J.Y.; Joung, H.; Nam, K.I.; Eom, G.H.; Choe, N.; Kim, H.S.; Kim, J.C.; Kook, H.; Seo, S.B.; Kook, H. (2009). Enhancer of polycomb1 acts on serum response factor to regulate skeletal muscle differentiation. *J Biol Chem* Vol. 284(24), pp. 16308-16316.

Kouzarides, T. (2007). Chromatin modifications and their function. *Cell* Vol. 128, pp. 693-705.

Krogan, N.J.; Keogh, M.C.; Datta, N.; Sawa, C.; Ryan, O.W.; Ding, H.; et al. (2003) A Snf2 family ATPase complex required for recruitment of the histone H2A variant Htz1. *Mol Cell* Vol. 12(6), pp. 1565-1576.

Krogan, N. J.; Baetz, K.; Keogh, M.C.; Datta, N.; Sawa, C.; Kwok, T. C.; Thompson, N. J.; Davey, M. G.; Pootoolal, J.; Hughes, T. R.; Emili, A.; Buratowski, S.; Hieter, P.; Greenblatt, J. F. (2004). Regulation of chromosome stability by the histone H2A variant Htz1, the Swr1 chromatin remodeling complex, and the histone acetyltransferase NuA4. *Proc Natl Acad Sci U S A* Vol. 101(37), pp.13513-13518.

Krogan, N.J.; Cagney, G.; Yu, H.; Zhong, G.; Guo, X.; Ignatchenko, A.; et al. (2006). Global landscape of protein complexes in the yeast Saccharomyces cerevisiae. *Nature* Vol. 440(7084), pp. 637-43.

Lauffart, B.; Howell, S.J.; Tasch, J.E.; Cowell, J.K.; Still, I.H. (2002). Interaction of the transforming acidic coiled-coil 1 (TACC1) protein with ch-TOG and GAS41/NuBI1 suggests multiple TACC1-containing protein complexes in human cells. *Biochem J* Vol. 363(Pt 1), pp.195-200.

Lauscher, J.C.; Loddenkemper, C.; Kosel, L.; Grone, J.; Buhr, H.J.; Huber, O. (2007). Increased pontin expression in human colorectal cancer tissue. *Hum Pathol* Vol. 38, pp. 978-985.

Le Masson, I.; Yu, D.Y.; Jensen, K.; Chevalier, A.; Courbeyrette, R.; Boulard, Y.; Smith, M.M.; Mann, C. (2003). Yaf9, a novel NuA4 histone acetyltransferase subunit, is required for the cellular response to spindle stress in yeast. *Mol Cell Biol* Vol. 23(17), pp. 6086-6102.

Li, H.; Cuenin, C.; Murr, R, Wang, Z.Q.; Herceg, Z. (2004). HAT cofactor Trrap regulates the mitotic checkpoint by modulation of Mad1 and Mad2 expression. *EMBO J* Vol. 23(24), pp. 4824-4834.

Li, W.; Zeng, J.; Li, Q.; Zhao, L.; Liu, T.; Bjorkholm, M.; Jia, J.; Xu, D. (2010). Reptin is required for the transcription of telomerase reverse transcriptase and over-expressed in gastric cancer. *Mol Cancer* Vol. 9, pp. 132

Lim, C.R.; Kimata, Y.; Ohdate, H.; Kokubo, T.; Kikuchi, N.; Horigome, T.; Kohno K. (2000). The Saccharomyces cerevisiae RuvB-like protein, Tih2p, is required for cell cycle progression and RNA polymerase II-directed transcription, *J Biol Chem* Vol. 275 (2000), pp. 22409-22417.

Lin, Y.Y.; Lu, J.Y.; Zhang, J.; Walter, W.; Dang, W.; Wan, J.; Tao, S. C.; Qian, J.; Zhao, Y.; Boeke, J.D.; Berger, S.L.; Zhu, H. (2009). Protein acetylation microarray reveals that NuA4 controls key metabolic target regulating gluconeogenesis. *Cell* Vol. 136 (6), pp.1073-1084.

Lin, Y.Y.; Qi, Y.; Lu, J.Y.; Pan, X.; Yuan, D.S.; Zhao, Y.; Bader, J.S.; Boeke, J.D. (2008). A comprehensive synthetic genetic interaction network governing yeast histone acetylation and deacetylation. *Genes Dev* Vol. 22(15), pp.2062-2074.

Liu, X.; Yang, H.; Zhang, X.; Liu, L.; Lei, M.; Zhang, Z.; Bao, X. (2009). Bdf1p deletion affects mitochondrial function and causes apoptotic cell death under salt stress. *FEMS Yeast Res* Vol. 9(2), pp. 240-246.

Loewith, R.; Meijer, M.; Lees-Miller, S.P.; Riabowol, K.; Young, D. (2000). Three yeast proteins related to the human candidate tumor suppressor p33(ING1) are associated with histone acetyltransferase activities. *Mol Cell Biol* 20(11), pp. 3807-3816.

Loukopoulos, P.; Shibata, T.; Katoh, H.; Kokubu, A.; Sakamoto, M.; Yamazaki, K.; Kosuge, T, Kanai, Y.; Hosoda, F.; Imoto, I.; Ohki, M.; Inazawa, J.; Hirohashi, S. (2007). Genome-wide array-based comparative genomic hybridization analysis of pancreatic adenocarcinoma: identification of genetic indicators that predict patient outcome. *Cancer Sci* Vol.; 98(3), pp. 392-400.

Lygerou, Z.; Conesa, C.; Lesage, P.; Swanson, R.N.; Ruet, A.; Carlson, M.; Sentenac, A.; Séraphin, B. (1994). The yeast BDF1 gene encodes a transcription factor involved in the expression of a broad class of genes including snRNAs. *Nucleic Acids Res* Vol. 22(24), pp. 5332-5340.

Martrat, G.; Maxwell, C.A.; Tominaga, E.; Porta-de-la-Riva, M.; Bonifaci, N.; Gómez-Baldó, L.; et al. (2011). Exploring the link between MORF4L1 and risk of breast cancer.*Breast Cancer Res* Vol. 13(2), pp.R40.

Matangkasombut, O.; Buratowski, R.M.; Swilling, N.W.; Buratowski, S. (2000). Bromodomain factor 1 corresponds to a missing piece of yeast TFIID. *Genes Dev* Vol. 14(8), pp.951-962.

Mattera, L.; Escaffit, F.; Pillaire, M.J.; Selves, J.; Tyteca, S, Hoffmann, J.S.; Gourraud, P.A.; Chevillard-Briet, M.; Cazaux, C.; Trouche, D. (2009). The p400/Tip60 ratio is critical for colorectal cancer cell proliferation through DNA damage response pathways. *Oncogene* Vol. 28(12), pp. 1506-1517.

Mitchell, L.; Lambert, J.P.; Gerdes, M.; Al-Madhoun, A.S.; Skerjanc, I.S.; Figeys, D.; Baetz, K. (2008). Functional dissection of the NuA4 histone acetyltransferase reveals its role as a genetic hub and that Eaf1 is essential for complex integrity. *Mol Cell Biol* Vol. 28(7), pp. 2244-2256.

Mizuguchi, G.; Shen, X.; Landry, J.; Wu, W. H. ; Sen, S.; Wu, C.. (2004). ATP-driven exchange of histone H2AZ variant catalyzed by SWR1 chromatin remodeling complex. Science Vol. 303, pp. 343-348.

Mohan, K.N.; Ding, F.; Chaillet, J.R. (2011). Distinct Roles of DMAP1 in Mouse Development. *Mol Cell Biol* Vol. 31(9), pp. 1861-1869.

Monden, T.; Wondisford, F.E.; Hollenberg, A. N. (1997). Isolation and characterization of a novel ligand-dependent thyroid hormone receptor-coactivating protein. *J Biol Chem* Vol. 272(47), pp. 29834-29841.

Monden, T.; Kishi, M.; Hosoya, T.; Satoh, T.; Wondisford, F.E.; Hollenberg, A.N.; Yamada, M.; Mori, M. (1999). p120 acts as a specific coactivator for 9-cis-retinoic acid receptor (RXR) on peroxisome proliferator-activated receptor-gamma/RXR heterodimers. *Mol Endocrinol* Vol. 13(10), pp. 1695-1703.

Mujtaba, S.; Zeng, L.; Zhou, M.M. (2007). Structure and acetyl-lysine recognition of the bromodomain. *Oncogene* Vol.;26(37), pp. 5521-5527.

Murr, R.; Loizou, J.I.; Yang, Y.G.; Cuenin, C.; Li, H.; Wang, Z.Q.; Herceg, Z. (2006). Histone acetylation by Trrap-Tip60 modulates loading of repair proteins and repair of DNA double-strand breaks. *Nat Cell Biol* Vol. 8(1), pp. 91-99.

Murr, R.; Vaissière, T.; Sawan, C.; Shukla, V.; Herceg, Z. (2007) Orchestration of chromatin-based processes: mind the TRRAP. *Oncogene* Vol. 26(37), pp. 5358-5372.

Nagashima, M.; Shiseki, M.; Pedeux, R.M.; Okamura, S.; Kitahama-Shiseki, M.; Miura, K.; Yokota, J.; Harris, C.C. (2003). A novel PHD-finger motif protein, p47ING3, modulates p53-mediated transcription, cell cycle control, and apoptosis. *Oncogene* Vol. 22(3), pp. 343-350.

Nakahata, S.; Saito, Y.; Hamasaki, M.; Hidaka, T.; Arai, Y.; Taki, T.; Taniwaki, M.; Morishita, K. (2009). Alteration of enhancer of polycomb 1 at 10p11.2 is one of the genetic events leading to development of adult T-cell leukemia/lymphoma. *Genes Chromosomes Cancer* Vol. 48(9), pp. 768-776.

Negishi, M.; Chiba, T.; Saraya, A.; Miyagi, S.; Iwama, A. (2009). Dmap1 plays an essential role in the maintenance of genome integrity through the DNA repair process. *Genes Cells* Vol. 14(11), pp.1347-1357.

Nishiu, M.; Yanagawa, R.; Nakatsuka, S.; Yao, M.; Tsunoda, T.; Nakamura, Y. Aozasa. K. (2002). Microarray analysis of gene-expression profiles in diffuse large B-cell lymphoma: identification of genes related to disease progression, Jpn J. *Cancer Res* Vol. 93, pp. 894–901.

Notaridou, M.; Quaye, L.; Dafou, D.; Jones, C.; Song, H.; Høgdall, E.; Kjaer, S.K.; Christensen, L.; Høgdall, C.; Blaakaer, J.; McGuire, V.; Wu, A.H.; et al. (2011). Common alleles in candidate susceptibility genes associated with risk and development of epithelial ovarian cancer. *Int J Cancer* Vol. 128(9), pp. 2063-2074.

Park, J.; Wood, M.A.; Cole, M.D. (2002). BAF53 forms distinct nuclear complexes and functions as a critical c-Myc-interacting nuclear cofactor for oncogenic transformation. *Mol Cell Biol* Vol. 22(5), pp.1307-1316.

Reid, J.L.; Moqtaderi, Z.; Struhl, K. (2004). Eaf3 regulates the global pattern of histone acetylation in Saccharomyces cerevisiae. *Mol Cell Biol* Vol. 24(2), pp.757-764.

Rountree, M.R.; Bachman, K.E.; Baylin, S.B. (2000). DNMT1 binds HDAC2 and a new co-repressor, DMAP1, to form a complex at replication foci. *Nat Genet* Vol. 25(3), pp. 269-277.

Saksouk, N.; Avvakumov, N.; Champagne, K.S.; Hung, T.; Doyon, Y.; Cayrou, C.; Paquet, E.; Ullah, M.; Landry, A.J.; Côté, V.; Yang, X.J.; Gozani, O.; Kutateladze, T.G.; Côté, J.

(2009). HBO HAT complexes target chromatin throughout gene coding regions via multiple PHD finger interactions with histone H3 tail. *Mol Cell* Vol. 33(2), pp. 257-265.

Saleh, A.; Schieltz, D.; Ting, N.; McMahon, S.B.; Litchfield, D.W.; Yates, J.R. 3rd; Lees-Miller, S.P.; Cole, M.D.; Brandl, C. J.(1998). Tra1p is a component of the yeast Ada.Spt transcriptional regulatory complexes. *J Biol Chem* Vol. 273(41), pp. 26559-26565.

Sanchez, R.; Zhou, M.M. (2011). The PHD finger: a versatile epigenome reader. *Trends Biochem Sci* [Epub ahead of print]

Sanchez-Carbayo, M.; Socci, N.D.; Lozano, J.; Saint, F. Cordon-Cardo, C. (2006). Defining molecular profiles of poor outcome in patients with invasive bladder cancer using oligonucleotide microarrays. *J Clin Oncol* Vol. 24, pp. 778-789.

Sardiu, M.E.; Cai, Y.; Jin, J.; Swanson, S.K.; Conaway, R.C.; Conaway, J.W.; Florens, L.; Washburn, M.P. (2008). Probabilistic assembly of human protein interaction networks from label-free quantitative proteomics. *Proc Natl Acad Sci U S A* Vol.105(5), pp.1454-1459.

Sen, G.L.; Reuter, J.A.,; Webster, D.E.; Zhu, L.; Khavari, P.A. (2010). DNMT1 maintains progenitor function in self-renewing somatic tissue. *Nature* 2010 Vol.; 463(7280), pp. 563-567.

Shen, X. Mizuguchi, G.; Hamiche, A.; Wu, C. (2000). A chromatin remodelling complex involved in transcription and DNA processing. *Nature* Vol. 406(6795), pp. 541-544

Stankunas, K.; Berger, J.; Ruse, C.; Sinclair, D.A.; Randazzo, F.; Brock, H.W. (1998). The enhancer of polycomb gene of Drosophila encodes a chromatin protein conserved in yeast and mammals. *Development* Vol. 125(20), pp. 4055-4066.

Sung, Y.H.; Choi, E.Y.; Kwon, H. (2001). Identification of a nuclear protein ArpN as a component of human SWI/SNF complex and its selective association with a subset of active genes. *Mol Cells* Vol. 11(1), pp. 75-81.

Tominaga, K.; Kirtane, B.; Jackson, J.G.; Ikeno, Y.; Ikeda, T.; Hawks, C.; Smith, J.R.; Matzuk, M.M.; Pereira-Smith, O.M. (2005). MRG15 regulates embryonic development and cell proliferation. *Mol Cell Biol* Vol. 25(8), pp. 2924-2937.

Tondeleir, D.; Vandamme, D.; Vandekerckhove, J.; Ampe, C.; Lambrechts, A. (2009). Actin isoform expression patterns during mammalian development and in pathology: insights from mouse models. *Cell Motil Cytoskeleton* Vol. 66(10), pp.798-815

Ueda, T.; Watanabe-Fukunaga, R.; Ogawa, H.; Fukuyama, H.; Higashi, Y.; Nagata, S.; Fukunaga, R. (2007). Critical role of the p400/mDomino chromatin-remodeling ATPase in embryonic hematopoiesis. *Genes Cells* Vol. 12(5), pp. 581-592.

Ullah, M.; Pelletier, N.; Xiao, L.; Zhao, S.P.; Wang, K.; Degerny, C.; Tahmasebi, S.; Cayrou, C.; Doyon, Y.; Goh, S.L.; Champagne, N.; Côté, J.; Yang, X.J. (2008). Molecular architecture of quartet MOZ/MORF histone acetyltransferase complexes. *Mol Cell Biol* Vol. 28(22), pp.6828-6843.

Wang, Y.; Dai, D.L.; Martinka, M.; Li, G. (2007). Prognostic significance of nuclear ING3 expression in human cutaneous melanoma. *Clin Cancer Res* Vol. 13(14), pp. 4111-4116.

Wei, X.; Walia, V.; Lin, J.C.; Teer, J.K.; Prickett, T.D.; Gartner, J.; Davis, S.; NISC Comparative Sequencing Program; Stemke-Hale, K.; Davies, M.A.; Gershenwald, J. E.; Robinson, W.; Robinson, S.; Rosenberg, S.A.; Samuels, Y. (2011). Exome sequencing identifies GRIN2A as frequently mutated in melanoma. *Nat Genet* Vol. 43(5), pp. 442-446.

Wu, W.H.; Alami, S.; Luk, E.; Wu, C.H.; Sen, S.; Mizuguchi, G.; Wei, D.; Wu, C. (2005). Swc2 is a widely conserved H2AZ-binding module essential for ATP-dependent histone exchange. *Nat Struct Mol Biol* Vol. 12(12), pp. 1064-1071.

Wurdak, H.; Zhu, S.; Romero, A.; Lorger, M.; Watson, J.; Chiang, C.Y.; Zhang, J.; Natu, V.S.; Lairson, L.L.; Walker, J.R.; Trussell, C.M.; Harsh, G.R.; Vogel, H.; Felding-Habermann, B.; Orth, A.P.; Miraglia, L.J.; Rines, D.R.; Skirboll, S.L.; Schultz, P.G. (2010). An RNAi screen identifies TRRAP as a regulator of brain tumor-initiating cell differentiation. *Cell Stem Cell* Vol. 6(1), pp. 37-47.

Yamada, H.Y.; Gorbsky, G.J. (2006) Cell-based expression cloning for identification of polypeptides that hypersensitize mammalian cells to mitotic arrest. *Biol Proced Online.* Vol. 8, pp.36-43.

Yamada, H.Y.; Rao, C.V. (2009). BRD8 is a potential chemosensitizing target for spindle poisons in colorectal cancer therapy. *Int J Oncol* Vol. 35(5), pp.1101-1109.

Yamaguchi, K.; Sakai, M.; Shimokawa, T.; Yamada, Y.; Nakamura, Y.; Furukawa, Y. (2010). C20orf20 (MRG-binding protein) as a potential therapeutic target for colorectal cancer.*Br J Cancer* Vol. 102(2), pp.325-31.

Yamaguchi, K.; Sakai, M.; Kim, J.; Tsunesumi, S.; Fujii, T.; Ikenoue, T.; Yamada, Y.; Akiyama, Y.; Muto, Y.; Yamaguchi, R.; Miyano, S.; Nakamura, Y.; Furukawa, Y. (2011). MRG-binding protein contributes to colorectal cancer development. *Cancer Sci* Vol. 102(8), pp.1486-1492.

Yuan, C.X.; Ito, M.; Fondell, J.D.; Fu, Z.Y.; Roeder, R.G. (1998). The TRAP220 component of a thyroid hormone receptor- associated protein (TRAP) coactivator complex interacts directly with nuclear receptors in a ligand-dependent fashion. *Proc Natl Acad Sci U S A* Vol. 95(14), pp. 7939-7944

Zeng L.; Zhou, M.M. (2002). Bromodomain: an acetyl-lysine binding domain. *FEBS Lett* Vol. 513(1), pp. 124-128.

Zhan, F.; Barlogie, B.; Arzoumanian, V.; Huang, Y.; Williams, D.R.; Hollmig, K.; Pineda-Roman, M.; Tricot, G.; van Rhee, F.; Zangari, M.; Dhodapkar, M. Shaughnessy Jr., J.D. (2007). Gene-expression signature of benign monoclonal gammopathy evident in multiple myeloma is linked to good prognosis. *Blood* Vol. 109, pp. 1692–1700.

Zhang, H.; Richardson, D.O.; Roberts, D.N.; Utley, R.; Erdjument-Bromage, H.; Tempst, P.; Côté, J, Cairns, B.R. (2004). The Yaf9 component of the SWR1 and NuA4 complexes is required for proper gene expression, histone H4 acetylation, and Htz1 replacement near telomeres. *Mol Cell Biol* Vol. 24(21), pp. 9424-9436.

Zhao, K.; Wang, W.; Rando, O.J.; Xue, Y.; Swiderek, K.; Kuo, A.; Crabtree, G.R. (1998). Rapid and phosphoinositol-dependent binding of the SWI/SNF-like BAF complex to chromatin after T lymphocyte receptor signaling. *Cell* Vol. 95(5), pp. 625-636.

7

Molecular Mechanisms
of Lymphatic Metastasis

M.C. Langheinrich[1], V. Schellerer[1], K. Oeckl[1],
M. Stürzl[2], E. Naschberger[2] and R.S. Croner[1]
[1]Department of Surgery, University Hospital Erlangen,
[2]Division of Molecular and Experimental Surgery, Department of Surgery,
University Hospital Erlangen,
Germany

1. Introduction

Colorectal cancer (CRC) is the third most common cancer worldwide. Considering the high rate of incidence and mortality of CRC it is critical to determine the mechanisms of its dissemination. Although one of the better characterised tumours the prognosis of patients decreases dramatically when lymphatic metastasis occurs. In addition, the main important prognostic factor of CRC is the stage of tumour at the time of diagnosis, which is defined by the TNM system from the American Joint Committee on Cancer and the International Union Against Cancer. Therefore, during surgical treatment not only the primary tumour but also the draining lymph nodes have to be removed. From multivariate analysis it is known, that the number of examined lymph nodes is an independent prognostic factor. In this context, a prognostic relevance has been demonstrated not only for N0-, but also for N1- and N2-status. Adjuvant chemotherapy is recommended for stage UICC III colon cancer. It has been shown to reduce tumour recurrence and improve overall survival (Schmiegel, Reinacher-Schick et al. 2008). The five-year survival rate drops significantly from the UICC stage I to IV (Table 1). Patients with an early stage tumour (UICC I) have an excellent prognosis and a five-year survival rate of 90%, compared to those with advanced tumours and lymph node metastasis, who have a five-year survival rate of 30-60%. Patients with distant metastasis have a five-year survival rate below 10%.

Thus the prognosis of CRC is significantly influenced by the occurrence of lymph node metastasis and in addition to its value as a prognostic indicator it also affects the therapeutically management of patients. The understanding of molecular mechanisms involved in lymphatic metastases may open the door for future treatment strategies.

2. The lymphatic system

2.1 Development of the lymphatic system

Aspects of the lymphatic fluid and the associated transport system were already mentioned by the ancient Greeks, but it was poorly considered until the 17th century. In 1622 the Italian physician Gasparo Asselli re-identified lymphatic vessels as "milky veins" in the gut of a

Stage			5-year survival rate
UICC	TNM	Dukes	
I a	T1N0M0	A	>90%
b	T2N0M0		
II a	T3N0M0	B	60-80%
b	T4N0M0		
III a	T1/2N1M0	C	30-60%
b	T3/4N1M0		
c	T1-4N2M0		
IV	T1-4N1-2M1	D	<10%

Table 1. UICC stage and 5-year cancer related survival of patients with CRC.

dog. The embryonic origin of lymphatic vessels remains further unclear. Since the beginning of the 20th century, two developmental theories -the centrifugal and the centripetal- have been controversial debated. The centrifugal theory by Sabin based upon dye and ink injection experiments in pigs. According to her view, lymphatic vessel formation occurs early during embryonic development from isolated primitive lymph sacs that originate from endothelial cells that bud from the veins. The peripheral lymphatic system originates from these primary lymph sacs by endothelial sprouting into the surrounding tissues and organs, where local capillaries are formed (Oliver and Detmar 2002). Simultaneously Huntington and McClure suggested an alternative model, the centripetal theory. In their opinion primary lymph sacs arise from mesenchymal precursor cells, independent of the veins and secondarily establish venous connections.

To date, the development of the lymphatic vasculature system has not been ultimately resolved. Recent molecular analyses describe a polarized expression of the homeobox transcription factor Prox-1 in anterior cardinal vein endothelial cells, which is required for specification of lymphatic endothelial cells (LECs). Prox-1 is a master regulator which drives the transcription of a variety of genes whose expression is associated with key LEC characteristics (Tammela, Petrova et al. 2005).

2.2 Structure and function of the lymphatic system

The lymphatic vascular system is a hierarchical network comprising blind-ended capillaries, collecting vessels, lymph nodes, lymphoid organs and circulation lymphocytes. A number of important physiological functions have been described. It maintains fluid homeostasis by absorbing and draining e.g. interstitial fluids, plasma proteins and cells extravasated from blood vessels and returning them back into the blood circulation (Butler, Isogai et al. 2009). Furthermore, the lymphatic system is also known to be an important part of the body´s immunological surveillance system (Wiig, Keskin et al. 2010). Lymphatic vessels are distributed to most organs, with the exceptions of the central nervous system, bone marrow, cartilage, cornea and epidermis. Due to its dual role, fluid absorption and lymph transport, the structure of lymphatic vessels differ from blood vessels (Schulte-Merker, Sabine et al.

2011). Lymph capillaries are characterized by loose intercellular junctions, no or an incomplete basement membrane. The wall of lymphatic endothelial cells (LECs) is joined to the extracellular matrix by anchoring filaments. These filaments help the vessels open and function. Collecting lymphatic vessels consist of pericytes, which reduce lymphatic fluid extravasation and they are surrounded by smooth muscle cells (Figure 1) (Shayan, Achen et al. 2006).

Tumour cells can take advantage of these structural characteristics to promote their dissemination to lymph nodes or other organs by the process of permeation into peritumoural lymphatics. In addition, LECs secrete chemotactic agents, which can attract tumours cells toward lymphatics, such as CCL21, whose receptor (CCR7) is expressed on some tumour cells (Shields, Emmett et al. 2007). Chemokines may mediate the tumour LEC interaction by increasing the interactive surface area (Ji 2006).

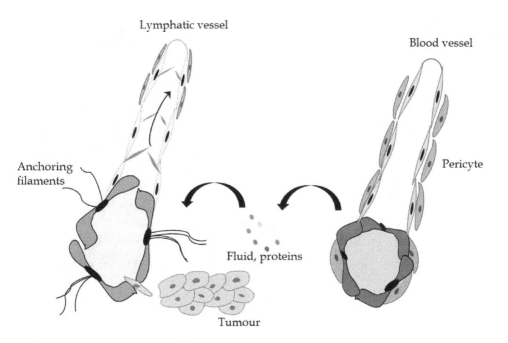

Fig. 1. Structure of lymphatic vessels compared against blood vessels. The initial lymphatics have no or an incomplete basement membrane and no pericytes, which makes them suitable for the uptake of tumour cells. Anchoring filaments attach LECs to the extracellular matrix (ECM) and prevent vessel collapse.

Gene expression profiles of LECs and blood endothelial cells (BECs) have been analysed and compared (Figure 2). The most obvious differences were detected in genes coding for pro-inflammatory cytokines/chemokines and their receptors, cytoskeletal and cell matrix organisation (Saharinen, Tammela et al. 2004). For example Interleukin (IL)-8, IL-6, the chemokine receptor CXCR4, ICAM-1, Integrin α5 are expressed in higher levels in the BECs.

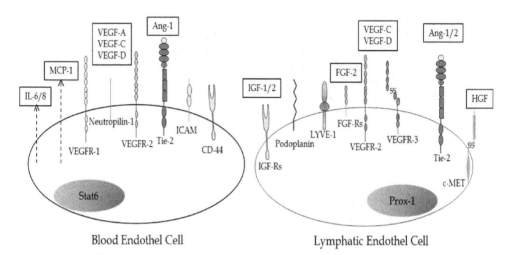

Blood Endothel Cell　　　　　　　　　　　　　Lymphatic Endothel Cell

Abbreviations: Stat6 (signal transducer and activator of transcription 6), MCP-1 (monocyte chemotactic protein-1), IL-6/8 (Interleukin-6/-8), ICAM (intracellular adhesion molecule), Ang-1 (Angiopoietin-1), VEGF/ R (Vascular endothelial growth factor/receptor), CD-44 (Cluster of Differentiation 44), IGF-1/2 (Insulin like growth factor 1/2), FGF-2 (Fibroblast growth factor 2), HGF (Hepatocyte growth factor), c-MET (mesenchymal epithelial transition factor), Tie-2 (angiopoietin receptor 2). Note that not all molecular markers are shown.

Fig. 2. Molecular characteristics of BECs and LECs.

3. Lymphangiogenesis

3.1 Lymphangiogenesis and cancer metastasis

Lymphangiogenesis takes place in a variety of physiological and pathophysiological processes, such as embryonic development, regeneration and wound healing on the one hand, and in lymph vascular malformations, inflammation and cancer on the other hand (Witte, Jones et al. 2006). Carcinogenesis is a complex multi-step process and despite the importance, that the lymphatic system provided one of the main routes for cancer progression, little information has been available about the molecular mechanisms by which the tumour cells gain access to the lymph system and are able to spread.

Traditionally, lymphatic metastasis of tumours was considered to be a passive process, where tumour cells metastasized to lymph nodes by utilizing pre-existing lymphatic vessels via open junctions or that lymphatic vessel entry occurred by tumour eroding. The process of new lymphatic formation (lymphangiogenesis) does not occur.

This view has been challenged (Achen and Stacker 2008). The identification of lymphatic specific markers, lymphangiogenic growth factors and their ligand receptor pathways, the isolation of lymphatic endothelial cells and the development of specific in vitro culture systems in the past decades led to a broader understanding of the molecular mechanisms that control lymphatic metastasis.

Yet there is mounting evidence that lymphangiogenesis does occur in tumours and that it promotes cancer progression. A shift in the balance between lymphangiogenic and anti-lymphangiogenic signalling, like in the process of angiogenesis, might lead to lymphangiogenesis. Therefore a wide range of interactions at the tumour host interface have to take place, which support tumour proliferation, migration and survival. These processes are controlled by growth factors, adhesion molecules, fibroblasts, blood vessels, cytokines and chemo attractants (Figure 3) (Cueni and Detmar 2006; Ji 2006). In the following section the most widely studied molecular mediators of lymphangiogenesis are reviewed.

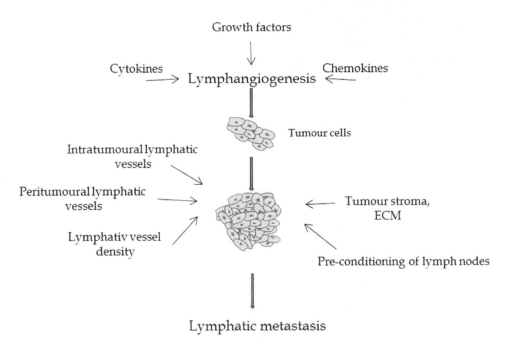

Fig. 3. Schematic overview of processes involved in tumour lymphangiogenesis and metastasis. Growth factors, cytokines, chemokines and tumour stroma contributes to tumour formation, growth, lymphangiogenesis and cancer progress. The tumour stroma consists of fibroblasts, ECM (extracellular matrix), blood vessels, lymphatic vessels and immune cells.

3.2 Molecular players in tumour lymphangiogenesis
3.2.1 Vascular endothelial growth factor

The human VEGF family of growth factors includes VEGF-A, -B, -C, -D and placental growth factor (PIGF). They bind with different specificity to three tyrosine kinase receptors: VEGFR-1 (fms-like tyrosine kinase 1), VEGFR-2 (human kinase insert domain receptor),

VEGFR-3 (fms-like tyrosine kinase 4) and two non-protein kinase co-receptors (neuropilin-1 and neuropilin-2). All VEGFRs have an extracellular binding region containing seven immunoglobulin-like domains (excepted VEGFR-3 who has only 6 domains), a single transmembrane helix and a conserved cytoplasmic domain that contains the catalytic core and regulatory sequences (Lohela, Bry et al. 2009). Activation of VEGFR by its ligands leads to receptor dimerization, autophosphorylation of tyrosine residues and initiation of signalling pathways (Roskoski 2008).

VEGF-C, VEGF-D and their ligand VEGFR-3 were the first discovered and most exensively studied lymphangiogenic factors (Baldwin et al. 2002; Nagy et al. 2002). After activation of VEGFR-3 by its ligands, autophosphorylation of tyrosine residues results in binding of the signalling adaptor proteins Shc (adaptor protein p66), Grb-2 (growth factor receptor-bound protein) and in activation of the ERK 1/2 (extracellular signal regulated kinase) signal transduction cascade in a protein kinase C dependent manner and via PI3K-Akt (phosphatidylinositol 3-kinase protein kinase B) signalling cascade (Figure 4). Binding of the adaptor protein CRK 1/2 initiates the MKK4-JNK 1/2 (mitogen-activated protein kinase kinase 4- Jun N-terminal kinase) pathway and results in induction of c-JNK (c-Jun N-terminal kinase) expression. The VEGFR-3 pathway mediates lymph endothelial growth, survival and migration (Wissmann and Detmar 2006).

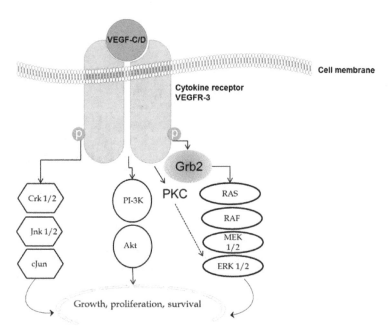

Fig. 4. The VEGF-C and VEGF-D pathways via VEGFR-3. Proteolytic processing, signal adaptor binding and activation of downstream signalling molecules results in lymph endothelial growth, proliferation and survival.

There are several studies, which suggested a correlation between the expression level of VEGF-C and lymph node metastasis (LNM) in e.g. CRC, gastric, prostate, esophageal and lung cancers (Achen and Stacker 2008). The mechanisms regulating the VEGF-C/VEGF-D expression in tumours are not fully revealed. It is known, that pro-inflammatory cytokines such as tumour necrosis factor (TNF) and Interleukins induce the expression of VEGF-C in tumour cells. The local ECM environment is assumed to trigger different VEGF receptors, resulting in signalling pathways which promote lymphangiogenesis.

In fact, the results of some studies showed that the expression levels of VEGF-D and VEGFR-3 in colorectal carcinoma tissues are significantly higher than in normal tissues (Omachi, Kawai et al. 2007). Furthermore, recent reports have linked the VEGF-C/VEGF-D expression to lymphatic metastasis and poor patient outcome (Nagahashi, Ramachandran et al. 2010; Lin, Lin et al. 2011). Our histopathological examination also revealed that VEGF-C was present in CRC tissue, whereas the surrounding tissue was negative.

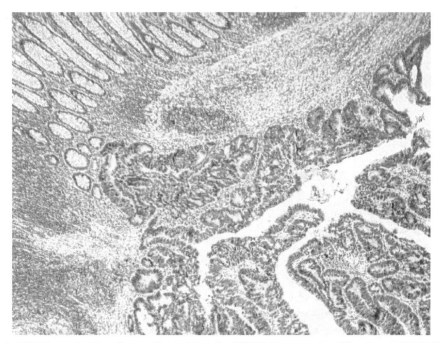

Fig. 5. CRC immunohistochemically staining for VEGF-C expression. The strong VEGF-C expression appears in the colon carcinoma tissue, while the surrounding tissue is negative.

VEGF-A is associated with angiogenesis, but it may also contribute to lymphangiogenesis. During angiogenesis VEGF-A induces proliferation and migration of endothelial cells, protease production and promotes cell survival. Fibroblasts, macrophages and endothelial cells are cells in the tumour microenvironment which are known to secrete VEGF-A. Evidence indicates that transforming growth factor α (TGFα) plays a role in regulating VEGF-A expression. The biological activity of VEGF-A is mainly mediated direct via activating of VEGFR-2 and indirectly by recruiting monocytes and neutrophils, which express VEGFR-1 and produce VEGF-C/VEGF-D.

A number of reports describe in CRC a correlation between VEGF-A expression levels and lymph node metastasis (Sundlisaeter, Dicko et al. 2007).

3.2.2 Prox-1

Prox-1 is a homeobox transcription factor. In several tissues, such as liver and pancreas Prox-1 is an important regulator of cell differentiation and oncogenesis. As mentioned before, the expression of Prox-1 is also essential for the lymphatic development and downstream signalling results in up-regulation of e.g. LYVE-1, VEGFR-3 and other lymphatic endothelial specific molecules.

Prox-1 expression is revealed to be significantly increased in CRC (Parr and Jiang 2003). The precise function must be further clarified.

3.2.3 Podoplanin

Podoplanin is a 38-kDa single transmembrane mucin-type glycoprotein and in normal human tissue it is expressed e.g. by osteoblasts, kidney podocytes and lung alveolar type 1 cells (Cueni, Hegyi et al. 2010). Due to its expression on lymphatic endothelial cells but not on blood vessels it is used as a specific marker for LECs.

Under normal conditions podoplanin is involved in the regulation of the shape of podocytes, LV formation and it is supposed to be involved in platelet aggregation. The expression of podoplanin is regulated by Prox-1 (Raica, Cimpean et al. 2008).

Since podoplanin expression is up-regulated in a number of different carcinomas such as vascular tumours, mesotheliomas and in squamous cell carcinomas, it is suggested that podoplanin is involved in carcinogenesis (Yamanashi et al. 2009). In addition, recent data in numerous of squamous cell carcinomas indicated that podoplanin is expressed at the invasive edge (Wicki and Christofori 2007). Podoplanin might favour tumour invasion via

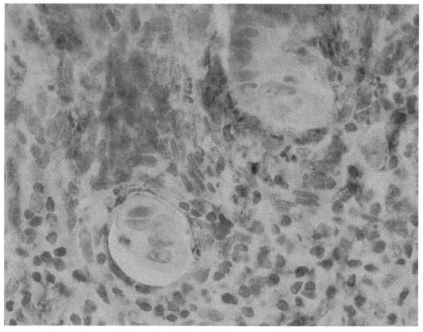

Fig. 6. Immunohistochemical detection of podoplanin positive lymphatic vessels, filled with cancer cells, in CRC.

its ability to remodel the cytoskeleton (Cueni, Hegyi et al. 2010). About the role of podoplanin in CRC little information is available. Lu et al. revealed, that the expression of podoplanin was significantly higher in patients with lymph node metastasis than in those without metastasis (Lu, Yang et al. 2007). While the group of Yamanashi suggested, that a positive podoplanin expression in stromal fibroblasts in patients with CRC is a significant indicator for a good prognosis (Yamanashi, Nakanishi et al. 2009). Figure 6 shows a lymphatic vessel stained with podoplanin and filled with a tumour cell embolus

3.2.4 LYVE-1

LYVE-1 is a homologue of the blood vascular endothelium specific hyaluronan receptor CD 44 and accordingly a member of the Link protein family. CD44 is directly involved in leucocyte migration (Jackson 2009). Lyve-1 is one of the most specific and widely used lymphatic endothelial markers (Hirakawa 2011). During embryogenesis it is expressed in cardinal vein endothelium and is involved in vascular development. On LECs LYVE-1 is expressed on the luminal and ab-luminal surface and functional studies demonstrated that it is able to act as an endocytic receptor for hyaluronan (Al-Rawi, Mansel et al. 2005). Hyaluronan is an important component of the extracellular matrix with versatile features for the interaction of cells during embryogenesis and woundhealing. LYVE-1 is also expressed by sinusoidal endothelial cells in the liver, spleen and by macrophages. Its exact function remains unclear.

3.2.5 Hepatocyte growth factor

Hepatocyte growth factor (HGF) belongs to the plasminogen-prothrombin gene superfamily. C-Met, the HGF receptor is a tyrosine kinase receptor and composed of an extracellular α chain and a transmembrane β chain. HGF activity has been reported to play a role in embryogenesis and organogenesis (Lee et al. 2010).

HGF is also supposed to be a potent lymphangiogenic factor. In this context HGF is involved in proliferation, migration, and tube formation of LECs (Cueni and Detmar 2006). The HGF downstream pathway is mediated via ERK 1/2 and PI3K and resulted in cell growth and inhibition of apoptosis. In many solid tumours c-Met is differently expressed. Novel investigations in CRC revealed an over expression of HGF and c-Met, and increased expression is associated with advanced disease stage and poor outcome (Kammula, Kuntz et al. 2007; Organ, Tong et al. 2011).

3.2.6 Fibroblast growth factors

The fibroblast growth factor family consists of structurally related ligands and four receptors (FGFR-1, FGFR-2, FGFR-3, FGFR-4), which consist the classical receptor tyrosine kinase structure: a extracellular Immunglobulin-like domain, a transmembrane domain and a intracellular tyrosine kinase domain, which initiated downstream signalling. The FGFs are involved in multi biological processes such as proliferation, survival, migration and differentiation during organogenesis and in adult life. A deregulation in human cancer has been found e.g. in breast cancer, prostate cancer, bladder cancer and cancer of the lung (Wesche, Haglund et al. 2011). FGF-2 is able to induce angiogenesis and lymphangiogenesis. Recent studies suggest that in LECs lymphangiogenic signalling is mediated through the

Akt-mammalian target of rapamycin (mTOR)-p70S6 kinase pathway (Matsuo, Yamada et al. 2007).

3.2.7 Angiopoietins

Ang-1 and Ang-2 are the more intensive analysed members of the angiopoietin family. Both bind to the Tie-2 receptor, which is expressed on the surface of LECs. The expression of Ang-1 and Ang-2 differs in human tissue. While Ang-1 is widely expressed in adult tissues, where it promotes vessel maturation and stabilization, Ang-2 expression occurs during vascular remodelling and via acting in conjugation with VEGF-A Ang-2 is supposed to be a stimulator of angiogenesis (Makinen, Norrmen et al. 2007).

About the role and function of the angiopoietins Ang-1/Ang-2 in lymphangiogenesis little information is known. Ang-1 is involved in LEC proliferation and lymphatic vessel sprouting. From analysis of pancreatic cancer, we know that Ang-2 drives lymphatic metastasis via a Tie-2 dependent manner and in a Tie-2 independent manner through enhancing the capacity of tumour cells for adherence to endothelial cells (Schulz, Fischer et al. 2011).

3.2.8 Insulin like growth factors

The insulin like growth factor system consists of the ligands insulin, insulin like growth factor 1 (IGF-1) and insulin like growth factor 2 (IGF-2) and acts via four receptors: the insulin receptor (IR), the type I IGF receptor, the type II IGF receptor and the hybrid IR/IGF-1R receptor. The IGF-IR receptor consists of two α and two β chains. IGF-IR ligand binding induces multiple downstream signal transduction pathways such as the MAPK, ERK and PI3-K pathway. It is well known, that IGF family members are frequently expressed in many solid tumours like CRC and breast cancer (Werner, Roberts et al. 1996; Reinmuth, Liu et al. 2002). In addition IGF-1R contributes to cancer development by regulation cell proliferation, differentiation and by preventing apoptosis. Other researchers investigated that IGF-1 and IGF-2 induce lymphangiogenesis (Bjorndahl, Cao et al. 2005) in a VEGFR-3 independent signalling pathway.

3.2.9 Chemokines

The chemokines, are a super family of chemotactic cytokines. They are key regulators of leukocyte, endothelial and epithelial cell migration and play a functional role in embryogenesis. Chemokines are low molecular weight proteins with cysteins at well conserved domains. According to the position of the cystein residue 4 chemokine subfamilies (CXC, CXC$_3$, CC, C) have been identified so far. The chemokine CXCL12 is supposed to be involved in lymphogenesis via its receptor CXCR4 and CCL21 mediates homing of lymphocytes and migration of dendritic cells into lymphatic vessel.

Nonetheless, it has been reported that chemokines and their receptors are expressed in a variety of human cancers such as melanoma, breast cancer, gastric cancer or prostate cancer (Hoon, Kitago et al. 2006). Recent findings about the direct role of chemokines in LNM in CRC, suggested an involvement of CXCR3, CXCL12/CXCR4 and CCL21/CCR7 (Kawada and Taketo 2011; Singh et al. 2011; Raman et al. 2010). In addition CXCL12 is supposed to be a prognostic factor for local recurrence and liver metastasis and CXCR4 expression was significantly positive in CRCs with high tumour stage and LNM.

Taken together, Table 2 summarizes factors which are involved in lymphangiogenesis.

Factor	Function during lymphangiogenesis
VEGF-C/VEGF-D via VEGFR-3	Growth factor/receptor: proliferation, migration, survival
VEGF-A via VEGFR-2	Activating VEGF-C/VEGF-D/VEGFR-3 signaling pathway
Prox-1	Transcription factor: LEC identity
Podoplanin	Cell motility
LYVE-1	Hyaluronan receptor
HGF	Growth factor: proliferation, migration, tube formation of LECs
FGF	LEC migration, proliferation
Ang-1/2	Growth factor
IGF	Growth factor: proliferation, differentiation and preventing apoptosis
Chemokines CCL21	Lymphocytes homing

Table 2. Molecules which are involved in lymphangiogenesis

3.3 Lymphatic vessel density and tumour progression

Since, microvessel density (MVD), a parameter for the ability of angiogenesis in tumours, is a prognostic marker in numerous cancers, the quantification of lymphatic vessel density (LVD) is of growing interest. Screening the literature, the prognostic significance of LVD in tumours remains controversial (Royston and Jackson 2009). Some studies reported that high LVD was associated with lymph node metastasis and patient outcome, while others could not confirm these findings (Gao, Knutsen et al. 2009). Furthermore, there is a debate about the dominant role of intratumoural vs. peitumoural lymphatic vessels. By some researchers it has been demonstrated that LVD in the intratumoural areas but not in peritumoural areas were associated with lymph node metastasis and poor outcome. Others reported that LVD in peritumoural areas was correlated to advanced tumour stage (Longatto-Filho, Pinheiro et al. 2008). In patients with colorectal cancer, a significant correlation between the number of intratumoural and peritumoural lymphatic vessels with the occurrence of lymph node metastases was evaluated (Matsumoto, Nakayama et al. 2007). These findings again underline the hypothesis of active lymphatic vessel formation within the tumour. These new lymphatic vessels may facilitate the drainage of tumour cells to regional lymph nodes.

3.4 Future perspectives

Further characterization of the exact molecular pathways which are involved in lymphatic metastasis is needed and essential for the development of new forecast estimates and individually oriented therapies. Gene expression profiling by microarray technique, which allows the investigation of thousands of differentially expressed genes, provide therefore a promising tool to further clarify the molecular signature for lymphatic metastasis in CRC. These signatures can provide new players which are responsible for lymphatic metastasis or identify patients with a high risk for the development of lymph node metastases. New treatment targets could be evaluated and high risk patients can be selected for individual treatment regiments. (Croner, Peters et al. 2005; Croner, Fortsch et al. 2008; Croner, Schellerer et al. 2010).

4. Conclusion

Metastasis via tumour cell invasion into lymphatic vessels and lymph nodes is a common feature of various carcinomas. Our knowledge of the mechanisms controlling lymphatic metastasis has increased significantly in the last decades since the identification of LEC specific markers such as LYVE-1, podoplanin and Prox-1. The visualisation of the lymphatic system led to a new understanding of tumour activities involved in lymphatic vessel differentiation and growth. Take together, lymphangiogenesis is a complex multi step process, which is regulated by numerous molecular players and additional studies are needed to devise new and more efficient strategies against CRC.

5. References

Achen, M. G. and S. A. Stacker (2008). "Molecular control of lymphatic metastasis." Ann N Y Acad Sci 1131: 225-234.

Al-Rawi, M. A., R. E. Mansel, et al. (2005). "Lymphangiogenesis and its role in cancer." Histol Histopathol 20(1): 283-298.

Bjorndahl, M., R. Cao, et al. (2005). "Insulin-like growth factors 1 and 2 induce lymphangiogenesis in vivo." Proc Natl Acad Sci U S A 102(43): 15593-15598.

Butler, M. G., S. Isogai, et al. (2009). "Lymphatic development." Birth Defects Res C Embryo Today 87(3): 222-231.

Croner, R. S., T. Fortsch, et al. (2008). "Molecular signature for lymphatic metastasis in colorectal carcinomas." Ann Surg 247(5): 803-810.

Croner, R. S., A. Peters, et al. (2005). "Microarray versus conventional prediction of lymph node metastasis in colorectal carcinoma." Cancer 104(2): 395-404.

Croner, R. S., V. Schellerer, et al. (2010). "One step nucleic acid amplification (OSNA) - a new method for lymph node staging in colorectal carcinomas." J Transl Med 8: 83.

Cueni, L. N. and M. Detmar (2006). "New insights into the molecular control of the lymphatic vascular system and its role in disease." J Invest Dermatol 126(10): 2167-2177.

Cueni, L. N., I. Hegyi, et al. (2010). "Tumor lymphangiogenesis and metastasis to lymph nodes induced by cancer cell expression of podoplanin." Am J Pathol 177(2): 1004-1016.

Gao, J., A. Knutsen, et al. (2009). "Clinical and biological significance of angiogenesis and lymphangiogenesis in colorectal cancer." Dig Liver Dis 41(2): 116-122.

Hirakawa, S. (2011). "Regulation of pathological lymphangiogenesis requires factors distinct from those governing physiological lymphangiogenesis." J Dermatol Sci 61(2): 85-93.

Hoon, D. S., M. Kitago, et al. (2006). "Molecular mechanisms of metastasis." Cancer Metastasis Rev 25(2): 203-220.

Jackson, D. G. (2009). "Immunological functions of hyaluronan and its receptors in the lymphatics." Immunol Rev 230(1): 216-231.

Ji, R. C. (2006). "Lymphatic endothelial cells, lymphangiogenesis, and extracellular matrix." Lymphat Res Biol 4(2): 83-100.

Ji, R. C. (2006). "Lymphatic endothelial cells, tumor lymphangiogenesis and metastasis: New insights into intratumoral and peritumoral lymphatics." Cancer Metastasis Rev 25(4): 677-694.

Kammula, U. S., E. J. Kuntz, et al. (2007). "Molecular co-expression of the c-Met oncogene and hepatocyte growth factor in primary colon cancer predicts tumor stage and clinical outcome." Cancer Lett 248(2): 219-228.

Lin, M., H. Z. Lin, et al. (2011). "Vascular endothelial growth factor-A and -C: expression and correlations with lymphatic metastasis and prognosis in colorectal cancer." Med Oncol 28(1): 151-158.

Lohela, M., M. Bry, et al. (2009). "VEGFs and receptors involved in angiogenesis versus lymphangiogenesis." Curr Opin Cell Biol 21(2): 154-165.

Longatto-Filho, A., C. Pinheiro, et al. (2008). "Peritumoural, but not intratumoural, lymphatic vessel density and invasion correlate with colorectal carcinoma poor-outcome markers." Virchows Arch 452(2): 133-138.

Lu, Y., Q. Yang, et al. (2007). "Expression analysis of lymphangiogenic factors in human colorectal cancer with quantitative RT-PCR." Cancer Invest 25(6): 393-396.

Makinen, T., C. Norrmen, et al. (2007). "Molecular mechanisms of lymphatic vascular development." Cell Mol Life Sci 64(15): 1915-1929.

Matsumoto, K., Y. Nakayama, et al. (2007). "Lymphatic microvessel density is an independent prognostic factor in colorectal cancer." Dis Colon Rectum 50(3): 308-314.

Matsuo, M., S. Yamada, et al. (2007). "Tumour-derived fibroblast growth factor-2 exerts lymphangiogenic effects through Akt/mTOR/p70S6kinase pathway in rat lymphatic endothelial cells." Eur J Cancer 43(11): 1748-1754.

Nagahashi, M., S. Ramachandran, et al. (2010). "Lymphangiogenesis: a new player in cancer progression." World J Gastroenterol 16(32): 4003-4012.

Oliver, G. and M. Detmar (2002). "The rediscovery of the lymphatic system: old and new insights into the development and biological function of the lymphatic vasculature." Genes Dev 16(7): 773-783.

Omachi, T., Y. Kawai, et al. (2007). "Immunohistochemical demonstration of proliferating lymphatic vessels in colorectal carcinoma and its clinicopathological significance." Cancer Lett 246(1-2): 167-172.

Organ, S. L., J. Tong, et al. (2011). "Quantitative Phospho-Proteomic Profiling of Hepatocyte Growth Factor (HGF)-MET Signaling in Colorectal Cancer." J Proteome Res 10(7): 3200-3211.

Parr, C. and W. G. Jiang (2003). "Quantitative analysis of lymphangiogenic markers in human colorectal cancer." Int J Oncol 23(2): 533-539.

Raica, M., A. M. Cimpean, et al. (2008). "The role of podoplanin in tumor progression and metastasis." Anticancer Res 28(5B): 2997-3006.

Reinmuth, N., W. Liu, et al. (2002). "Blockade of insulin-like growth factor I receptor function inhibits growth and angiogenesis of colon cancer." Clin Cancer Res 8(10): 3259-3269.

Royston, D. and D. G. Jackson (2009). "Mechanisms of lymphatic metastasis in human colorectal adenocarcinoma." J Pathol 217(5): 608-619.

Saharinen, P., T. Tammela, et al. (2004). "Lymphatic vasculature: development, molecular regulation and role in tumor metastasis and inflammation." Trends Immunol 25(7): 387-395.

Schmiegel, W., A. Reinacher-Schick, et al. (2008). "[Update S3-guideline "colorectal cancer" 2008]." Z Gastroenterol 46(8): 799-840.

Schulte-Merker, S., A. Sabine, et al. (2011). "Lymphatic vascular morphogenesis in development, physiology, and disease." J Cell Biol 193(4): 607-618.

Schulz, P., C. Fischer, et al. (2011). "Angiopoietin-2 drives lymphatic metastasis of pancreatic cancer." FASEB J.

Shayan, R., M. G. Achen, et al. (2006). "Lymphatic vessels in cancer metastasis: bridging the gaps." Carcinogenesis 27(9): 1729-1738.

Shields, J. D., M. S. Emmett, et al. (2007). "Chemokine-mediated migration of melanoma cells towards lymphatics--a mechanism contributing to metastasis." Oncogene 26(21): 2997-3005.

Sundlisaeter, E., A. Dicko, et al. (2007). "Lymphangiogenesis in colorectal cancer--prognostic and therapeutic aspects." Int J Cancer 121(7): 1401-1409.

Tammela, T., T. V. Petrova, et al. (2005). "Molecular lymphangiogenesis: new players." Trends Cell Biol 15(8): 434-441.

Werner, H., C. T. Roberts, Jr., et al. (1996). "Regulation of insulin-like growth factor I receptor gene expression by the Wilms' tumor suppressor WT1." J Mol Neurosci 7(2): 111-123.

Wesche, J., K. Haglund, et al. (2011). "Fibroblast growth factors and their receptors in cancer." Biochem J 437(2): 199-213.

Wicki, A. and G. Christofori (2007). "The potential role of podoplanin in tumour invasion." Br J Cancer 96(1): 1-5.

Wiig, H., D. Keskin, et al. (2010). "Interaction between the extracellular matrix and lymphatics: consequences for lymphangiogenesis and lymphatic function." Matrix Biol 29(8): 645-656.

Wissmann, C. and M. Detmar (2006). "Pathways targeting tumor lymphangiogenesis." Clin Cancer Res 12(23): 6865-6868.

Witte, M. H., K. Jones, et al. (2006). "Structure function relationships in the lymphatic system and implications for cancer biology." Cancer Metastasis Rev 25(2): 159-184.

Yamanashi, T., Y. Nakanishi, et al. (2009). "Podoplanin expression identified in stromal fibroblasts as a favorable prognostic marker in patients with colorectal carcinoma." Oncology 77(1): 53-62.

8

Characterization of the Cell Membrane During Cancer Transformation

Barbara Szachowicz-Petelska[1], Izabela Dobrzyńska[1],
Stanisław Sulkowski[2] and Zbigniew A. Figaszewski[1,3]
[1]Institute of Chemistry, University in Bialystok,
[2]Department of General Pathomorphology, Medical University of Bialystok,
[3]Faculty of Chemistry, University of Warsaw,
Poland

1. Introduction

Colorectal cancer is one of the most common cancers diagnosed worldwide. The development of colorectal cancer, like many types of cancer is a multistage process that involves many different pathways. In particular, deregulation of cell-cell communication plays an important role. Moreover, cell-cell comunication is indispensable for the maintenance of homeostasis in a multicellular organism. *Gap*-type junctions are one of the most common and perhaps most interesting, mediators of intercellular communications. Digestive tract gap junctions are also important and are flanked by various cell types within each layer of the wall. The composition and organisation of gap junction channel subunits plays a critical role in determining the properties of these channels, including conductance properties and pH sensitivity. Structurally, gap junctions are composed of transmembrane proteins which form structures called connexons, with a single connexon consistings of six peripherally arranged subunits of integral membrane proteins known as connexins. Correspondingly, normal human epithelial cells in the colon have been found to express the connexins, Cx32 and Cx43. Moreover, in our previous studies Cx26 expression was detected in normal colon epithelium as well as in colorectal cancer tissues (Contreras et al., 2002, Cascio, 2005, van Zeijl et al., 2007).

A number of biological and chemical substances affect the function of gap junctions. For example junctions can be inhibited following the phosphorylation of connexin proteins or following exposure to agents that disrupt the accumulation of connexin or mediate local damage to cellular membranes. The function of membrane channels also require the presence of particular species of lipid in the surrounding membrane. Locke and Harris were the first to identify endogenous phospholipids tightly associated with connexin channels and these results suggested that specific phospholipids are associated with different connexin isoforms to form connexin-specific regulatory networks and/or structural interactions with lipid membranes. Ongoing studies of connexin channel function and cell biology to characterize lipid-protein interactions and membrane biophysics are providing valuable insight into these processes (Locke & Harris, 2009).

Phenomena associated with changes in cell membranes are suspected to play an important role during the cancer transformation. At physiological pH, the cell membrane surface is negatively charged, which is determined based on the number of negative and positive charge carriers present (i.e., phosphates, carboxyl and amino groups of proteins and phospholipids). Furthermore, electrical properties of a membrane are determined by acid-base and complex formation equilibria at the membrane and in response to surrounding medium components. For example, membrane components including – proteins, phospholipids, and free fatty acids contribute to this equilibria. Correspondingly, we hypothesis that the electrical charge of tumor cells can indirectly represent changes that have occurred during cell transformation and may indicate tumor cell status.

2. The cell membrane

Biological membranes are essential boundaries within a living cell. The cell membranes separate the interior of the cell from its microenvironment and also participate in intercellular communication.

2.1 Electric properties of cell membranes

For a biological membrane, its electrical charge and difference in potential between the membrane and surrounding solution are key properties. Cell membrane charge has been found to increase during tumorigenesis and decrease during necrosis (Dołowy, 1984). Correspondingly, investigations of factors that influence membrane electric charge during cancer transformation have been performed. These factors include determining pH, acidic (C_{TA}) and basic (C_{TB}) functional group concentrations and their average association constants with hydrogen (K_{AH}) or hydroxyl (K_{BOH}) ions (Dobrzyńska et al., 2006).

The electrical properties of a membrane are determined by acid-base and complex formation equilibria. Both membrane and surrounding medium components contribute to this equilibria, with the former including proteins, phospholipids and fatty acids (Gennis, 1989; Tien, 1974). As a result, we hypothesise that the electrical charge of tumor cells can be indirectly estimated from changes detected in tumor cells that are concomitant with their transformation during tumorigenesis.

2.1.1 Surface charge density cell membrane

Surface charge density dependence on pH of normal and tumor large intestine cell membrane are similarly shaped (Fig. 1). For example, an increase in positive surface charge density is observed at low pH values until a plateau is reached. Conversely, at high pH values, the proportion of negative charges present increases until it reaches a plateau. Overall, an increase in negative charge at low pH values as well as in positive charge at high pH is observed in human large intestine tumor cells compared to unaffected cells (Szachowicz-Petelska et al., 2002).

2.1.2 Theory

The dependence of surface charge density of a cell membrane on pH of electrolyte solution can be described according to four equilibria factors. Two equilibria concern negative groups and involve sodium and hydrogen ions, and two other equilibria refer to positive groups and involve hydroxide and chloride ions. These factors can then be expressed as follows written in the form:

$$A^- + H^+ \Leftrightarrow AH \tag{1}$$

$$A^- + Na^+ \Leftrightarrow ANa \tag{2}$$

$$B^+ + OH^- \Leftrightarrow BOH \tag{3}$$

$$B^+ + Cl^- \Leftrightarrow BCl \tag{4}$$

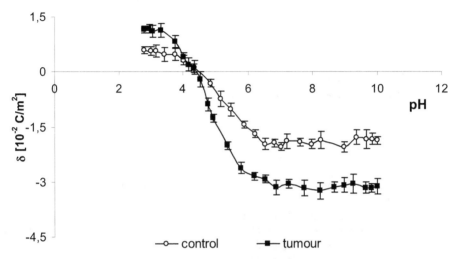

Fig. 1. The dependence of surface charge density on pH for normal and colorectal cancer cell membranes from several patients.

An association constant of the H^+ Na^+, OH^- and Cl^- ions with functional groups can be expressed according to the following equations:

$$K_{AH} = \frac{a_{AH}}{a_{A^-} \cdot a_{H^+}} \tag{5}$$

$$K_{ANa} = \frac{a_{ANa}}{a_{A^-} \cdot a_{Na^+}} \tag{6}$$

$$K_{BOH} = \frac{a_{BOH}}{a_{B^+} \cdot a_{OH^-}} \tag{7}$$

$$K_{BCl} = \frac{a_{BCl}}{a_{B^+} \cdot a_{Cl^-}} \tag{8}$$

Here:

K_{AH}, K_{ANa}, K_{BOH} and K_{BCl} represent association constants,

a_{A^-}, a_{AH}, a_{ANa}, a_{B^+}, a_{BOH} and a_{BCl} represent surface concentrations, that are present on the membrane surface,

and a_{H^+}, a_{Na^+}, a_{OH^-} and a_{Cl^-} represent corresponding concentrations in solution.

Surface charge density (δ) is expressed as follows:

$$\delta = (a_{B^+} - a_{A^-}) \cdot F \tag{9}$$

where F=96487 [C/mol] - Faraday constant.
And functional group concentration balances can be expressed as follows:

$$C_{TA} = a_{A^-} + a_{AH} + a_{ANa} \tag{10}$$

$$C_{TB} = a_{B^+} + a_{BOH} + a_{BCl} \tag{11}$$

where C_{TA} and C_{TB} represent the total surface concentrations functional groups.
Elimination of a_{A^-}, a_{AH}, a_{B^+}, and a_{BOH} values from above equations yields the following formula:

$$\frac{\delta}{F} = \frac{C_{TB} \cdot a_{H^+}}{a_{H^+}(1 + K_{BCl} \cdot a_{Cl^-}) + K_{BOH} \cdot K_w} - \frac{C_{TA}}{K_{AH} \cdot a_{H^+} + K_{ANa} \cdot a_{Na^+} + 1} \tag{12}$$

It is difficult to carry out the regression function of Eqn. (12) to determine the C_{TA}, C_{TB}, K_{AH} and K_{BOH} constants.
Simplifying to one fraction and making transformations described in this work (Dobrzyńska et al., 2006), we can receive the equation of a straight line for high and low ion concentration H^+, from which C_{TA}, C_{TB}, K_{AH} and K_{BOH} values can be established.
The coefficients could be determined using linear regression and C_{TA}, C_{TB}, K_{AH} and K_{BOH} values could be calculated. However, in determining each values, there are points that would need to be considered in the regression, both for high and low H^+ concentration ranges.

2.1.3 Parameters characterizing the cell membrane
In this study C_{TA}, C_{TB} and K_{BOH} values for a cell membrane were found to be affected by cancer cell transformation, and were higher than the same parameters assayed in unmodified cells (Figs. 2-4). Meanwhile K_{AH} was found to decrease in cancer cells versus normal cells (Fig. 3).
In normal cells, the aminophospholipids such as phoshatidylserine (PS) and phosphatidylethanolamine (PE) are asymmetrically distributed across the plasma membrane e.g., they primarily localize to the cell's inner membrane leaflet (Stafford & Thorpe, 2011; Marconescu & Thorpe, 2008). This membrane lipid asymmetry is maintained by a group of P-type ATPases known as aminophospholipid translocases (APTLs). These APTLs catalyze the active transport of PS and PE from the external side to the internal side of the leaflet of the plasma membrane (Devaux, 1992). The distribution of PS, a component of the skeleton, has been shown to undergo changes, which could cause an increase in the proportion of negatively charged groups present at high pH values. As a result, anionic phospholipids present on tumor vessels could potentially represent tumor-specific markers for targeting and imaging (Ran et al., 2002).
Hypoxia/reoxygenation and acidity-induced exposure of anionic phospholipids, most likely phosphatidylserine and phosphatidylethanolamine (Zhao et al., 1998; Ran et al., 2002). According to previous studies both hypoxia and acidity can exist in a tumor. In particular,

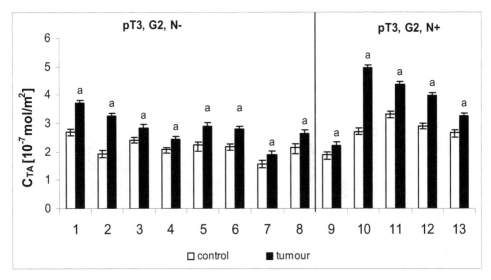

Fig. 2. The concentration of acidic functional groups present on pT3 stage, G2 grade human colorectal cancer cell membranes associated with metastasis (N+) and not associated with metastasis (N-). [a] $p < 0.05$, compared with control.

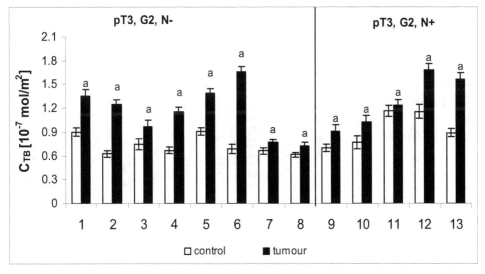

Fig. 3. The concentration of basic functional groups present on pT3 stage, G2 grade human colorectal cancer cell membranes associated with metastasis (N+) and not associated with metastasis (N-). [a] $p < 0.05$, compared with control.

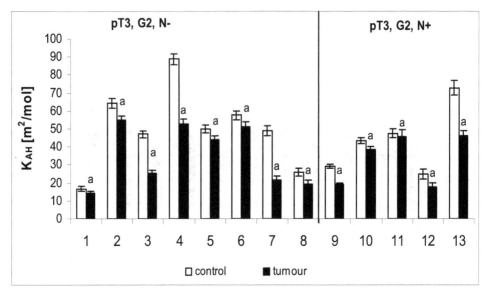

Fig. 4. The average association constant for hydrogen ions associated with pT3 stage, G2 grade human colorectal cancer cell membranes associated with metastasis (N+) and not associated with metastasis (N-). [a] $p < 0.05$, compared with control.

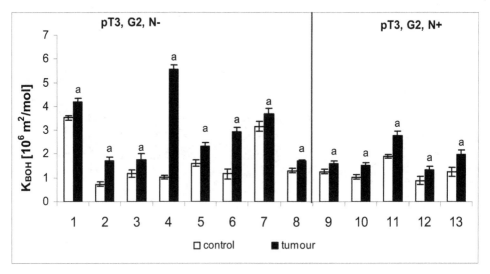

Fig. 5. The average association constant for hydroxyl ions associated with pT3 stage, G2 grade human colorectal cancer cell membranes associated with metastasis (N+) and not associated with metastasis (N-). [a] $p < 0.05$, compared with control.

hypoxia represents an important cellular stressor that can trigger a survival program by which cells attempt to adapt to a new environment. Typically, these adaptations will largely affect cell metabolism and/or stimulation of oxygen delivery (Bos et al., 2004).

Cell membrane charge is also affected by sialic acid present in glycolipids and glycoproteins. It has previously been hypothesized that sialic acid influences the concentrations of acid and basic groups present on the cell surface as well as association constants of positively and negatively charged groups during cancer transformation. An increase in the content of sialic acid in glycolipids and glycoproteins has been confirmed in, and increased sialic acid content has been found to provoke an increase in the surface concentration of acid groups (Erbil et al., 1986; Narayanan, 1994; Wang, 2005).

2.2 The compounds present in the cell membranes of human colorectal cancer

Neoplasms produce and secrete agents at trace levels inside of cells. These agents can include carcinogenic antigens, hormones, metabolites, growth factors, enzymes and cytokines (Skrzydlewska et al., 2005; Koda et al., 2004). In malignant cells, the ultrastructural architecture of the cell membrane is altered, partially as a result of changes in the quantities of membrane components present. Correspondingly, the transport of agents through the cell membrane is affected, thereby altering the biological properties of a cell. In many cases, expression levels of proteins, phospholipids and free unsaturated fatty acids are also affected due to enzyme disorders associated with biosynthesis processes that are altered. It is hypothesized that quantitation of the changes in the levels of phospholipids and structural proteins at the cell surface can reflect the extent of disintegration and impairment of genomic functioning that has occurred as a result of mutations associated with malignant transformation (Baldassarre et al., 2004; Tsunada et al., 2003).

Changes in membrane composition have the potential to affect cell growth and interactions between cells (including cells of the immune system), as well as the function of proteins and other components present at the cell membrane. For example, the immune system depends on interactions between different cell types for its function and these interactions are mediated by the membrane composition of the cells involved (Yaqoob, 2003). Moreover, immune cell activation (e.g., cell proliferation, phagocytosis) and tumor growth (malignancy) are processes associated with an increased rate of *de novo* synthesis and turnover of membrane phospholipids (Field & Schley, 2004).

2.2.1 Changes in the phospholipids composition of human colorectal cancer cell membranes

Phospholipids are an integral part of a cell membrane and determine its structure. Accordingly, different biological conditions are associated with differences in membrane phospholipids composition particularly during cancer transformation (Dobrzyńska et al., 2005; Szachowicz-Petelska et al., 2007).

For example, most cases of colorectal cancer involve an increase in the concentration of all phospholipid types at the cell membrane, including: phosphatidylinositol (PI), phosphatidylserine (PS), phosphatidylethanolamine (PE) and phosphatidylcholine (PC) (Table 1).

Previous studies have shown that an increase in the concentration of phospholipids in the cell membrane is associated with human colon cancer cells (Dueck et al., 1996) and murine mammary tumor cells (Monteggia et al., 2000). Moreover, this increase has been proposed to be the result of enhanced cell membrane synthesis related to accelerated neoplasm cell replication (Ruiz-Cabello & Cohen, 1992). Furthermore, the mechanisms involved can vary

Patient no	Type of phospholipid	Phospholipid content detected (mg/g tissue)	
		Control	Tumor
1.	PI	0.010 ± 0.002	0.225 ± 0.020[a]
	PS	0.016 ± 0.003	0.100 ± 0.010[a]
	PE	0.550 ± 0.010	0.890 ± 0.030[a]
	PC	0.675 ± 0.011	1.100 ± 0.061[a]
2.	PI	0.012 ± 0.003	0.239 ± 0.040[a]
	PS	0.028 ± 0.002	0.151 ± 0.022[a]
	PE	0.510 ± 0.020	0.740 ± 0.081[a]
	PC	0.116 ± 0.010	1.237 ± 0.099[a]
3.	PI	0.074 ± 0.008	0.081 ± 0.007
	PS	0.086 ± 0.006	0.131 ± 0.010[a]
	PE	0.494 ± 0.021	0.902 ± 0.051[a]
	PC	0.648 ± 0.024	1.240 ± 0.085[a]
4.	PI	0.087 ± 0.009	0.248 ± 0.020[a]
	PS	0.097 ± 0.007	0.097 ± 0.006
	PE	0.901 ± 0.050	0.932 ± 0.050
	PC	1.139 ± 0.061	1.245 ± 0.089[a]
5.	PI	0.064 ± 0.005	0.109 ± 0.010[a]
	PS	0.086 ± 0.004	0.114 ± 0.015[a]
	PE	0.498 ± 0.012	0.768 ± 0.080[a]
	PC	0.677 ± 0.018	1.054 ± 0.095[a]
6.	PI	0.020 ± 0.002	0.056 ± 0.006[a]
	PS	0.024 ± 0.002	0.096 ± 0.009[a]
	PE	0.432 ± 0.012	0.951 ± 0.092[a]
	PC	0.707 ± 0.019	1.368 ± 0.101[a]
7.	PI	0.009 ± 0.001	0.030 ± 0.015[a]
	PS	0.010 ± 0.011	0.021 ± 0.010
	PE	0.419 ± 0.023	0.828 ± 0.052[a]
	PC	0.675 ± 0.034	1.182 ± 0.065[a]
8.	PI	0.036 ± 0.012	0.136 ± 0.016[a]
	PS	0.042 ± 0.015	0.103 ± 0.050[a]
	PE	0.468 ± 0.028	0.895 ± 0.039[a]
	PC	0.686 ± 0.039	1.287 ± 0.070[a]

Table 1. The phospholipid content of pT3 stage, G2 grade human colorectal cancer cell membranes not associated with metastasis (N-). [a] $p < 0.05$, compared with control.

depending on the cell type, cell growth phase and malignancy status. For example, the greatest changes in the content of PC and PE have been observed in the G_1 phase of the cell cycle, during which activity of the enzymes controlling biosynthesis, catabolism and metabolism of phospholipids is maximal (Jackowski et al., 1996; Jackowski et al., 1994). As shown in Table 1 the PC content detected in normal mucosa in lesions of colorectal cancer cells and in other cancer cells was found to be higher than that of other phospholipids. These observations are consistent with the results of previous studies.

Patient no	Type of phospholipid	Phospholipid content detected (mg/g tissue)	
		Control	Control
9.	PI	0.044 ± 0.002	0.225 ± 0.011[a]
	PS	0.043 ± 0.002	0.145 ± 0.009[a]
	PE	0.642 ± 0.011	0.909 ± 0.019[a]
	PC	0.783 ± 0.012	1.406 ± 0.025[a]
10.	PI	0.150 ± 0.009	0.160 ± 0.008
	PS	0.055 ± 0.003	0.055 ± 0.003
	PE	0.540 ± 0.012	0.545 ± 0.013
	PC	0.925 ± 0.022	1.555 ± 0.028[a]
11.	PI	0.044 ± 0.002	0.144 ± 0.009[a]
	PS	0.025 ± 0.001	0.075 ± 0.005[a]
	PE	0.381 ± 0.018	0.396 ± 0.011
	PC	0.475 ± 0.020	1.281 ± 0.016[a]
12.	PI	0.018 ± 0.001	0.113 ± 0.008[a]
	PS	0.031 ± 0.003	0.110 ± 0.007[a]
	PE	0.551 ± 0.018	0.592 ± 0.013[a]
	PC	0.698 ± 0.021	0.933 ± 0.026[a]
13.	PI	0.026 ± 0.003	0.039 ± 0.003[a]
	PS	0.013 ± 0.001	0.026 ± 0.002[a]
	PE	0.433 ± 0.019	0.546 ± 0.014[a]
	PC	0.770 ± 0.030	1.240 ± 0.019[a]

Table 2. The phospholipid content of pT3 stage, G2 grade human colorectal cancer cell membranes associated with metastasis (N+). [a] $p<0.05$, compared with control.

Differences in membrane phospholipid content can also affect the potential for metastasis (Podo, 1999; Dobrzyńska et al., 2005). For example, malignant neoplasm cells associated with a greater number of metastases were characterized by a higher PC/PE ratio than malignant neoplasm cells with fewer metastases (Table 2).

2.2.2 Changes in the membrane free unsaturated fatty acid composition of human colorectal cancer cells

Free fatty acids are present in cell membranes, with the former present at low levels and the latter having a strong influence on the structure, properties and functions of the cell membrane. Polyunsaturated free fatty acids (PUFAs) also participate in the normal functioning of a cell, particularly by contributing to intracellular cell signaling. In addition, PUFAs represent nutritional components of a human diet and can indirectly affect tumorigenesis. For example, long-chain n-3 fatty acids have been shown to alter co-stimulatory molecules and activation markers, as well as calcium signaling and protein kinase C translocation at the cell membrane of immune cells (Hughes & Pinder, 2000). Similarly, the incorporation of n-3 fatty acids in the membrane of other cell types has been shown to alter membrane permeability, membrane fluidity and hormone and growth factor binding (Hashimoto et al., 1999; Lund et al., 1999). In colorectal cancer cells, reduced levels of PUFAs have been detected in the membrane, concomitant with increased levels of arachidonic and oleic acids, and lower levels of linoleic and α-linolenic acids (Table 3) (Szachowicz-Petelska et al., 2002, 2007).

Moreover, decreased levels of linoleic and α-linolenic acids have been detected in the plasma and erythrocytes of colorectal cancer patients. These changes are probably due to metabolic alterations caused by the illness and not necessarily by malnutrition (Baro et al., 1998). In addition, two clinical investigations have reported a significant increase in plasma and tissue concentrations of arachidonic acid (AA) in colorectal cancer patients compared with control patients (Neoptolemos et al., 1991; Hendrickse et al., 1994). This increase may be related to an enhancement of lipid peroxidation, which is a feature of rapidly growing cells (Skrzydlewska et al., 2001, 2005). Alternatively, increased AA levels could be due to elevated desaturase activity involving linoleic acid (LA) and α-linolenic acid (ALA), possibly leading to increased formation of prostaglandins and other lipoxygenase products (Dommels et al., 2002).

Other classes of unsaturated fatty acids include the palmitoleic (n-7) and oleic (n-9) family, both of which can be produced by most cells in humans and, thus, are not essential (Pandian et al., 1999). Levels of oleic acids have been found to be increased in colon cancer cells (Table 3). Furthermore, a significant elevation in the concentration of oleic acid has been detected in the plasma of colorectal cancer patients (Baro et al., 1998). Correspondingly, an almost statistically significant increase in the intake of oleic acid was found in another study of high-risk subjects for colorectal cancer (Schloss et al., 1997). These results may be due to changes in oleic acid metabolism as part of the pathogenic process. It has also been shown that human colon tumor growth is promoted by oleic acid (Calder et al., 1998) via mechanisms of increased fatty acid oxidation and a disturbance of membrane enzymes (Suziki et al., 1997).

Work by Rakheja et al., demonstrated that an overall reduction in free unsaturated fatty acids was associated with cancer cell membranes, while another recent report detected an elevated proportion of saturated versus unsaturated total fatty acids in colonic adenocarcinoma (Rakheja et al., 2005). In the latter case, the increase in saturated total fatty acids was attributed to elevated levels of the enzyme fatty acid synthase (Rashid et al., 1997). Furthermore, saturated fatty acids may be targeted to lipid raft microdomains, which are rich in cholesterol, sphingolipids and phospholipids with saturated fatty acid side chains (Swinnen et al., 2003; Rakheja et al., 2005). Recently, an increased intake of dietary n-3 fatty acids has been shown to decrease levels of sphingomyelin, cholesterol and caveolin-1 collectively, suggesting that n-3 fatty acids can modulate the composition of lipid rafts (Martin et al., 2005). Moreover, polyunsaturated fatty acids have been proposed to play a role in cancer therapy and to perturb membrane lipids rafts, thereby affecting cell functions (Hardman, 2004; Ma et al., 2004).

Under pathological conditions, such as hypoxia/reoxygenation, byproducts of AA that are generated can reduce gap junction-mediated coupling (Martinez & Saez, 2000). Dommels et. al., demonstrated that short-term incubation with LA, α-ALA or AA did not influence gap junctional intercellular communication (GJIC), yet long-term incubation with LA and α-ALA did inhibit GJIC of colon cells. Although the exact mechanisms mediating the inhibition of GJIC remain unclear, it is hypothesized that the associated cytotoxicity releated to the disruption of gap junctions is mediated by lipid peroxidation products. This hypothesis is supported by the observation that incubation with PUFAs, such as AA, can completely abolish GJIC (Dommels et. al., 2002).

Patient no	Type of fatty acid	Fatty acid content detected (mg/g tissue)	
		Control	Control
1.	18:2n-6	0.059 ± 0.005	0.014 ± 0.002[a]
	18:3n-3	0.045 ± 0.002	0.032 ± 0.005[a]
	16:1	0.032 ± 0.009	0.027 ± 0.007
	20:4n-6	0.036 ± 0.008	0.050 ± 0.010
2.	18:2n-6	0.028 ± 0.005	0.014 ± 0.005[a]
	18:3n-3	0.086 ± 0.010	0.071 ± 0.011
	16:1	0.021 ± 0.005	0.028 ± 0.005
	20:4n-6	0.064 ± 0.007	0.071 ± 0.008
3.	18:2n-6	0.033 ± 0.006	0.011 ± 0.003[a]
	18:3n-3	0.055 ± 0.005	0.039 ± 0.008[a]
	16:1	0.022 ± 0.003	0.022 ± 0.004
	20:4n-6	0.044 ± 0.009	0.061 ± 0.007[a]
4.	18:2n-6	0.022 ± 0.004	0.003 ± 0.001[a]
	18:3n-3	0.034 ± 0.006	0.028 ± 0.005
	16:1	0.016 ± 0.003	0.016 ± 0.003
	20:4n-6	0.028 ± 0.005	0.031 ± 0.006
5.	18:2n-6	0.014 ± 0.004	0.007 ± 0.001[a]
	18:3n-3	0.034 ± 0.006	0.017 ± 0.003[a]
	16:1	0.010 ± 0.002	0.014 ± 0.002
	20:4n-6	0.027 ± 0.004	0.041 ± 0.006[a]
	18:1	0.058 ± 0.007	0.075 ± 0.008[a]
6.	18:2n-6	0.016 ± 0.004	0.003 ± 0.001[a]
	18:3n-3	0.024 ± 0.005	0.019 ± 0.004
	16:1	0.005 ± 0.001	0.008 ± 0.001[a]
	20:4n-6	0.024 ± 0.004	0.035 ± 0.005[a]
	18:1	0.011 ± 0.002	0.027 ± 0.004[a]
7.	18:2n-6	0.009 ± 0.002	0.002 ± 0.001[a]
	18:3n-3	0.019 ± 0.004	0.009 ± 0.002[a]
	16:1	0.005 ± 0.001	0.005 ± 0.001
	20:4n-6	0.015 ± 0.003	0.026 ± 0.005[a]
	18:1	0.009 ± 0.002	0.019 ± 0.004[a]
8.	18:2n-6	0.057 ± 0.008	0.007 ± 0.001[a]
	18:3n-3	0.071 ± 0,009	0.036 ± 0.005[a]
	16:1	0.028 ± 0.005	0.043 ± 0.004[a]
	20:4n-6	0.064 ± 0.007	0.071 ± 0.007
	18:1	0.019 ± 0.004	0.056 ± 0.006[a]

18:2n-6, linoleic acid;18:3n-3, α-linolenic acid;16:1, palmitoleic acid;20:4n-6, arachidonic acid;18:1, oleic acid.

Table 3. PUFA content of pT3 stage, G2 grade human colorectal cancer cells not associated with metastasis (N-). [a] p<0.05, compared with control.

2.2.3 Changes in membrane proteins of human colorectal cancer cells

Currently, membrane proteins are classified into five groups according to their putative functions. These include: 1) receptor proteins associated with various extracellular ligands such as growth factors and hormones, 2) channel proteins that mediate the transportation of ions and small molecules across the membrane, 3) various enzyme proteins such as phospholipases and phosphatases, 4) regulatory proteins associated with functional proteins such as p21 and 5) cellular adhesion proteins such as cell - CAMs. In the latter case, most CAMs belong to one of four protein families: immunoglobulin (Ig), superfamily (IgSF), integrins, cadherins or selectins.

Structural changes in membrane proteins are associated with changes in the electrical potential of tumor cell membranes. These changes also correspond with altered biological properties exhibited by tumor cells. For example, a decrease in levels of E-cadherin expression in colorectal cancer cells has been shown to affect the diversification of cells in a tumor as well as the probability that tumor cells will contribute to distant metastasis.

While characterization of membrane proteins of tumor cells has made progress and provided valuable insight into the role of the cell membrane in tumorigenesis, additional studies are still needed to elucidate tumor-specific mechanisms associated with these changes (Kojima, 1993).

3. Conclusions

A higher proportion of phospholipids present in cell membranes results in a larger number of functional groups present at the cell surface and these can include: amino, carboxy and phosphate functional groups. Correspondingly, in acidic medium (e.g., a low pH), the charge associated with the phospholipid population at the cell surface is mainly determined by the amino groups present. In contrast, carboxy and phosphate groups present in a basic medium (e.g., a high pH) are key. For large intestine cell membranes, the main component of the outer layer is PC and at higher concentrations, PC can provoke an increase in both C_{TA} and C_{TB} values. In addition, when cells undergo transformation the association constant of negatively charged groups present (e.g., K_{AH}) decreases while the association constant of positively charged groups (e.g., K_{BOH}) increases.

Anionic phospholipids associated with tumor vessels also potentially represent markers for tumor vessel targeting and imaging (Ran et al., 2002). In addition, alterations in the distribution of PS, a component of the skeleton, can cause an increase in C_{TA} values.

Therefore, an evaluation of the membrane status of tumor cells may be an important consideration in future studies of tumor biology.

4. References

Baro, L.; Hermoso, J.C.; Nunez, M.C.; Jimenez-Rios, J.A. & Gil, A. (1998). Abnormalities in plasma and red cell fatty acid profiles of patients with colorectal cancer. *British Journal of Cancer* Vol.77, No.11, pp. 1978-1983, ISSN 0007-0920

Bos, R.; van Diest, P.J.; van der Groep, P.; Shvarts, A.; Greijer, A.E. & van der Wall, E. (2004). Expression of hypoxia-inducible factor-1α and cell cycle proteins in invasive breast cancer are estrogen receptor related. *Breast Cancer Research*. Vol.6, No.4, (June 2004), pp. R450-R459, ISSN 1465-5411

Calder, P.C.; Davis, J.; Yaqoob, P.; Pala, H.; Thies, F. & Newsholme, E.A. (1998). Dietary fish oil suppresses human colon tumour growth in athymic mice. *Clinical Science* Vol.94, No.3, (March 1998), pp. 303-311, ISSN 0143-5221

Cascio, M. (2005). Connexins and their environment: effects of lipids composition on ion channels. *Biochimica et Biophysica Acta.* Vol.1711, (December 2004), pp. 142-153, ISSN 0006-3002

Contreras, J.E.; Sanchez, H.A.; Eugenin, E.A.; Speidel, D.; Theis, M.;Willecke, K.; Bukauskas, F.F.; Bennett, M.V.L. & Saez, J.C. (2002). Metabolic inhibition induces opening of unopposed connexin 43 gap junction hemichannels and reduces gap junctional communication in cortical astrocytes in culture. *Proceedings of the National Academy of Sciences of the United States of America.* Vol.99, No.1, (November 2001), pp. 495-500, ISSN 0027-8424

Devaux, P.F. (1992). Protein involvement in transmembrane lipid asymmetry. *Annual Review of Biophysics and Biomolecular Structure.* Vol.21, (June 1992), pp. 417-439, ISSN 1056-8700

Dobrzyńska, I., Skrzydlewska, E. Figaszewski, Z. (2006). Parameters characterizing acid-base equilibria between cell membrane and solution and their application to monitoring the effect of various factors on the membrane. *Bioelectrochemistry.* Vol.69, No.2, (February 2006), pp. 142-147, ISSN 1567-5394

Dobrzyńska, I.; Szachowicz-Petelska, B.; Figaszewski, Z. & Sulkowski, S. (2005). Changes in electric charge and phospholipid composition in human colorectal cancer cells. *Molecular and Cellular Biochemistry.* Vol.276, No.1-2, (August 2005), pp. 113-119, ISSN: 0300-8177

Dołowy, K. (1984). Bioelectrochemistry of cell surface. *Progress in Surface Science.* Vol.15, No.3, pp. 245-368, ISSN 0079-6816

Dommels, Y.E.M.; Alink, G.M.; Linssen, J.P. & van Ommen, B. (2002). Effects of n-6 and n-3 polyunsaturated fatty acids on gap junctional intercellular communication during spontaneous differentiation of the human colon adenocarcinoma cell line Caco-2. *Nutrition and Cancer.* Vol.42, No.1, pp. 125-130, ISSN 0163-5581

Dueck, D.A.; Chan, M.; Tran, K.; Wong, J.T.; Jay, F.T.; Littman, C.; Stimpson, R. & Choy, P.C. (1996). The modulation of choline phosphoglyceride metabolism in human colon cancer. *Molecular and Cellular Biochemistry.* Vol.162, No.2, pp. 97-103, ISSN: 0300-8177

Erbil, K.M.; Sen, S.E.; Zincke, H. & Jones, J.D. (1986). Significance of serum protein and lipid-bound sialic acid as a marker for genitourinary malignancies. *Cancer.* Vol.57, No.7, (April 1986), pp. 1389-1394, ISSN 1097-0142

Field, C.J. & Schley, P.D. (2004). Evidence for potential mechanisms for the effect of conjugated linoleic acid on tumor metabolism and immune function: lessons from n-3 fatty acids. *American Journal of Clinical Nutrition.* Vol.79, No.6, (June 2004), 1190S-1198S, ISSN 0002-9165

Gennis, R.B. (1989). *Biomembranes: Molecular structure and functions.* Springer-Verlag, ISBN 0-387-96760-5, New York, USA.

Hardman, W.E. (2004). (n-3) fatty acids and cancer therapy. *Journal of Nutrition.* Vol.134, No.12, (December 2004), 3427S-3430S, ISSN 0022-3166

Hashimoto, M.; Hossain, S.; Yamasaki, H.; Yazawa, K. & Masumura, S. (1999). Effects of eicosapentaenoic acid and docosahexaenoic. acid on plasma membrane fluidity of aortic endothelial cells. *Lipids* Vol.34, No.12, (December 1999), pp. 1297-1304, ISSN 0024-4201

Hendrickse, C.W.; Kelly, R.W.; Radley, S.; Donovan, I.A.; Keighley, M.R. & Neoptolemos, J.P. (1994). Lipid peroxidation and prostaglandins in colorectal cancer. *British Journal of Surgery.* Vol.81, No.8, (August 1994), pp. 1219-1223, ISSN 0007-1323

Hughes, D.A. & Pinder, A.C. (2000). n-3 polyunsaturated fatty acids inhibit the antigen-presenting function of human monocytes. *American Journal of Clinical Nutrition.* Vol.71, No.1, (January 2000), 357S-360S, ISSN 0002-9165

Jackowski, S. (1996). Cell cycle regulation of membrane phospholipids metabolism. *Journal of Biological Chemistry.* Vol.271, (August 1996), pp. 20219-20222, ISSN 0021-9258

Jackowski, S. (1994). Coordination of membrane phospholipids synthesis with the cell cycle. *Journal of Biological Chemistry.* Vol.269, (February 1994), pp. 3858-3867, ISSN 0021-9258

Koijma, K. (1993). Molecular aspects of the plasma membrane in tumor cells. *Nagoya Journal of Medical Science* Vol.56, No.1-4, (November 1993), pp.1-18 , ISSN 00277622

Locke, D. & Harris, A.L. (2009). Connexin channels and phospholipids: association and modulation. *BMC Biology.* Vol.7, (August 2009), pp. 52-76, ISSN 1741-7007

Lund, E.K.; Harvey, L.J.; Ladha, S.; Clark, D.C. & Johnson, I.T. (1999). Effects of dietary fish oil supplementation on the phospholipid composition and fluidity of cell membranes from human volunteers. *Annals of Nutrition and Metabolism.* Vol.43, No.5, pp. 290-300, ISSN 0250-6807

Ma, D.W.; Seo, J.; Switzer, K.C.; Fan, Y.Y.; McMurray, D.N.; Lupton, J.R. & Chapkin, R.S. (2004). n-3 PUFA and membrane microdomains: a new frontier in bioactive lipid research. *The Journal of Nutritional Biochemistry.* Vol.15, No.11, (November 2004), pp. 700-706, ISSN 0955-2863

Marconescu, A. & Thorpe, P.E. (2008). Coincident exposure of phosphatidylethanolamine and anionic phospholipids on the surface of irradiated cells. *Biochimica et Biophysica Acta.* Vol.1778, pp. 2217-2224, ISSN 0006-3002

Martin, R.E.; Elliott, M.H.; Brush, R.S. & Anderson, R.E. (2005). Detailed characterization of the lipid composition of detergent-resistant membranes from photoreceptor rod outer segment membranes. *Investigative Ophthalmology & Visual Science.* Vol.46, No.4, (April 2005), pp. 1147-1154, ISSN 0146-0404

Monteggia, E.; Colombo, I.; Guerra, A. & Berra, B. (2000). Phospholipid distribution in murine mammary adenocacinomas induced by activated neu oncogene. *Cancer Detection and Prevention.* Vol.24, No.3, pp.207-211, ISSN 0361-090X

Narayanan, S. (1994). Sialic acid as a tumor marker. Annals of Clinical and Laboratory Science. Vol.24, No.4, (July-August 1994), pp. 376-384, ISSN 0091-7370

Neoptolemos, J.P.; Husband, D.; Imray, C.; Rowley, S. & Lawson, N. (1991). Arachidonic acid and docosahexaenoic acid are increased in human colorectal cancer. *Gut.* Vol.32, No.3, (March 1991), pp. 278-281, ISSN 0017-5749

Podo, F. (1999). Tumour phospholipid metabolism. *NMR in Biomedicine.* Vol.12, No.7, (November 1999), pp. 413-439, ISSN 0952-3480

Rakheja, D.; Kapur, P.; Hoang, M.P.; Roy, L.C. & Bennett, M.J. (2005). Increased ratio of saturated to unsaturated C18 fatty acids in colonic adenocarcinoma: implications for cryotherapy and lipid raft function. *Medical Hypotheses.* Vol.65, No.6, (August 2005), pp. 1120-1123, ISSN 0306-9877

Ran, S.; Downes, A. & Thorpe, P.E. (2002). Increased exposure of anion phospholipids on the surface of tumor blood vessels. *Cancer Research.* Vol.62, (November 2002), pp. 6132-6140, ISSN 0008-5472

Rashid, A.; Pizer, E.S.; Moga, M.; Milgraum, L.Z.; Zahurak, M.; Pasternack, G.R.; Kuhajda, F.P. & Hamilton, S.R. (1997). Elevated expression of fatty acid synthase and fatty acid synthetic activity in colorectal neoplasia. *The American Journal of Pathology.* Vol.150, No.1, (January 1997), pp. 201-208, ISSN 0002-9440

Ruiz-Cabello, J. & Cohen, J.S. (1992). Phospholipids metabolites as indicators of cancer cell function. *NMR in Biomedicine.* Vol.5, No.5, (September-October 1992), pp. 226-233, ISSN 0952-3480

Schloss, I.; Kidd, M.S.G.; Young, G.O. & O'Keefe, S.J. (1997). Dietary factors associated with a low risk of colon cancer in coloured west coast fishermen. *South African Medical Journal.* Vol.87, No.2, (February 1997), pp. 152-8, ISSN 0256-9574

Skrzydlewska, E.; Stankiewicz, A.; Sulkowska, M.; Sulkowski, S. & Kasacka, I, (2001). Antioxidant status and lipid peroxidation in colorectal cancer. *Journal of Toxicology and Environmental Health A.* 12, Vol.64, No.3, (October 2001), pp. 213-22, ISSN 1528-7394

Skrzydlewska, E.; Sulkowski, S.; Koda, M.; Zalewski, B.; Kanczuga-Koda, L. & Sulkowska, M. (2005). Lipid Peroxidation and antioxidant status in colorectal cancer. *World Journal of Gastroenterology* Vol.11, No.3, (January 2005), pp. 403-406, ISSN 1007-9327

Stafford, J.H. & Thorpe P.E. (2011). Increased exposure of phosphatidylethanolamine on the surface of tumor vascular endothelium. *Neoplasia.*Vol.13, No.4, pp. 299-308, ISSN 0004-3664

Suziki, I.; Iigo, M.; Ishikawa, C.; Kuhara, T.; Asamoto, M.; Kunimoto, T.; Moore, M.A.; Yazawa, K.; Araki, E. & Tsuda, H. (1997). Inhibitory effects of oleic acid and DHA on lung metastasis by colon-carcinoma-26 cells are associated with reduced matrix metalloproteinase-2 and -9 activities. *International Journal of Cancer.* Vol.73, pp. 607-612, ISSN 0020-7136

Swinnen, J.V.; van Veldhoven, P.P.; Timmermans, L.; Schrijver, E.D.; Brusselmans, K.; Vanderhoydonc, F.; Van de Sande, T.; Heemers, H.; Heyns, W. & Verhoeven, G. (2003). Fatty acid synthase drives the synthesis of phospholipids partitioning into detergent-resistant membrane microdomains. *Biochemical and Biophysical Research Communications.* Vol.302, No.4, (March 2003), pp. 898-903, ISSN 0006-291X

Szachowicz-Petelska, B.; Dobrzyńska, I.; Sulkowski, S. & Figaszewski, Z. (2010). Characterization of the cell membrane during cancer transformation. *Journal of Environmental Biology.* Vol.31, (September 2010), pp. 845-850, ISSN: 0254-8704

Szachowicz-Petelska, B.; Sulkowski, S. & Figaszewski, Z. (2007). Altered membrane free unsaturated fatty acid composition in human colorectal cancer tissue. *Molecular and Cellular Biochemistry.* Vol.294, No.1-2, (January 2007), pp. 237-242, ISSN: 0300-8177

Szachowicz-Petelska, B.; Dobrzyńska, I.; Sulkowski, S. & Figaszewski, Z. (2002). Changes in physico-chemical properties of human large intestine tumour cells membrane. *Molecular and Cellular Biochemistry.* Vol.238, No.1-2, (September 2002), pp. 41-47, ISSN: 0300-8177

Tien, H.T. (1974). *Bilayer Lipid Membranes (BLM): Theory and Practice.* Marcel Dekker Inc., ISBN 0-8247-6048-4, New York, USA

Wang, P.H. (2005). Altered glycosylation in cancer: sialic acid and sialyltransferases. *Journal of Cancer Molecules*. Vol.1, No.2, pp. 73-81, ISSN 1817-4256

Van Zeijl, L.; Ponsioen, B.; Giepmans, B.N.C.; Ariaens, A.; Postma, F.R.; Varnai, P.; Balla, T.; Divecha, N.; Jalink, K. & Moolenaar, W.H. (2007). Regulation of connexin43 gap junctional communication by phosphatidylinositol 4,5-bisphosphate. *The Journal of Cell Biology*. Vol.177, No.5, (June 2007), pp. 881-891, ISSN 0021-9525

Zhao, J.; Zhou, Q.; wiedmer, T. & Sims, P.J. (1998). Level of expression of phospholipid scramblase regulates induced movement of phosphotidylserine to the cell surface. *Journal of Biological Chemistry*. Vol.273, No.12, (March 1998), pp. 6603-6606, ISSN 0021-9258

9

Emergent Concepts from the Intestinal Guanylyl Cyclase C Pathway

Mehboob Ali and Giovanni M. Pitari
Division of Clinical Pharmacology,
Thomas Jefferson University, Philadelphia, PA,
USA

1. Introduction

Cancer is one of the world's top killers accounting for 7.4 million deaths, or 13% of all deaths (World Health Organization [WHO], 2011). Colorectal cancer is the third most common and deadly cancer worldwide (Jemal et al., 2011). An unequal geographic distribution of the disease burden exists, with less developed areas of the world exhibiting the lowest incidence and mortality (Pitari et al., 2003). In contrast, populations dwelling in western countries are at increased risk to develop and die of colorectal cancer. In the US, 141,210 new cases are estimated to be diagnosed in 2011 and 49,380 patients are expected to die for this disease, representing an intolerable socio-economical toll (Siegel et al., 2011).

Promises derive from substantial advancements in early detection and prevention strategies, which have contributed to reduce colorectal cancer incidence and mortality rates in recent years (Siegel et al., 2011). However, new chemotherapeutic approaches have not emerged and terminal clinical stages of the disease remain incurable. Specifically, invasion and metastatic disease progression, traditionally unnameable to surgical resection, are largely refractory to pharmacological therapy. About 90% of patients with distant metastasis die of the disease within 5 years from diagnosis (Siegel et al., 2011). Moreover, racial and educational health-disparities exist in which minorities and less educated individuals of the affected population exhibit the worst clinical prognosis and the highest mortality, in part reflecting their more advanced stages at diagnosis compared to other patient segments (Siegel et al., 2011). Together, these considerations underscore the enormous impact that therapeutic target discovery might have on western societies, especially if they would translate into innovative, curative pharmacological approaches that will prolong the survival of patients with colorectal cancer.

Crucial systems regulating the intestinal crypt-villus axis are also important determinants of the carcinogenetic process (Aoki et al., 2003; Fodde et al., 2001; Korinek et al., 1998). Among these, the signalling pathway orchestrated by the surface receptor guanylyl cyclase C (GCC) has recently emerged as both an integral component of intestinal mucosa homeostasis and a negative regulator of the malignant cell phenotype. GCC, expressed in the epithelial layer of the gastrointestinal wall, and its endogenous ligands guanylin and uroguanylin control fluid balance and renewal crypt dynamics by operating sophisticated biochemical circuits in both the small and large intestine. Intriguingly, a bacterial mimicry of endogenous hormones exists, the E. coli heat-stable enterotoxin (ST), which may confer both harmful (watery diarrhea) and beneficial (colorectal cancer resistance) effects to exposed individuals (Lucas et al., 2000; Pitari et al., 2001). In this model, the uneven epidemiological distribution of colon cancer incidence across different geographic areas of the world reflect, in part, inverse differences in the prevalence of enterotoxigenic E. coli infections (Pitari et al., 2003). Moreover, an unexplained mutation early in colorectal tumorigenesis leads to the loss of guanylin and uroguanylin expression, producing a dormant GCC pathway in neoplastic cells (Fig. 1) (Pitari et al., 2007).

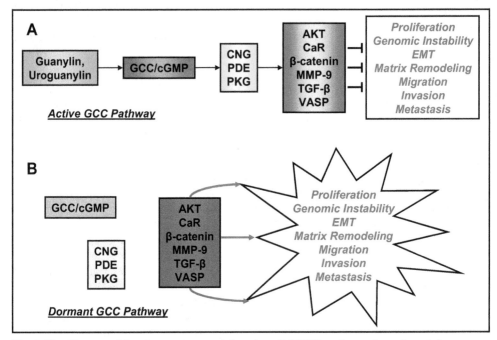

Fig. 1. Significance of the dormant guanylyl cyclase C (GCC) pathway for colorectal carcinogenesis.
Selected GCC signalling components with reported impact on tumorigenesis are depicted. A) In normal intestinal physiology, the GCC pathway is constitutively activated by paracrine hormonal regulation with the endogenous GCC agonists guanylin and uroguanylin. The active GCC pathway promotes signalling by proximal cGMP effectors cyclic nucleotide-gated channel (CNG), phosphodiesterases (PDE) and protein kinase G (PKG) that, in turn, affect the function of key distal effectors, including the v-akt murine thymoma viral oncogene homolog (AKT), Ca^{2+}-sensing receptor (CaR), β-catenin, matrix metalloproteinase 9 (MMP-9), transforming growth factor β (TGF-β), and vasodilator-stimulated phosphoprotein (VASP). As a result, tumorigenic forces are restrained and normal intestinal mucosa homeostasis is maintained. B) During neoplastic transformation the GCC pathway becomes dormant, principally because of the loss of endogenous hormone expression. Loss of signalling between GCC and the proximal cGMP effectors deregulates the distal components of the pathway, thereby producing an oncogenic system favouring colorectal cancer progression and metastasis. EMT, epithelial-mesenchymal transition.

This chapter will details the consequences at the functional and cellular level of the silenced GCC signalling for colorectal tumor formation and progression. Key molecular effectors comprising the GCC pathway with high clinical translational significance will be presented and their potential impacts for both diagnostic and therapeutic advances discussed.

2. GCC and the intestinal crypt-villus axis

GCC is a member of membrane-bound guanylyl cyclases (GCA to GCG), enzymes which catalyze the formation of cyclic guanosine monophosphate (cGMP) from GTP. Although they exhibit unique physicochemical and antigenic properties, particulate guanylyl cyclases are homodimeric transmembrane domain proteins sharing conserved cytoplasmic portions with tyrosine kinase-like and cyclase catalytic domains (Lucas et al., 2000). The amino acid sequence of GCC considerably diverges from the other isoforms in the extracellular domain, which represents the ligand binding domain for the E. coli heat-stable enterotoxin ST and the endogenous peptides guanylin and uroguanylin (Lucas et al., 2000). Beyond selected dopaminergic neurons in the central nervous system (Gong et al., 2011), in mammals GCC expression is principally restricted to brush-border membranes of epithelial cells lining the intestinal inner surface from the duodenum to the rectum, uniformly distributed along the crypt-villus axis (Lucas et al., 2000). This unique anatomical distribution subserves the functional role of GCC as a critical regulator of the intestinal mucosa homeostasis. In particular, the signalling pathway regulated by GCC and its second messenger cGMP contributes to the control of epithelial self-renewal and maturation dynamics underlying the integrity of the crypt-villus axis (Pitari et al., 2007).

2.1 The GCC pathway

Modulation of intracellular cGMP concentrations represents the fundamental event of a variety of signal transduction circuits shaping cellular behaviour. Synthesis (by guanylyl cyclases) and breakdown (by phosphodiesterases) are recognized as the major mechanisms defining cGMP levels in tissues. In intestinal epithelial cells, GCC is the principle source of cGMP (Lucas et al., 2000). GCC activity defines the type, intensity and duration of biological responses mediated by cGMP through unique physical, spatial and temporal dynamics at intestinal mucosal surfaces. The most important modality to regulate GCC activity is by ligand binding to its extracellular domain, which induces an intramolecular conformational change that is transmitted down to the cytoplasmic C-terminus catalytic domain. In this way, cellular cGMP levels can be raised numerous folds over basal states (Lucas et al., 2000; Schulz et al., 1989). Furthermore, the three ligand peptides know to induce GCC activation in mammalian cells exhibit different affinities and potencies for GCC, resulting in different patterns of cGMP concentrations/effects. The exogenous ligand ST, produced by E. coli and responsible for life-threatening diarrhoeagenic syndromes, is the most potent GCC agonist and consists of 18 amino acids with three intrachain disulfide bonds (Guarino et al., 1989). In contrast the endogenous paracrine hormones, guanylin and uroguanylin, are 15-16 amino acid long with two intrachain disulfide bonds and uneven tissue distributions and physico-chemical characteristics. Thus, while uroguanylin is a more potent (~100 fold) and abundant GCC agonist at acidic pH of proximal intestinal tracts, guanylin is more potent (~4 fold) as a GCC agonist at basic pH and is highly expressed in the colon and rectum (Forte, 1999; Hamra et al., 1997). Finally, elegant spatio-temporal constrains along the crypt-villus axis represent additional determinants of cGMP signalling by GCC. At the tissue level, maximal GCC activity and the dependant cGMP functions are imposed at the epithelial crypt/villus interface by increased GCC ligand expression (Cohen et al., 1995; Whitaker et al., 1997). In addition at the cellular level, compartmentalization of GCC-ligand interactions at luminal membrane borders establishes an increasing baso-apical cGMP gradient, wherein highest nucleotide concentrations are ensured at microvillus cell domains (Lucas et al., 2000).

Beyond GCC activation, the functional consequences of cGMP rises in intestinal epithelial cells reflect the specific expression and compartmentalization of downstream target molecules. Two evolutionarily distinct allosteric binding sites for cGMP exist in eukaryotic cells: one is present in cGMP- (PKG) and cAMP- (PKA) dependent protein kinases and in the cyclic nucleotide gated (CNG) cation channels, while the other is expressed in cGMP-regulated phoshodiesterases (PDEs). These proteins represent the intracellular receptors for cGMP and permit the selective transmission of information in a cell-(and subcellular-) specific manner. PKGs are Ser/Thr protein kinases comprising the soluble type I, widely distributed across tissues and including the isoforms Iα and Iβ, and the particulate type II, mainly expressed in the intestine (Pfeifer et al., 1999). PKA is a tetrameric kinase preferentially activated by cAMP (Chao et al., 1994). CNG channels are heterotetrameric proteins of α- and β-subunits, which mediate membrane Na$^+$ and Ca^{2+} influx by cGMP in intestine as well as different other tissues (Bielet al., 1999). Further, cGMP-regulated PDEs (eg, PDE2, PDE5) are hydrolytic enzymes specialized in cleaving the cyclic nucleotide phosphodiester bond, thereby terminating correspondent biological activities (Corbin & Francis, 1999; Francis et al., 2011). Cyclic GMP binding to the consensus site of these intracellular targets results in regulation of important downstream effectors which control specific biochemical networks and cellular functions. Molecules distal to cGMP with paramount significance for intestinal cell biology include ions, ion channels, cytoskeleton regulators and enzymes. For instance, cGMP binding to two allosteric sites present at the amino-terminal region of PKG II fully activates the enzyme and induces phosphorylation and opening of the cystic fibrosis transmembrane conductance regulator (CFTR), a pivotal mechanism underlying control of intestinal fluid homeostasis (Pfeifer et al., 1999). For an in depth discussion on the regulation of the various biochemical cGMP-dependent targets, such as the CFTR channel, the reader is referred to other comprehensive reviews (Browning et al., 2010; Lucas et al., 2000; Steinbrecher & Cohen, 2011). Here, the focus will be on those molecular elements of the GCC and cGMP pathway that affect the epithelial cell phenotype, including its proliferative, morphogenetic and migratory attributes that greatly influence the crypt-villus homeostasis and the process of neoplastic transformation.

2.2 Regulation of the intestinal epithelial cell phenotype

The human intestinal mucosa is characterized by minute tubular invaginations called crypts, of maximal length in large intestinal tracts. In addition, the small intestinal mucosa exhibits lumenal protrusions of multi- (villi) and sub-cellular (microvilli) dimensions devoted to digestive activities. As a result, the inner intestinal surface is enormously expanded to optimally serve fundamental processes, from food processing and absorption to pathogen protection and immune system control (Montgomery et al., 1999). In this context, the complexity of those processes, constantly exposing the organism to potentially harmful external factors, is reflected by the sophisticated functional organization adopted by the columnar monolayer of epithelial cells lining the intestine. First, a self-renewal epithelial ability is conferred by multipotent stem cells located at crypt bottoms, ensuring weekly cycles of cellular replacement to eliminate damaged or aging cells worn out by the demanding intestinal functions (Potten & Loeffler, 1990). Also, intriguing maturation dynamics are operating that turn proliferating progenitor cells into differentiated, cell cycle-arrested epithelial cells with specialized functions, mostly populating the upper crypt and villus areas. They include a) the enterocytes, absorptive cells with food digestive functions (Montgomery et al., 1999), b) goblet cells, mucus-producing cells with detergent activities (Koldovsky et al., 1995), c) enteroendocrine cells, hormone-secreting cells comprising an intestinal endocrine system (Koldovsky et al., 1995), and d) Paneth cells, which secrete antimicrobial peptides and growth factors and are uniquely located at crypt bases (Bry et al., 1994). Further, incompletely understood check-up mechanisms constantly detect genetic or epigenetic defects and direct epithelial cells to the appropriate maintenance (e.g., cell resistance), self-repair (e.g., DNA excision repair) or death (e.g., apoptosis, autophagy) program (Potten & Loeffler, 1990). Finally, the spatio-temporal coordination of this variety of processes is ensured by the migratory nature of the epithelial monolayer that physically maps the proliferation-differentiation transition at crypt/villus (small intestine) or lower/upper crypt (colon) interfaces, and drives the shedding of senescent cells at mucosal tips (Montgomery et al., 1999).

The GCC signalling pathway represents one of the elaborate homeostatic mechanisms evolved to direct the integration of each component supporting the intestinal epithelial cell phenotype. Indeed, targeted deletion of guanylin expression induces expansion of the proliferating crypt compartment and accelerated cell migration in mouse colon, presumably as a consequence of reduced GCC activation and cGMP-dependent signalling (Steinbrecher et al., 2002). In agreement with this notion, elimination of GCC in mice produces hyperplastic colonic crypts, populated by a higher number of fast-cycling and fast-migrating progenitor cells, associated with impaired cell maturation and death dynamics, with fewer Paneth and goblet cells but increased apoptotic events (Li et al., 2007a). Moreover, compound mice in which the expression of uroguanylin or GCC has been disrupted exhibit similar structural alterations in the crypt-villus axis, with loss of tight junction-mediated intestinal barrier function and increased mucosal permeability (Han et al., 2011). Of relevance, intestine-specific expression of GCC is under the control of the caudal homeobox gene Cdx2, a transcriptional factor regulating development and cell fate specification of intestinal epithelial cells (Park et al., 2000). The Cdx2 gene product binds a consensus site present in the GCC proximal promoter and stimulates GCC transcription in an intestine-specific fashion (Di Guglielmo et al., 2001). Thus, it is tempted to speculate that GCC expression and the dependant cGMP signalling are part of the universal developmental program supporting the integrity of the intestinal crypt-villus axis.

Molecular mechanisms underlying effects of the GCC pathway on the intestinal cell phenotype have only recently been investigated. In one paradigm, lumenal Ca^{2+} is the key distal mediator of GCC activity (Pitari et al., 2003, 2008). The role of dietary Ca^{2+} as antiproliferative agent and promoter of differentiation and cell death along the epithelial crypt-villus axis is well defined (Lipkin & Newmark, 1995; Whitfield, 1992), and Ca^{2+}-deficient diets induce larger proliferative compartments in mouse colonic crypts (Rozen et al., 1989). One key molecular target for antiproliferative effects by dietary Ca^{2+} is the Ca^{2+}-sensing receptor (CaR), a G protein-coupled receptor present at apical membranes of intestinal epithelial cells (Sheinin et al., 2000). Binding of Ca^{2+} to the N-terminal extracellular domain of CaR initiates discreet intracellular events mediated by the second messengers inositol 1,4,5-triphosphate (IP3) and diacylglycerol (DAG), which result in mobilization of intracellular Ca^{2+} and protein kinase C (PKC) activation, respectively (Berridge et al., 2000; Gama et al., 1997; Rhee, 2001). Intriguingly, elimination of GCC expression in mice is associated with loss of CaR from enterocyte brush borders (Pitari et al., 2008). Moreover, expression of CaR and GCC ligands is maximal at upper-crypt areas (Chakrabarty et al., 2005; Cohen et al., 1995; Whitaker et al., 1997), where epithelial cells stop proliferation and enter the maturation program, suggesting that CaR activity may be subordinated to GCC signalling along the crypt–villus axis (Pitari et al., 2008). Further, lumenal Ca^{2+} (1-3 mM) triggering cell cycle arrest at colonic mid-crypts (Whitfield et al., 1995) opposes pro-proliferative β–catenin activity and favour p21- and p27-mediated differentiation (Chakrabarty et al., 2003, 2005), molecular effectors also regulated by cGMP signalling in the intestine (Lin et al., 2010; Liu et al., 2001). Thus, GCC signalling may promote the proliferation-differentiation transition of intestinal epithelial cells through CaR regulation (Pitari et al., 2008). This is important as CaR is also the receptor for other polyvalent cations (i.e., Gd^{3+}, Mg^{2+}, Ni^{2+}) and polyamines (i.e., spermine, spermidine, putrescine) produced by commensal colonic bacteria (Hofer & Brown, 2003), pointing to a crucial role of the GCC-CaR pathway as regulator of a variety of antiproliferative signals in intestine (Pitari et al., 2008). In addition, lumenal Ca^{2+} may mediate intestinal GCC actions through CaR-independent mechanisms, including ionic currents by CNG channels (Biel et al., 1999; Pitari et al., 2003, 2008). Cyclic GMP-gated Ca^{2+} current through CNG is a major regulator of signal generation and transmission in excitable cells (Ames et al., 1999; Zufall et al., 1997). Of relevance, in colon cancer cells GCC signalling slows cell cycle progression, in part, by inducing cGMP-dependent CNG channel activation, intracellular Ca^{2+} influx and cytosolic Ca^{2+} rises (Pitari et al., 2003).

Another model proposes the v-akt murine thymoma viral oncogene homolog (AKT) as the master biological effector of the GCC pathway (Lin et al., 2010). AKT regulates survival and metabolic circuits in proliferating intestinal cells, and AKT over activation promotes crypt hyperplasia and tumorigenesis in mouse intestine (Sakatani et al., 2005). Importantly, elimination of GCC expression in mice results in hyperactivation of AKT signalling pathways, associated with expanded crypt compartments populated by glycolytic cells with accelerated G_1-S cell cycle transition (Lin et al., 2010). Conversely, loss of GCC and cGMP signalling restricts the differentiated villus compartment and diminishes mitochondria-dependent oxidative metabolism in intestinal epithelial cells (Lin et al., 2010). Investigations employing genetic and pharmacologic manipulation of AKT confirmed that GCC signalling through cGMP control the proliferative cell metabolism by decreasing the function of AKT (Lin et al., 2010). Thus, AKT-dependent regulation of cell survival and glycolytic metabolism along the crypt-villus axis, at the basis of intestinal mucosa development and homeostasis, may be conditionally regulated by the activity of the GCC pathway, whose increasing crypt-villus gradient directly correlates with differentiation and oxidative phosphorylation.

2.3 Regulation of epithelium-stroma interactions
Beyond the epithelium, the intestinal wall also encompasses mesenchymal and a smooth muscle layers. The intestinal mesenchymal compartment comprises mucosal and submucosal layers of connective tissues, composed of both acellular (e.g., glycoproteins,

hyaluronic acid, proteoglycans, collagen I and III) and cellular components (e.g., fibroblasts, myofibroblasts, leukocytes, endothelial cells). The basement membrane, a balanced mix of matrix components (e.g., nidogen, laminin, collagen IV, perlecan), physically separates the enterocytes from the underlying mesenchyme. The basement membrane and all the other mesenchymal components significantly contribute to the dynamic renewal of intestinal epithelial cells. Indeed, intestinal epithelium-stroma interactions contribute to maintain the crypt-villus homeostasis through direct cell-matrix and cell-cell contacts or paracrine signalling (Montgomery et al., 1999; Pinchuk et al., 2010). In contrast, corrupted epithelium-stroma interactions promote the initiation and progression of an array of intestinal pathologies (Kraus & Arber, 2009; Suzuki et al., 2011).

Studies with targeted deletion of GCC in mice revealed striking morphogenetic alterations affecting the extra-epithelial layers of the intestine (Gibbons et al., 2009). Indeed, the intestinal wall of these mice is significantly enlarged compared to mice with normal GCC expression. The mesenchymal compartment exhibits hypertrophy as a result of both exaggerated activation of its cellular elements and increased deposition of its interstitial matrix components (Gibbons et al., 2009). In particular, an increased ratio of activated myofibroblasts over quiescent fibroblasts is present in mice with loss of GCC signalling, an alteration which contributes to the establishment of a reactive stromal environment characterized by overexpression of collagen I, tenascin C and matrix metalloproteinase 9 (MMP-9) (Gibbons et al., 2009). In part, these alterations appear to be the consequence of an increased interstitial activity of the profibrinogenic transforming growth factor β (TGF-β), as GCC signalling through cGMP inhibits TGF-β secretion and function in intestinal epithelial cells and opposes stromal remodelling underlying inflammatory processes (Gibbons et al., 2009). Further, intestinal smooth muscle layers of mice lacking GCC signalling exhibit hyperplasia and hypertrophy, which represent important contributors of the transmural gut enlargement in these animals (Gibbons et al., 2009). Thus, the GCC pathway operating in intestinal mucosal cells exerts strong developmental and functional influences on the underlying stroma, presumably by regulating discreet hormonal circuits supporting epithelial-mesenchymal crosstalk (Pitari et al., 2007). Given the established role of the intestinal mesenchyme in inflammation and tumorigenesis (Kraus & Arber, 2009; Pinchuk et al., 2010; Suzuki et al., 2011), it is possible to speculate that dysregulation of GCC signalling in intestinal epithelial cells may favour the emergence of a reactive stromal environment promoting pathological processes.

3. GCC and intestinal transformation

Colorectal carcinogenesis comprises a pathological continuum turning pre-cancerous lesions into invasive malignant tumors. The process begins with single (epi)genetic mutations driven by carcinogenic insults that disrupt the physiological epithelial cell phenotype (Gryfe et al., 1997; van Engeland et al., 2011). As a result, the balance of migration, proliferation, differentiation and cell death along the colonic crypt-surface axis is perturbed and neoplastic cells with limitless replicative potential emerge. Remodelling of the surrounding stroma also participates to the promotion and progression of transformation, imposing cell non-autonomous drivers of tumorigenesis such us angiogenesis and inflammation (Kraus & Arber, 2009; Suzuki et al., 2011). Ultimately, malignant cells lose their epithelial characteristics and acquire a mesenchymal phenotype that enables them to translocate and establish new colonies at distant sites, such as the liver, lung and peritoneum (Nicolson, 1988; Polyak & Weinberg 2009; Suzuki et al., 2011).

The paracrine hormone hypothesis of colorectal cancer suggests that sporadic intestinal tumorigenesis is a process initiated by loss of endogenous GCC ligand expression, which induces a state of guanylinopenia and uroguanylinopenia (Pitari et al., 2007). Indeed, extensive studies have demonstrate that early in transformation intestinal epithelial cells acquire a mysterious mutation that renders pre-cancerous adenomatous lesions devoid of guanylin and uroguanylin (Birkenkamp-Demtroder et al., 2002; Cohen et al., 1998; Notterman et al., 2001; Steinbrecher et al., 2000). Those reports suggest that guanylin and uroguanylin, organized in a tail-to-tail configuration on human chromosome 1p, are the most commonly lost gene products in colorectal cancer in both animals and humans, exhibiting mutational frequency rates comparable to that of APC. Conversely, GCC is retained in colorectal cancer cells, which often exhibit higher GCC expression levels compared to normal epithelial tissues (Schulz et al., 2006; Witek et al., 2005). Increased GCC in the context of reduced guanylin and uroguanylin expression probably reflects the common pharmacological paradigm of receptor upregulation following specific ligand deprivation. More importantly, dysregulation of GCC signalling with an intact, but silent (for failure of ligand-dependent activation), intracellular molecular pathway produces a dormant cGMP-regulated system, which might be pathognomonically associated with neoplastic disease progression (Pitari et al., 2007). In this model, colorectal carcinogenesis following paracrine GCC ligand insufficiency reflects the central role of GCC in coordinating processes maintaining epithelial cell homeostasis and the crypt-villus axis, including the proliferation-differentiation balance, migration, metabolic programming and mesenchymal development (Li et al., 2007a; Pitari et al., 2007).

3.1 Regulation of the colon cancer cell phenotype

Neoplastic cell transformation ensues from the stepwise accumulation of mutations that produce hyper functioning oncogenes and silenced tumor suppressors (Bishop & Weinberg, 1996). Universally, the final combination of all the mutations and signalling deregulations occurring in cancers has similar functional consequences, the promotion of tumor cell growth and dissemination, and the evasion of host mechanisms of elimination (e.g., immuno-surveillance) (Hanahan & Weinberg, 2000). In intestinal tumorigenesis, acquisition of these malignant traits resembles a pathological amplification of the crypt stem cell phenotype, which self-perpetuates through relentless rounds of cell proliferation and migration (Montgomery et al., 1999; Potten & Loeffler, 1990). Conversely, invasive cancer cells progressively lose the morphology and metabolism of the differentiated epithelium, acquiring the ancestral functional plasticity of pluripotent stem cells. Indeed, overexpression of molecules (Wnt, β-catenin, Tcf) that support the crypt cell compartment (Gregorieff & Clevers, 2005; Korinek et al., 1998), or disruption of gene products (the adenomatous polyposis coli gene APC, Smad, CDX-2) restricting it (Aoki et al., 2003; Fodde et al., 2001; Tang et al., 2005) promotes intestinal tumorigenesis in animal models. In close agreement with these observations, the majority of sporadic human colorectal cancers exhibits a perturbed APC signalling as the initial mutational event, which crystallizes crypt-like nuclear proliferative programs driven by the β-catenin/Tcf complex (Fodde et al., 2001).

Since it regulates crypt compartments and the proliferation-differentiation balance along the crypt-villus axis (Li et al., 2007a; Pitari et al., 2007), dormancy of the GCC signalling pathway contributes to neoplastic transformation in the intestine (Li et al., 2007a; Pitari et al., 2007). Indeed, the increased migration and proliferation induced by loss of GCC signalling in mucosal colonocytes (Li et al., 2007a) represents a significant oncogenic stress (Aoki et al., 2003; Spruck et al., 1999) that creates the pre-neoplastic intestinal crypt (Pitari et al., 2007). Accordingly, cell cycle progression and growth of human colon cancer cells, experimental mimicry of the GCC dormancy characterizing the human disease because they express GCC but not the endogenous ligands (Lucas et al., 2000; Pitari et al., 2001), are greatly impaired upon reactivation of GCC signalling with exogenous supplementation of its specific agonists (Pitari et al., 2001, 2003, 2005, 2008). Ligand-dependent GCC activation restores lost cGMP-regulated circuits and imposes cancer cytostasis by reducing nuclear DNA synthesis and the G_1/S transition (Lin et al., 2010; Pitari et al., 2001). Antiproliferation by GCC, in part, is mediated by extracellular Ca^{2+} actions at cancer cell membrane surfaces, through its dependant effects on CaR activation and CNG channel-mediated Ca^{2+} influx (Pitari et al., 2003; Pitari et al., 2008). In addition, reactivation of GCC signalling through cGMP opposes the Wnt/β-catenin/Tcf4 signalling axis, the regulator of the proliferative crypt phenotype and tumor promoter in intestine (Pinto & Clevers 2005; Reya & Clevers 2005; van Es et al., 2005), by directly inhibiting β-catenin stability (Liu et al., 2001; Thompson et al., 2000). Underscoring the significance of the dormant GCC pathway in colon cancer, elimination of GCC in mice significantly enhances intestinal tumor initiation and progression (Li et al., 2007b). Mice deficient of GCC signalling exhibit enhanced sensitivity to tumorigenesis induced by Apc[Min/+] and the carcinogen azoxymethane, reflected by increased tumor incidence, multiplicity, and burden (Li et al., 2007b). A principal mechanism by which GCC promotes colorectal tumorigenesis is the perturbation of regulators of G_1/S cell cycle transition, including increased expression of oncogenes cyclin D_1 and pRb, and decreased activity of tumor suppressor p27 (Li et al., 2007b). Beyond hyperproliferation, GCC-deficient mice also exhibit increased genomic instability in their intestinal mucosa cells. In particular, an increased incidence of DNA breaks, loss of heterozygosity and point mutations in genes central to tumorigenesis, including APC and β-catenin, are observed along the crypt-villus axis (Li et al., 2007b). Although it remains unclear, the molecular mechanism mediating maintenance of the genome by GCC, including damage detection or mutational repair, appears to be distinct from that regulating proliferation (Li et al., 2007b). Rather, proliferative restriction and genomic quality control reflect two reinforcing systems by which the GCC pathway opposes intestinal carcinogenesis (Li et al., 2007b; Pitari et al., 2007). While accelerated G_1/S cell cycle transition favours inheritance and amplification of genetic mutations (Aoki et al., 2003; Spruck et al., 1999), instability involving tumor suppressors or oncogenes further deregulates the cancer cell cycle (Spruck et al., 1999).

Another consequence of a dormant GCC pathway in colorectal transformation is the promotion of the cancer cell metabolism (Lin et al., 2010). As discussed above, intestinal crypt stem cells principally rely on glycolysis to produce ATP and support their metabolism. Activation of GCC signalling restricts the glycolytic crypt compartment and favours the acquisition of mitochondria-mediated oxidative phosphorylation by differentiated epithelial cells in villi (Lin et al., 2010). Importantly, neoplastic cells utilize glycolytic ATP as their source of energy, even in the context of optimal environmental oxygen levels (Capuano et al., 1997; Kroemer, 2006; Pelicano et al., 2006). Dr. Otto Warburg first described this malignant paradox suggesting that cancer cells undergo metabolic reprogramming, wherein they switch from oxidative phosphorylation to aerobic glycolysis to produce ATP (Warburg, 1956). This malignant transition provides a competitive advantage to cancer cells that have a readily accessible supply of energy and substrates to support proliferation, adapt to the hypoxic tumor microenvironment, and promote invasion. Of relevance, restoration of GCC signalling by exogenous ligand administration increases the number, size and function of mitochondria in human colon cancer cells (Lin et al., 2010). Tumor reversion to mitochondria-dependent oxidative metabolism is associated with concurrent reduction in rate-limiting glycolytic enzymes, and reflects modulation of AKT and its downstream effectors (e.g., mTOR) by GCC signalling reactivation (Lin et al., 2010). Thus, while GCC signalling in human colon cancer cells induces expression of critical transcription factors required for mitochondrial biogenesis (PGC1α, mtTFA, NRF1), inhibition of glycolysis by GCC results in a reduced ability of tumors to uptake glucose and produce lactate (Lin et al., 2010). Importantly, elimination of AKT rescues the tumorigenic intestinal phenotype of mice deficient in GCC signalling (Lin et al., 2010), underscoring the central role of metabolic circuits in mediating inhibition of colorectal carcinogenesis by GCC. Together, these observations suggest that the dormant GCC pathway, produced by hormone deprivation early in transformation (Birkenkamp-Demtroder et al., 2002; Cohen et al., 1998; Notterman et al., 2001; Steinbrecher et al., 2000), can be envisioned as a loss-of-function mutation of a tumor suppressor system, which promotes crypt stem-like proliferation and metabolism and favours genomic instability and the development of the colon cancer cell phenotype.

3.2 Regulation of the colon tumor microenvironment

The tumor microenvironment is recognized as a major determinant of cancer formation, growth and dissemination (Fidler, 2001; Kraus & Arber, 2009; Suzuki et al., 2011). Both cellular and acellular components comprising the tumor stroma contribute to intestinal transformation, reflecting the intimate crosstalk between tumor epithelial cells and the underneath mesenchyme (Kraus & Arber, 2009; Suzuki et al., 2011; Witz & Levy-Nissenbaum, 2006). Thus, interstitial matrix remodelling, secretion of paracrine factors by stromal cells, lymphocyte-mediated immunoresponses, and neo-angiogenesis significantly influence cancer development (Fidler, 2001; Kraus & Arber, 2009; Suzuki et al., 2011). Among the molecular mediators of cancer-mesenchyme interactions, the matrix metalloproteinases (MMPs) play an essential role (Zucker & Vacirca, 2004). MMPs are a family of zinc-dependent metalloendopeptidases that cleave interstitial matrix components, growth factors, chemokines and cell surface receptors creating a nurturing niche for cancer growth and invasion (Cox & O'Byrne, 2001; Curran & Murray, 2000; McCawley & Matrisian, 2001). Depending on their substrate specificities, MMPs are divided into collagenases, gelatinases, stromelysins, and matrilysins (Stamenkovic, 2003).

The soluble collagenase MMP-9 has been conclusively linked with colorectal carcinogenesis (Chu et al., 2011; Lubbe et al., 2006; Nascimento et al., 2010; Zucker & Vacirca 2004; Zuzga et al., 2008). Structurally, MMP-9 (92-kDa protein) consists of a pro-peptide sequence, a catalytic domain containing the zinc binding site and fibronectin type II-like repeats, which promote MMP-9 binding to gelatin and elastin (Fridman et al., 2003; Shipley et al., 1996). Although enzymatic-independent signalling also has been reported (Bjorklund et al., 2004; Librach et al., 1991), the catalytic activity of MMP-9 is the principal mediator of tumor matrix remodelling (Fridman et al., 2003; Lubbe et al., 2006). In this way, MMP-9 degrades basement membrane collagen type IV, allowing intestinal tumor epithelial cells to invade the adjacent stromal compartment (Fridman et al., 2003). Moreover, MMP-9 promotes tumor angiogenesis by specifically processing and releasing TGF-β and VEGF from cancer cell surfaces and the interstitial matrix, respectively (Bergers et al., 2000; Qian et al., 1997; Yu & Stamenkovic, 2000). Given its crucial role in those pathological processes, MMP-9-dependent proteolytic activity is considered a driving force conferring the migratory and invasive phenotype to cancer cells and favouring tumor progression (Bergers et al., 2000; Fridman et al., 2003; Lubbe et al., 2006; Yu & Stamenkovic, 2000). Consequently, MMP-9 activity needs to be tightly controlled in biological tissues. Indeed, normally MMP-9 is a silent protease, secreted by cancer cells as a pro-zymogen that is activated only upon cleavage of its 10-kDa N-terminal pro-peptide by various proteases (e.g., MMP-2, MMP-3, MMP-13, plasmin, thrombin) (Ahmed et al., 2003; Fridman et al., 2003; Ramos-DeSimone et al., 1999). Endogenous inhibitors of MMP-9 also exists (e.g., the tissue inhibitor of matrix metalloproteinase 1) which bind to both the pro- and the active-form of MMP-9 and neutralize its proteolytic activity (Goldberg et al., 1992; Stamenkovic, 2003).

Beyond inhibition of catalytic activity, regulation of zymogen expression and secretion represents additional effective modalities to contain tumorigenic MMP-9 functions (St-Pierre et al., 2003; Zhang et al., 2006). Cyclic GMP inhibits the synthesis and secretion of MMP-9 in various cell systems (Akool el et al., 2003; Gurjar et al., 1999). Accordingly, restoration of ligand-dependent GCC signalling though cGMP induces a compartmental redistribution of colon cancer cell MMP-9, in which intracellular retention results in reciprocal extracellular depletion of that collagenase (Lubbe et al., 2009). As a consequence, MMP-9 proteolytic activities at the pericellular tumor space are suppressed, with abrogation of MMP-9-dependent interstitial matrix remodelling and cell spreading (Lubbe et al., 2009). Conversely, mutational dormancy of the GCC pathway early in transformation (Birkenkamp-Demtroder et al., 2002; Cohen et al. 1998; Notterman et al., 2001; Steinbrecher et al., 2000) may permit the emergence of a pro-tumorigenic stromal environment characterized by increased MMP-9 secretion, break-down of epithelial basement membranes by MMP-9 catalytic activity and disruption of homeostatic epithelial-mesenchymal interactions. It has been proposed that GCC effect on spatiotemporal MMP-9 dynamics in colon cancer cells has a profound impact on the overall tumor phenotype, because by disrupting its surface localization, membrane anchoring and focal catalytic activity it suppresses oncogenic MMP-9 functions (Lubbe et al., 2009).

4. GCC and colorectal cancer metastasis

Cancer metastasis consists in the dissemination of tumor cells to distant locations (Fidler, 2003). Clinically, metastasis coincides with the most terminal disease stages, incurable conditions associated with poor prognosis and survival (Mehlen & Puisieux, 2006; Siegel et al., 2011). Pathogenetically, it comprises a sequence of distinct, individual processes including cancer cell invasion of the primary site, intravasation and distribution through blood or lymphatic vessels, and colonization of target organs (Fidler, 2003; Folkman, 1986; Nicolson, 1988). Following organ seeding, tumor cells have to migrate into and invade tissue parenchyma (Wanget al., 2004; Steeg, 2006), resist to local immune defences and establish a nurturing micro-environment to develop and growth (Fidler, 2003; Folkman, 1986). In colon cancer, preferred organs of metastatic colonization include the liver, lung and peritoneum.

Once colorectal cancer has spread to these organs, the risk of mortality increases dramatically, and ~90% of patients diagnosed with distant metastasis die within 5 years from diagnosis (Siegel et al., 2011). Indeed, the management of patients with colorectal cancer metastasis is characterized by the highest incidence of therapeutic failure, in which surgery is not practicable (Pihlet al., 1981; Shapiro, 1992) and adjuvant chemotherapy is ineffective (increasing median survival only few months) (Meyerhardt & Mayer, 2005).

The functional phenotype of metastatic cells is unique and very selective. It has been calculated that of intravasated tumor cells, only a minute fraction remains viable after 24 hour, and >99.99% are eliminated before reaching their target organ (Fidler, 1970). This metastatic inefficiency reflects the scarcity of cancer cell clones exhibiting the full molecular machinery to execute all the individual steps comprising the metastatic process (Fidler, 1970; Weiss, 1990). In that context, since its inception primary colorectal cancer consists of biologically heterogeneous cell subpopulations, among which are present those possessing the ability to migrate and spread to distant parenchyma (Fidler, 2003; Heppner, 1984). Intriguingly as demonstrated by extensive immune detection and mRNA analyses of clinical specimens, GCC is uniformly expressed in metastatic colon tumors regardless of anatomical location (Carrithers et al., 1994; Carrithers et al., 1996; Waldman et al., 1998). Moreover, the structural and functional integrity of GCC and its principal downstream effectors appears to be preserved in metastasis, as colorectal cancer cells at extra-intestinal sites exhibit identical binding characteristics to, and signalling activation by, the exogenous ligand ST to those of normal intestinal cells (Carrithers et al., 1994; Schulz et al., 2006; Witek et al., 2005). However away from its primary organ, GCC is a ligand-starved receptor with an intracellular dormant pathway, as normal mucosal cells in intestine are the principal producers of endogenous hormones guanylin and uroguanylin (Forte, 1999). Thus, the loss of GCC ligand expression early in transformation (Birkenkamp-Demtroder et al., 2002; Cohen et al., 1998; Notterman et al., 2001; Steinbrecher et al., 2000) may be part of the exclusive phenotypic mutations conferring a pro-metastatic evolutionary advantage to selected colon cancer clones (Lubbe et al., 2009; Pitari et al., 2007; Zuzga et al., 2011).

4.1 Control of invasive cell shape

To successfully execute the metastatic program, transformed cells require a dynamic actin cytoskeleton. Thus, a hallmark of metastasis is the abandon of the static epithelial cell polarity and the acquisition of plastic membrane borders with specialized actin-based organelles promoting locomotion and invasion (Fidler, 2003; Steeg, 2006). Similarly to lymphocytes or neutrophils at inflammatory sites, cancer cells constantly remodel their actin to assume atypical morphological architectures, a process often referred to as epithelial-mesenchymal transition (Polyak & Weinberg, 2009). Changes in cell shapes reflect profound molecular rearrangements at tumor surfaces, including loss of E-cadherin-dependent cell-cell contacts and transient assembly of integrin-driven cell-matrix adhesions (Avizienyte et al., 2004, 2005; Polyak & Weinberg, 2009). These processes permit *de novo* development of membrane protrusions, such as filopodia and lamellipodia for probing the matrix during spreading and migration, and invadopodia for focal proteolytic matrix degradation in invasion (Linder, 2007; Yamaguchi & Condeelis, 2007).

In general, common molecular regulators coordinate tumor cytoskeletal remodelling by transducing external signals into actin processes. In colon cancer cells, tyrosine kinase receptors (e.g., EGF receptor, Eph receptors, Met receptors), G protein-coupled receptors (e.g., cholecystokinin receptors) and cytokine receptors (e.g., chemokine receptors, TGF-β receptor) have been established as important inducers of the metastatic cell morphology (Dienstmann & Tabernero 2010; Dong et al., 2009; Fulton, 2009; Kitamura et al., 2010; Larsen & Dashwood, 2010; Ongchin et al., 2009; Yuet al., 2006). They activate the intracellular signalling system controlling cytoskeletal actin (e.g., focal adhesion kinases, rho-GTPases, Arp2/3 complex), which assembles the membrane protrusive structures mediating invasion (Linder, 2007; Yamaguchi & Condeelis, 2007). Normally restricted at intestinal epithelial brush borders (Lucas et al., 2000), GCC is ideally positioned to affect those molecular networks and exert spatio-temporal control of actin remodelling. Indeed, ligand-dependent GCC signalling through cGMP appears to act as a suppressor of metastatic cell morphology in intestine (Lubbe et al., 2009; Zuzga et al., 2011). Thus, colon cancer cells assume a rounded shape upon GCC signalling activation, with elimination of F-actin rich filopodia and lamellipodia (Lubbe et al., 2009). The number and length of cancer cell invadopodia also significantly decreases after activation of the GCC pathway (Zuzga et al., 2011). Importantly, failure to form protrusive structures forces tumor cells to aggregate into compact colonies devoid of spreading and invading abilities (Lubbe et al., 2009; Zuzga et al., 2011). Together, these observations suggest that the GCC pathway is one of the intrinsic homeostatic systems that maintain the stable epithelial cell polarity, shape and tight junctions, which form the essential mucosal barrier between the intestine and the external environment (Han et al., 2011). This notion is further supported by the inhibitory role that GCC signalling exerts on known inducers of epithelial-mesenchymal transition (Polyak & Weinberg, 2009), including the reactive stromal environment (with enhanced TGF-β and MMP-9 activities) (Gibbons et al., 2009) and the stem cell-promoting PI3K/AKT system (Lin et al., 2010). Hence, dysregulation of GCC signalling in intestinal tumorigenesis may enable the epithelial-mesenchymal transition required for cancer cell dissemination (Lubbe et al., 2009).

A key intracellular effector of the GCC pathway that regulates colon cancer cell shape is the vasodilator-stimulated phosphoprotein (VASP) (Zuzga et al., 2011). Ena/VASP family proteins control F-actin geometry supporting cell motility (Krause et al., 2003). VASP promotes filopodia and lamellipodia formation and extension by organizing molecular complexes comprising G-actin, F-actin and actin regulatory proteins (Krause et al., 2003). It functions by protecting actin barbed ends from binding to capping proteins, thereby permitting filament elongation (Bear et al., 2002; Mejillano et al., 2004). Three critical domains enable VASP to intimately interact with the actin cytoskeleton (Krause et al., 2003), including 1) the N-terminus Ena/VASP homology 1 (EVH1), which binds to focal adhesion proteins vinculin and zyxin, 2) the central prolin-rich region, which contains a consensus binding motif for the G-actin-binding protein profilin, and 3) the C-terminus EVH2, which binds to both G- and F-actin and mediates VASP oligomerization. Importantly, Ser239 within the EVH2 VASP domain is a preferred phosphorylation site for PKG, functioning as a biological marker for cGMP signalling in intestinal (Deguchi et al., 2002) and other cells (Krause et al., 2003; Yaroslavskiy et al., 2005). Cyclic GMP-dependent VASP phosphorylation inhibits membrane protrusion formation in normal cells (Krause et al., 2003; Lindsay et al., 2007). Accordingly, in colorectal cancer cells VASP Ser239 phosphorylation induced by ligand activation of GCC signalling through cGMP and PKG induces rapid disassembly (less than 10 minutes) of invasive and migratory membrane organelles (Zuzga et al., 2011). Herein, GCC promotes VASP removal from tumor membrane protrusions with subsequent collapse of the F-actin infrastructure supporting filopodia and invadopodia (Zuzga et al., 2011). However, colorectal cancer cells expressing a mutant VASP construct not-phosphorylatable at Ser239 are resistant to GCC effects on VASP intracellular distribution and membrane protrusions (Zuzga et al., 2011). These findings are the most significant because they uncover the novel paradigm of a single intracellular biochemical reaction, VASP Ser239 phosphorylation, as an invasion suppressive mechanism for colon cancer (Zuzga et al., 2011). Hence, the loss of this mechanism during colorectal tumorigenesis, reflecting silencing of the GCC-cGMP-VASP system following hormonal deprivation (Birkenkamp-Demtroder et al., 2002; Cohen et al., 1998; Notterman et al., 2001; Steinbrecher et al., 2000), may favour the acquisition of the metastatic cell morphology, characterized by dissolution of normal cell-matrix and cell-cell contacts, increased actin polymerization dynamics, and enhanced formation of membrane protrusions (Zuzga et al., 2011).

4.2 Control of cancer cell dissemination

Relocation of cancer cells to distant sites requires acquisition of novel motor abilities, enabling them to spread through remodelled matrix surfaces at both primary and secondary tissues. In primary tumors, cancer cell spreading in the direction of blood vessels initiates the migratory journey of the intravasation process (Fidler et al., 1978; Fidler, 2003). In secondary organs, tumor cell adhesion and spreading onto vascular endothelial surfaces starts cancer invasion of target parenchyma (Im et al., 2004; Wang et al., 2004). In this context, polarized cell spreading drives cancer cell migration in the direction of invasion by permitting the establishment of specialized cell-matrix contacts at membrane protrusions, which mediates actin cytoskeleton-driven anchorage and traction of the cell body (Small et al., 1996). Thus, regulators of the cytoskeleton, adhesion receptors and extracellular proteases, which universally control spreading and migration in cells, are key players underlying cancer dissemination (Yamaguchi & Condeelis, 2007). Since its signalling through cGMP and VASP controls actin cytoskeletal dynamics and membrane protrusions in colon cancer cells (Zuzga et al., 2011), the GCC pathway may exert substantial impacts on those processes underlying formation of distant metastasis. Consistent with this hypothesis, elimination of GCC signalling in mice accelerates cell migration along the intestinal crypt-villus axis (Li et al., 2007a). Of relevance, basal GCC activity appears insufficient to restraining epithelial cell motility, as demonstrated by the increased migration of intestinal mucosa cells in mice with targeted ligand (guanylin) deletion (Steinbrecher et al., 2002). These observations suggest a model in which loss of hormone expression at the beginning of colorectal tumorigenesis (Birkenkamp-Demtroder et al., 2002; Cohen et al., 1998; Notterman et al., 2001; Steinbrecher et al., 2000) results in the acquisition of increased migratory abilities by transformed cells, driven by the accelerated formation of locomotory organelles mediating cell spreading and invasion (Zuzga et al., 2011).

A significant regulator of colorectal cancer cell migration and dissemination is the MMP-9 secreted by tumor epithelial cells (Lubbe et al., 2006). Beyond matrix degradation, this MMP-9 promotes the spreading and migration of colon cancer cells along two dimensional surfaces (Lubbe et al., 2006). Moreover, the catalytic activity of cancer cell MMP-9 is required for optimal colon tumor cell seeding of target mouse organs (Lubbe et al., 2006), an effect probably reflecting remodelling of the tumor pericellular microenvironment by MMP-9 (Fridman et al., 2003). Accordingly, inhibitors of MMP-9 suppress the formation of colorectal liver metastasis in an animal model (Aparicio et al., 1999). The significance of

MMP-9 for colon cancer metastasis is further underscored by its universal role in regulating migration and invasion across different cell types (Buisson et al., 1996; Leppert et al., 1995; Sanceau et al., 2003; Schultz et al., 1988; Yu & Stamenkovic, 1999). Importantly, ligand-dependent GCC signalling through cGMP suppresses the function of the MMP-9 produced by colorectal cancer cells (Lubbe et al., 2009). Activation of the GCC pathway suppresses tumor cell spreading, migration and dissemination by specifically inhibiting the secretion of cancer cell MMP-9 in the extracellular space (Lubbe et al., 2009). Further, colon tumor cells treated with GCC ligands fail to form metastatic colonies on mouse diaphragms following intraperitoneal injections (Lubbe et al., 2009). This effect also depends on the ability of GCC to inhibit cancer cell MMP-9, as demonstrated by the resistance of cells overexpressing MMP-9 to GCC-mediated inhibition of peritoneal metastasis (Lubbe et al., 2009). Conceivably, a silent GCC pathway in colorectal carcinogenesis (Birkenkamp-Demtroder et al., 2002; Cohen et al., 1998; Notterman et al., 2001; Steinbrecher et al., 2000) facilitates colon tumor invasion and metastatic dissemination by removing a key inhibitory mechanism restraining the oncogenic activity of cancer cell MMP-9.

5. The GCC pathway as a source of novel clinical targets

As discussed above, the loss of ligand-dependent GCC signalling produces a dormant GCC/cGMP pathway, which has significant impacts on the initiation, progression and metastasis of colorectal cancer. Conversely, deregulation of that pathway and its individual molecular components uncovers novel targets with unexploited clinical potential for improved diagnosis and therapy of patients. Thus, detection of hormone downregulation in colon biopsies could indicate presence of intestinal carcinogenesis and demand appropriate follow-up (Cohen et al., 1998; Notterman et al., 2001). The selective expression of GCC in colorectal tumor cells at metastatic sites (Carrithers et al., 1994, 1996; Waldman et al., 1998), suggests its utility as a diagnostic marker and specific target for delivering imaging and therapeutic agents *in vivo* (Gali et al., 2001; Wolfe et al., 2002). Indeed, clinical trials are confirming the value of GCC as a diagnostic marker for molecular staging of patients and prognostic indicator of colorectal cancer recurrence (Mejia et al., 2010; Waldman et al., 2009). Moreover, the structural preservation of GCC and its intracellular effectors offers the GCC hormone replacement therapy as a novel clinical paradigm for the prevention and treatment of colorectal cancer (Pitari et al., 2007). In this context, oral administration of uroguanylin prevents polyp formation in an animal model of intestinal tumorigenesis (Shailubhai et al., 2000). Further, the resistance to colon cancer initiation and progression exhibited by populations living in the developing world (Pitari et al., 2003; Shailubhai et al., 2000), where enterotoxigenic infections are highest, suggests that replacement therapy with the exogenous GCC ligand ST, the enterotoxin produced by E. coli, might be an effective treatment for colorectal cancer patients (Pitari et al., 2007). This latter consideration is supported by observations that ST is the most potent GCC agonist available (Lucas et al., 2000), and the only ligand successfully investigated to fully restore the tumor suppressor activities of the GCC pathway in colorectal cancer cells (Lubbe et al., 2009; Pitari et al., 2001, 2003, 2005, 2007; Zuzga et al.,2011).

Distal components of the GCC pathway also could be exploited in original clinical applications against colon cancer. As expected for its significance in intestinal mucosa homeostasis, the intracellular GCC signalome comprises a complex molecular network

(Pitari et al., 2007), probably still incomplete and in which each of the molecular elements may deserve critical translational evaluations. For some of these, preclinical testing is currently ongoing that is revealing emerging features as promising colorectal cancer bio-targets (Table 1). One model is the CaR, whose surface expression in colon cancer cells is conditionally regulated by activation of GCC signalling (Pitari et al., 2008). The dormant GCC pathway probably contributes to the reduced CaR expression observed in colorectal tumors (Chakrabarty et al., 2003; Kallay et al., 2003), a mutational event with clinical potential as a diagnostic marker of disease progression (Pitari et al., 2008). Moreover, CaR activation by extracellular Ca^{2+} inhibits cell proliferation (Chakrabarty et al., 2003), and dietary Ca^{2+} supplementation has been proposed as a chemopreventive strategy for colon cancer (Cho et al., 2004). Since restoration of the GCC pathway with exogenous ST administration potentiates antitumorigenic CaR signalling in human colon carcinoma cells (Pitari et al., 2008), combinatorial therapies including dietary Ca^{2+} and GCC ligand replacement may represent promising clinical regimens for the prevention and treatment of colorectal cancer.

Protein	Alteration in Colorectal Tumorigenesis	Diagnostic Target	Therapeutic Target	Ref.
CaR	Reduced expression	Tumor formation	Inhibition of tumor growth	(Chakrabarty et al., 2003; Kallay et al., 2003; Pitari et al., 2008)
MMP-9	Increased cancer cell secretion	Distant metastasis	Metastasis prevention	(Lubbe et al., 2009; Zuzga et al., 2008)
VASP	Loss of Ser phosphorylation	Invasion, metastasis	Local invasion prevention	(Zuzga et al., 2011)

Table 1. Examples of emergent colon cancer molecular targets from the GCC pathway.

Another intriguing effector of the GCC pathway is MMP-9, whose cancer cell compartmentalization depends on intracellular cGMP signalling (Lubbe et al., 2009). A silent GCC network may favour increased release and proteolytic activity of MMP-9 at the tumor pericellular space (Lubbe et al., 2009), thereby promoting matrix remodelling and invasion (Curran & Murray, 1999). Importantly, colon cancer cell MMP-9 behaves as a selective prognostic and predictive biomarker for disease stage stratification and therapeutic regimen selection in patients (Bendardaf et al., 2010; Zuzga et al., 2008). Reactivation of the GCC pathway with ST, in turn, is one successful strategy to specifically inhibit MMP-9 in tumor epithelial cells, without collateral damage in normal tissue, that has been suggested for the chemoprevention of colorectal cancer metastasis (Lubbe et al., 2009). Further, recent studies are indicating VASP as yet another GCC target with attractive translational applications for patients with colon cancer (Zuzga et al., 2011). VASP is a crucial actin-binding protein controlling membrane protrusion geometry, cell adhesion and migration (Bear et al., 2002; Krause et al., 2003; Mejillano et al., 2004). Dormancy of the GCC pathway in tumorigenesis depletes colon cancer cells of the cGMP-dependent VASP Ser phosho-species, molecular regulators of VASP activity at dynamic membrane regions (Krause et al., 2003). Thus, loss of VASP Ser phosphorylation may represent a novel prognostic biomarker of colon cancer progression (Zuzga et al., 2011). Conversely, reconstitution of VASP Ser phosphorylation could be exploited as an original paradigm for the chemoprevention of cancer migration and invasion, because the potent GCC ligand ST suppresses the malignant cell morphology and its pathological functions in colon cancer (Zuzga et al., 2011).

6. Conclusion

A novel paradigm is emerging in which colorectal cancer, one of the top cancer killers in the world, is pathogenetically conditioned by a dormant GCC pathway, developed early in tumorigenesis following specific ligand downregulation. Indeed, GCC and its paracrine hormones restrict the proliferative crypt phenotype and promote the normal epithelial cell morphology by orchestrating an articulated intracellular network comprising interconnected, but functionally distinct molecular effectors. Silencing of the pathway for loss of agonist-induced GCC/cGMP signalling alters the activity of those molecules with profound consequences for the initiation and progression of colorectal transformation (Fig. 1). Virtually all the key processes underlying carcinogenesis and metastasis are enhanced by dysregulation of the GCC pathway components, including proliferation, survival, genetic instability, migration, matrix remodelling and invasion. At the same time, the dormant pathway creates unexplored opportunities for novel diagnostic applications. This is because the biochemical deregulation that ensues from the silent cGMP-dependent machinery can be traced by analysis of the single pathway components at the molecular level. As a result, novel molecular fingerprints of colorectal carcinogenesis are emerging from the GCC pathway that can be exploited as clinical prognostic or predictive indicators of disease.

Restoration of the lost function by the GCC pathway in colorectal tumors also is proving its great translational value. Preclinical studies indicate that, though dormant, the pathway is largely intact and can be reconstituted simply by ligand replacement. Thus, administration of bacterial enterotoxin STs, potent GCC agonists, suppresses proliferation, migration, matrix degradation, invasion and metastasis by colorectal cancer cells. Altogether, these findings support the notion that oral replacement therapy with GCC ligands could represent a novel strategy for both the chemoprevention and cure of colorectal cancer. Additional therapies targeting the individual pathway components, either alone or in combination, also are being developed with the goal to improve clinical efficacy and selectivity. However, information from clinical testing is still missing and important questions remain to be addressed before this knowledge could be applied to the patient bed. In particular, general gastrointestinal toxicity worries need to be dissipated as GCC ligands such as ST are known for their potent diarrheagenic effects. Also, the temporal profile of GCC-targeted therapy will require complete characterization, including estimation of duration of treatments and effects. Finally, pharmacokinetics evaluation will need to be performed to accurately define dosing and timing regimens. In summary, the intestinal GCC pathway is an exciting potential source of novel diagnostic and therapeutic targets that could significantly affect the clinical management and disease outcome of patients with colorectal cancer.

7. Acknowledgment

This work was supported by grants to GMP from the National Institute of Health (R03CA133950), the Elsa U. Pardee Foundation and the American Institute for Cancer Research. The National Institute of Health specifically disclaims responsibility for any analyses, interpretations or conclusions.

8. References

Ahmed, N., Oliva, K., Wang, Y., Quinn M., & Rice, G. (2003). Downregulation of urokinase plasminogen activator receptor expression inhibits Erk signalling with concomitant suppression of invasiveness due to loss of uPAR-beta1 integrin complex in colon cancer cells. *Br J Cancer,* Vol.89, No.2, (July 2003), pp. 374-384, PMID 12865932

Akool el, S., Kleinert, H., Hamada, F.M., Abdelwahab, M.H., Forstermann, U., Pfeilschifter, J., & Eberhardt, W. (2003). Nitric oxide increases the decay of matrix metalloproteinase 9 mRNA by inhibiting the expression of mRNA-stabilizing factor HuR. *Mol Cell Biol,* Vol.23, No.14, (July 2003), pp. 4901-4916, PMID 12832476

Ames, J.B., Dizhoor, A.M., Ikura, M., Palczewski, K., & Stryer, L. (1999). Three-dimensional structure of guanylyl cyclase activating protein-2, a calcium-sensitive modulator of photoreceptor guanylyl cyclases. *J Biol Chem,* Vol.274, No.27, (July 1999), pp. 19329-19337, PMID 10383444

Aoki, K., Tamai, Y., Horiike, S., Oshima, M., & Taketo, M. M. (2003). Colonic polyposis caused by mTOR-mediated chromosomal instability in Apc+/Delta716 Cdx2+/- compound mutant mice. *Nat Genet,* Vol.35, No.4, (Dec 2003), pp. 323-330, PMID 14625550

Aparicio, T., Kermorgant, S., Dessirier, V., Lewin, M & Lehy T. (1999). Matrix metalloproteinase inhibition prevents colon cancer peritoneal carcinomatosis development and prolongs survival in rats. *Carcinogenesis,* Vol.20, No.8, (Aug 1999), pp. 1445-1451, PMID 10426790

Avizienyte, E., Fincham, V.J., Brunton, V.G., & Frame, M.C. (2004). Src SH3/2 domain-mediated peripheral accumulation of Src and phospho-myosin is linked to deregulation of E-cadherin and the epithelial-mesenchymal transition. *Mol Biol Cell,* Vol.15, No.6, (June 2004), pp. 2794-2803, PMID 15075377

Avizienyte, E., Brunton, V.G., Fincham, V.J., & Frame M.C. (2005). The SRC-induced mesenchymal state in late-stage colon cancer cells. *Cells Tissues Organs,* Vol.179, No.1-2, (June 2005), pp. 73-80, PMID 15942195

Bear, J.E., Svitkina, T.M., Krause, M., Schafer, D.A., Loureiro, J.J., Strasser, G.A., Maly, I.V., Chaga, O.Y., Cooper, J.A., Borisy, G.G., & Gertler, F.B. (2002). Antagonism between Ena/VASP proteins and actin filament capping regulates fibroblast motility. *Cell,* Vol.109, No.4, (May 2002) pp. 509-521, PMID 12086607

Bendardaf, R., Buhmeida, A., Hilska, M., Laato, M., Syrjanen, S., Syrjanen, K., Collan Y., & Pyrhonen S. (2010). MMP-9 (gelatinase B) expression is associated with disease-free survival and disease-specific survival in colorectal cancer patients. *Cancer Invest,* Vol.28, No.1, (Jan 2010), pp. 38-43, PMID 20001295

Bergers, G., Brekken, R., McMahon, G., Vu, T.H., Itoh, T., Tamaki, K., Tanzawa, K., Thorpe, P., Itohara, S., Werb, Z., & Hanahan, D. (2000). Matrix metalloproteinase-9 triggers the angiogenic switch during carcinogenesis. *Nat Cell Biol,* Vol.2, No.10, (Oct 2000), pp. 737-744, PMID 11025665

Berridge, M.J., Lipp, P., & Bootman, M.D. (2000). The versatility and universality of calcium signalling. *Nat Rev Mol Cell Biol,* Vol.1, (Oct 2000), pp. 11-21, PMID 11413485

Biel, M., Zong, X., Ludwig, A., Sautter, A., & Hofmann, F. (1999). Structure and function of cyclic nucleotide-gated channels. *Rev Physiol Biochem Pharmacol,* Vol.135, pp. 151-171, PMID 9932483

Birkenkamp-Demtroder, K., Christensen, L.L., Olesen, S.H., Frederiksen, C.M., Laiho, P., Aaltonen, LA., Laurberg, S., Sorensen, F.B., Hagemann, R., & TF, O.R. (2002). Gene expression in colorectal cancer. *Cancer Res,* Vol.62, No.15, (Aug 2002), pp. 4352-4363, PMID 12154040

Bishop, JM.,&Weinberg, RA. (Eds.). (1996). *Molecular Oncology,* SA Inc., New York

Bjorklund, M., Heikkila, P., & Koivunen, E. (2004). Peptide inhibition of catalytic and noncatalytic activities of matrix metalloproteinase-9 blocks tumor cell migration and invasion. *J Biol Chem,* Vol.279, No.28, (July 2004), pp. 29589-29597, PMID 15123665

Browning, D.D., Kwon, I.K., & Wang, R. (2010). cGMP-dependent protein kinases as potential targets for colon cancer prevention and treatment. *Future Med Chem,* Vol.2, No.1, (Jan 2010), pp. 65-80, PMID21426046

Bry, L., Falk, P., Huttner, K., Ouellette, A., Midtvedt, T., & Gordon, J.I. (1994). Paneth cell differentiation in the developing intestine of normal and transgenic mice. *Proc Natl Acad Sci U S A,* Vol.91, No.22, (Oct 1994), pp. 10335-10339, PMID 7937951

Buisson, A.C., Zahm, J.M., Polette, M., Pierrot, D., Bellon, G., Puchelle, E., Birembaut, P., & Tournier, J.M. (1996). Gelatinase B is involved in the in vitro wound repair of human respiratory epithelium. *J Cell Physiol,* Vol.166, No.2, (Feb 1996), pp. 413-426, PMID 8592002

Capuano, F., Guerrieri, F., & Papa, S. (1997). Oxidative phosphorylation enzymes in normal and neoplastic cell growth. *J Bioenerg Biomembr,* Vol.29, No.4, (Aug 1997), pp. 379-384, PMID 9387098

Carrithers, S.L., Parkinson, S.J., Goldstein S., Park, P., Robertson, D.C., & Waldman, S.A. (1994). Escherichia coli heat-stable toxin receptors in human colonic tumors. *Gastroenterology,* Vol.107, No.6, (Dec 1994) pp. 1653-1661, PMID 7958675

Carrithers, S.L., Barber, M.T., Biswas, S., Parkinson, S.J., Park, P.K., Goldstein, S.D., & Waldman, S.A. (1996). Guanylyl cyclase C is a selective marker for metastatic colorectal tumors in human extraintestinal tissues. *Proc Natl Acad Sci U S A,* Vol.93, No.25, (Dec 1996), pp. 14827-14832, PMID 8962140

Chakrabarty, S., Radjendirane, V., Appelman, H., & Varani, J. (2003). Extracellular calcium and calcium sensing receptor function in human colon carcinomas: promotion of E-cadherin expression and suppression of beta-catenin/TCF activation. *Cancer Res,* Vol.63, No.1, (Jan 2003), pp. 67-71, PMID 12517779

Chakrabarty, S., Wang, H., Canaff, L., Hendy, G.N., Appelman, H. & Varani, J. (2005). Calcium sensing receptor in human colon carcinoma: interaction with Ca(2+) and 1,25-dihydroxyvitamin D(3). *Cancer Res,* Vol. 65, No.2, (Jan 2005), pp. 493-498, PMID 15695393

Chao, A.C., de Sauvage, F.J., Dong, Y.J., Wagner, J.A., Goeddel, D.V., and Gardner, P. (1994). Activation of intestinal CFTR Cl- channel by heat-stable enterotoxin and guanylin via cAMP-dependent protein kinase. *EMBO J,* Vol.13, No.5, (March 1994), pp. 1065-1072, PMID 7510634

Cho, E., Smith-Warner, S.A., Spiegelman, D., Beeson, W.L., van den Brandt, P.A., Colditz, G.A., Folsom, A.R., Fraser, G.E., Freudenheim, J.L., Giovannucci, E., Goldbohm, R.A., Graham, S., Miller, A.B., Pietinen, P., Potter, J.D., Rohan, T.E., Terry, P., Toniolo, P., Virtanen, M.J., Willett, W.C., Wolk, A., Wu, K., Yaun, S.S., Zeleniuch-Jacquotte A., & Hunter, D.J. (2004). Dairy foods, calcium, and colorectal cancer: a pooled analysis of 10 cohort studies. *J Natl Cancer Inst,* Vol.96, No.13, (July 2004) pp. 1015-1022, PMID 15240785

Chu, D., Zhao, Z., Zhou, Y., Li, Y., Li, J., Zheng, J., Zhao, Q., & Wang, W. (2011). Matrix Metalloproteinase-9 Is Associated with Relapse and Prognosis of Patients with Colorectal Cancer. *Ann Surg Oncol*, (Epub ahead of print), PMID 21455597

Cohen, M.B., Witte, D.P., Hawkins J.A., & Currie, M.G. (1995). Immunohistochemical localization of guanylin in the rat small intestine and colon. *Biochem Biophys Res Commun*, Vol.209, No.3, (April 1995), pp. 803-808, PMID 7733972

Cohen, M.B., Hawkins, J.A., & Witte, D.P. (1998). Guanylin mRNA expression in human intestine and colorectal adenocarcinoma. *Lab Invest*, Vol.78, No.1, (Jan 1998), pp. 101-108, PMID 9461126

Corbin, J.D., & Francis, S.H. (1999). Cyclic GMP phosphodiesterase-5: target of sildenafil. *J Biol Chem*, Vol.274, No.20, (May 1999), pp. 13729-13732, PMID 10318772

Cox, G., & O'Byrne, K.J. (2001). Matrix metalloproteinases and cancer. *Anticancer Res*, Vol.21, No.6B, (Nov-Dec 2001), pp. (4207-4219), PMID 11908674

Curran, S., & Murray, G.I. (1999). Matrix metalloproteinases in tumour invasion and metastasis. *J Pathol*, Vol.189, No.3, (Nov 1999) pp. 300-308, PMID 10547590

Curran, S., & Murray, G.I. (2000). Matrix metalloproteinases: molecular aspects of their roles in tumour invasion and metastasis. *Eur J Cancer*, Vol.36, No.13 Spec no, (Aug 2000), pp. 1621-1630, PMID 10959048

Deguchi, A.J., Soh, W., Li, H., Pamukcu, R., Thompson, W.J., & Weinstein, I.B. (2002). Vasodilator-stimulated phosphoprotein (VASP) phosphorylation provides a biomarker for the action of exisulind and related agents that activate protein kinase G. *Mol Cancer Ther*, Vol.1, No.10, (Aug 2001), pp. 803-809, PMID 12492114

Di Guglielmo, M.D., Park, J., Schulz, S., & Waldman, S.A. (2001). Nucleotide requirements for CDX2 binding to the cis promoter element mediating intestine-specific expression of guanylyl cyclase C. *FEBS Lett*, Vol.507, No.2, (Oct 2001), pp. 128-132, PMID 11684084

Dienstmann, R. ,& Tabernero, J. (2010). Necitumumab, a fully human IgG1 mAb directed against the EGFR for the potential treatment of cancer. *Curr Opin Investig Drugs*, Vol.11, No.12, (Dec 2010), pp. 1434-1441, PMID 21154125

Dong, Y., Wang, J., Sheng, Z., Li, G., Ma, H., Wang, X., Zhang, R., Lu, G., Hu, Q., Sugimura, H., & Zhou, X. (2009). Downregulation of EphA1 in colorectal carcinomas correlates with invasion and metastasis. *Mod Pathol*, Vol.22, No.1, (Jan 2009) pp. 151-160, PMID 19011600

Fidler, I.J. (1970). Metastasis: guantitative analysis of distribution and fate of tumor embolilabeled with 125 I-5-iodo-2'-deoxyuridine. *J Natl Cancer Inst*, Vol.45, No.4, (Oct1 970), pp. 773-782, PMID 5513503

Fidler, I.J., Gersten, D.M., & Hart, I.R. (1978). The biology of cancer invasion and metastasis. *Adv Cancer Res*, Vol.28, pp. (149-250), PMID 360795.

Fidler, I.J. (2001). Seed and soil revisited: contribution of the organ microenvironment to cancer metastasis. *Surg Oncol Clin N Am*, Vol.10, No.2, (April 2001), pp. 257-269, PMID 11382586

Fidler, I.J. (2003). The pathogenesis of cancer metastasis: the 'seed and soil' hypothesis revisited. *Nat Rev Cancer*, Vol.3, No.6, (Jun 2003), pp. 453-458, PMID 12778135

Fodde, R., Kuipers, J., Rosenberg, C., Smits, R., Kielman, M., Gaspar, C., van Es, J.H., Breukel, C., Wiegant, J., Giles, R.H., & Clevers, H. (2001). Mutations in the APC tumour suppressor gene cause chromosomal instability. *Nat Cell Biol*, Vol.3, No.4, (April 2001), pp. 433-438, PMID 11283620

Folkman, J. (1986). How is blood vessel growth regulated in normal and neoplastic tissue? G.H.A. Clowes memorial Award lecture. *Cancer Res*, Vol.46, No.2, (Feb 1986), pp. 467-473, PMID 2416426

Forte, L.R. (1999). Guanylin regulatory peptides: structures, biological activities mediated by cyclic GMP and pathobiology. *Regul Pept*, Vol.81, No.1-3, (May 1999), pp. 25-39, PMID 10395405

Francis, S.H., Blount M.A., & Corbin, J.D. (2011). Mammalian cyclic nucleotide phosphodiesterases: molecular mechanisms and physiological functions. *Physiol Rev*, Vol.91, No.2, (Apr 2011), pp. 651-690, PMID 21527734

Fridman, R., Toth, M., Chvyrkova, I., Meroueh, S.O., & Mobashery, S. (2003). Cell surface association of matrix metalloproteinase-9 (gelatinase B). *Cancer Metastasis Rev*, Vol.22, No.2-3, (Jun-Sep 2003), pp. 153-166, PMID 12784994

Fulton, A.M. (2009). The chemokine receptors CXCR4 and CXCR3 in cancer. *Curr Oncol Rep*, Vol.11, No.2, (Mar 2009), pp. 125-131, PMID 19216844

Gali, H., Sieckman, G.L., Hoffman, T.J., Owen, N.K., Chin, D.T., Forte, L.R., & Volkert, W.A. (2001). In vivo evaluation of an 111In-labeled ST-peptide analog for specific-targeting of human colon cancers. *Nucl Med Biol*, Vol.28, No.8, (Nov 2001), pp. 903-909, PMID 11711309

Gama, L., Baxendale-Cox, L.M., & Breitwieser, G.E. (1997). Ca2+-sensing receptors in intestinal epithelium. *Am J Physiol*, Vol.273, No.4Pt1, (Oct 1997), pp. C1168-C1175, PMID 9357760

Gibbons, A.V., Snook, A.E., Li, P., Lin, J.E., DeGodoy, M., Rattan, S.C., Dasgupta, A., Schulz, S., Pitari, G.M., & Waldman, S.A. (2009). The intestinal tumor susceptibility gene product GUCY2C coordinates epithelial-mesenchymal interactions opposing the tumorigenic stromal niche through TGF-β_1, *Proceedings of American Association for Cancer Research Annual Meeting*, Denver (CO), Apr 2009

Goldberg, G.I., Strongin, A., Collier, I.E., Genrich, L.T., & Marmer, B.L. (1992). Interaction of 92-kDa type IV collagenase with the tissue inhibitor of metalloproteinases prevents dimerization, complex formation with interstitial collagenase, and activation of the proenzyme with stromelysin. *J Biol Chem*, Vol.267, No.7, (March 1992), pp. 4583-4591, PMID 1311314

Gong, R., Ding, C., Hu, J., Lu, Y., Liu, F., Mann, E., Xu, F., Cohen, MB., & Luo M. (2011). Role for the Membrane Receptor Guanylyl Cyclase-C in Attention Deficiency and Hyperactive Behavior. *Science*, (Epub ahead of print), PMID 21835979

Gregorieff, A., & Clevers, H. (2005). Wnt signaling in the intestinal epithelium: from endoderm to cancer. *Genes Dev*, Vol. 19, No.8, (April 2005), pp. 877-890, PMID 15833914

Gryfe, R., Swallow, C., Bapat, B., Redston, M., Gallinger, S., & Couture, J. (1997). Molecular biology of colorectal cancer. *Curr Probl Cancer*, Vol.21, No.5, (Sept-Oct 1997), pp. 233-300, PMID 9438104

Guarino, A., Guandalini,S., Alessio,M., Gentile,F., Tarallo,L., Capano,G., Migliavacca,M., & Rubino,A. (1989). Characteristics and mechanism of action of a heat-stable enterotoxin produced by Klebsiella pneumoniae from infants with secretory diarrhea. *Pediatr Res*, Vol.25, No.5, (May 1989), pp. 514-518, PMID 2470015

Gurjar, M.V., Sharma, R.V., & Bhalla, R.C. (1999). eNOS gene transfer inhibits smooth muscle cell migration and MMP-2 and MMP-9 activity. *Arterioscler Thromb Vasc Biol*, Vol.19, No.12, (Dec 1999) pp. 2871-2877, PMID 10591663

Hamra, F.K., Eber, S.L., Chin, D.T., Currie, M.G., & Forte, L.R. (1997). Regulation of intestinal uroguanylin/guanylin receptor-mediated responses by mucosal acidity. *Proc Natl Acad Sci U S A*, Vol.94, No.6, (March 1997), pp. 2705-2710, PMID 9122260

Han, X., Mann, E., Gilbert, S., Guan, Y., Steinbrecher, K.A., Montrose, M.H., & Cohen, M.B. (2011). Loss of guanylyl cyclase C (GCC) signaling leads to dysfunctional intestinal barrier. *PLoS One*, Vol.6, No.1, (Jan 2011), pp. e16139, PMID 21305056

Hanahan, D., & Weinberg, R.A. (2000). The hallmarks of cancer. *Cell*, Vol.100, No.1, (Jan 2000), pp. 57-70, PMID 10647931

Heppner, G.H. (1984). Tumor heterogeneity. *Cancer Res*, Vol.44, No.6, (Jun 2000), pp. 2259-2265, PMID 6372991

Hofer, A.M., & Brown, E.M. (2003). Extracellular calcium sensing and signalling. *Nat Rev Mol Cell Biol*, Vol.4, No.7, (July 2003), pp. 530-538, PMID, 12838336

Im, J.H., Fu, W., Wang, H., Bhatia, S.K., Hammer, D.A., Kowalska, M.A., & Muschel, R.J. (2004). Coagulation facilitates tumor cell spreading in the pulmonary vasculature during early metastatic colony formation. *Cancer Res*, Vol.64, No.23, (Dec 2004), pp. 8613-8619, PMID 15574768

Jemal, A., Bray, F., Center, M.M., Ferlay, J., Ward, E. & Forman, D. (2011). Global cancer statistics. *CA Cancer J Clin*, Vol.61, No.2, (March-Apr 2011), pp. 69-90, PMID 21296855

Kallay, E., Bonner, E., Wrba, F., Thakker, R.V., Peterlik, M., & Cross, H.S. (2003). Molecular and functional characterization of the extracellular calcium-sensing receptor in human colon cancer cells. *Oncol Res*, Vol.13, No.12, pp. 551-559, PMID 12899245

Kitamura, T., Fujishita, T., Loetscher, P., Revesz, L., Hashida, H., Kizaka-Kondoh, S., Aoki, M., & Taketo, M.M. (2010). Inactivation of chemokine (C-C motif) receptor 1 (CCR1) suppresses colon cancer liver metastasis by blocking accumulation of immature myeloid cells in a mouse model. *Proc Natl Acad Sci U S A*, Vol.107, No.29, (July 2010), pp. 13063-13068, PMID

Koldovsky, O., Dobiasova, M., Hahn, P., Kolinska, J., Kraml, J., & Pacha, J. (1995). Development of gastrointestinal functions. *Physiol Res*, Vol.44, No.6, pp. 341-348, PMID 20616008

Korinek, V., Barker, N., Moerer, P., van Donselaar, E., Huls, G., Peters, P.J., & Clevers, H. (1998). Depletion of epithelial stem-cell compartments in the small intestine of mice lacking Tcf-4. *Nat Genet*, Vol. 19, No.4, (Aug 1998), pp. 379-383, PMID 8798267

Kraus, S., & Arber, N. (2009). Inflammation and colorectal cancer. *Curr Opin Pharmacol*, Vol.9, No.4, (Aug 2009), pp. 405-410, PMID 19589728

Krause, M., Dent, E.W., Bear, J.E., Loureiro, J.J., & Gertler, F.B. (2003). Ena/VASP proteins: regulators of the actin cytoskeleton and cell migration. *Annu Rev Cell Dev Biol*, Vol.19, pp. 541-564, PMID 14570581

Kroemer, G. (2006). Mitochondria in cancer. *Oncogene*, Vol.25, No.34, (Aug 2003) pp. 4630-4632, PMID 16892077

Larsen, C.A., & Dashwood, R.H. (2010). (-)-Epigallocatechin-3-gallate inhibits Met signaling, proliferation, and invasiveness in human colon cancer cells. *Arch Biochem Biophys*, Vol.501, No.1, (Sep 2010), pp. 52-57, PMID 20361925

Leppert, D., Hauser, S.L., Kishiyama, J.L., An, S., Zeng, L., & Goetzl, E.J. (1995). Stimulation of matrix metalloproteinase-dependent migration of T cells by eicosanoids. *FASEB J*, Vol.9, No.14, (Nov 1995), pp. 1473-1481, PMID 7589989

Li, P., Lin, J.E., Chervoneva, I., Schulz, S., Waldman, S.A., & Pitari, G.M. (2007a). Homeostatic control of the crypt-villus axis by the bacterial enterotoxin receptor guanylyl cyclase C restricts the proliferating compartment in intestine. *Am J Pathol*, Vol.171, No.6, (Dec 2007), pp. 1847-1858, PMID 17974601

Li, P., Schulz, S., Bombonati, A., Palazzo, J.P., Hyslop, T.M., Xu, Y., Baran, A.A., Siracusa, L.D., Pitari, G.M., & Waldman, S.A. (2007b). Guanylyl cyclase C suppresses intestinal tumorigenesis by restricting proliferation and maintaining genomic integrity. *Gastroenterology*, Vol.133, No.2, (Aug 2007), pp. 599-607, PMID

Librach, C.L., Werb, Z., Fitzgerald, M.L., Chiu, K., Corwin, N.M., Esteves, R.A., Grobelny, D., Galardy, R., Damsky, C.H., & Fisher, S.J. (1991). 92-kD type IV collagenase mediates invasion of human cytotrophoblasts. *J Cell Biol*, Vol.113, No.2, (April 1991), pp. 437-449, PMID 1849141

Lin, J.E., Li, P., Snook, A.E., Schulz, S., Dasgupta, A., Hyslop, T.M., Gibbons, A.V., Marszlowicz, G., Pitari, G.M., & Waldman, S.A. (2010). The hormone receptor GUCY2C suppresses intestinal tumor formation by inhibiting AKT signaling. *Gastroenterology*, Vol.138, No.1, (Jan 2010), pp. 241-254, PMID 19737566

Linder, S. (2007). The matrix corroded: podosomes and invadopodia in extracellular matrix degradation. *Trends Cell Biol*, Vol.17, No.3, (March 2007), pp. 107-117, PMID 17275303

Lindsay, S.L., Ramsey, S., Aitchison, M., Renne, T., & Evans, T.J. (2007). Modulation of lamellipodial structure and dynamics by NO-dependent phosphorylation of VASP Ser239. *J Cell Sci*, Vol.120, No.Pt17, (Sep 2007), pp. 3011-3021, PMID 17684063

Lipkin, M., & Newmark, H. (1995). Calcium and the prevention of colon cancer. *J Cell Biochem Suppl*, Vol.22, pp. 65-73, PMID 8538212

Liu, L., Li, H., Underwood, T., Lloyd, M., David, M., Sperl, G., Pamukcu, R., & Thompson, W.J. (2001). Cyclic GMP-dependent protein kinase activation and induction by exisulind and CP461 in colon tumor cells. *J Pharmacol Exp Ther*, Vol.299, No.2, (Nov 2001), pp. 583-592, PMID 11602670

Lubbe, W.J., Zhou, Z.Y., Fu, W., Zuzga, D., Schulz, S., Fridman, R., Muschel, R.J., Waldman, S.A., & Pitari, G.M. (2006). Tumor epithelial cell matrix metalloproteinase 9 is a target for antimetastatic therapy in colorectal cancer. *Clin Cancer Res*, Vol.12, No.6, (March), pp. 1876-1882, PMID 16551873

Lubbe, W.J., Zuzga, D.S., Zhou, Z., Fu, W., Pelta-Heller, J., Muschel, R.J., Waldman, S.A., & Pitari, G.M. (2009). Guanylyl cyclase C prevents colon cancer metastasis by regulating tumor epithelial cell matrix metalloproteinase-9. *Cancer Res*, Vol.69, No.8, (April 2009), pp. 3529-3536, PMID 19336567

Lucas, K.A., Pitari, G.M., Kazerounian, S., Ruiz-Stewart, I., Park, J., Schulz, S., Chepenik, K.P., & Waldman, S.A. (2000). Guanylyl cyclases and signaling by cyclic GMP. *Pharmacol Rev*, Vol.52, No.3, (Sep 2000), pp. 375-414, PMID 10977868

McCawley, L.J., & Matrisian, L.M. (2001). Tumor progression: defining the soil round the tumor seed. *Curr Biol*, Vol.11, No.1, (Jan 2001), pp. R25-R27, PMID 11166192

Mehlen, P., & Puisieux, A. (2006). Metastasis: a question of life or death. *Nat Rev Cancer*, Vol.6, No.6, (Jun 2006), pp. 449-458, PMID 16723991

Mejia, A., Schulz, S., Hyslop, T., Weinberg, D.S., & Waldman, S.A. (2010). Molecular staging estimates occult tumor burden in colorectal cancer. *Adv Clin Chem*, Vol.52, pp. 19-39, PMID 21275338

Mejillano, M.R., Kojima, S., Applewhite, D.A., Gertler, F.B., Svitkina, T.M., & Borisy, G.G. (2004). Lamellipodial versus filopodial mode of the actin nanomachinery: pivotal role of the filament barbed end. *Cell*, Vol.118, No.3, (Aug 2004), pp. 363-373, PMID 15294161

Meyerhardt, J.A., & Mayer, R.J. (2005). Systemic therapy for colorectal cancer. *N Engl J Med*, Vol.352, No.5, (Feb 2005), pp. 476-487, PMID 15689586

Montgomery, R.K., Mulberg, A.E., & Grand, R.J. (1999). Development of the human gastrointestinal tract: twenty years of progress. *Gastroenterology*, Vol.116, No.3, (March 1999), pp. 702-731, PMID 10029630

Nascimento, C.F., Gama-De-Souza, L.N., Freitas, V.M., & Jaeger, R.G. (2010). Role of MMP9 on invadopodia formation in cells from adenoid cystic carcinoma. Study by laser scanning confocal microscopy. *Microsc Res Tech*, Vol.73, No.2, (Feb), pp. 99-108, PMID 19658178

Nicolson, G.L. (1988). Cancer metastasis: tumor cell and host organ properties important in metastasis to specific secondary sites. *Biochim Biophys Acta*, Vol.948, No.2, (Nov 1998), pp. 175-224, PMID 3052592

Notterman, D.A., Alon, U., Sierk, A.J., & Levine, A.J. (2001). Transcriptional gene expression profiles of colorectal adenoma, adenocarcinoma, and normal tissue examined by oligonucleotide arrays. *Cancer Res*, Vol.61, No.7, (April 2001), pp. 3124-3130, PMID 11306497

Ongchin, M., Sharratt, E., Dominguez, I., Simms, N., Wang, J., Cheney, R., LeVea, C., Brattain, M., & Rajput, A. (2009). The effects of epidermal growth factor receptor activation and attenuation of the TGF beta pathway in an orthotopic model of colon cancer. *J Surg Res*, Vol.156, No.2, (Oct 2009), pp. 250-256, PMID 19524264

Park, J., Schulz, S., & Waldman, S.A. (2000). Intestine-specific activity of the human guanylyl cyclase C promoter is regulated by Cdx2. *Gastroenterology*, Vol.119, No.1, (July 2000) pp. 89-96, PMID 10889158

Pelicano, H., Martin, D.S., Xu, R.H., & Huang, P. (2006). Glycolysis inhibition for anticancer treatment. *Oncogene*, Vol.25, No.34, (Aug 2006), pp. 4633-4646, PMID 16892078

Pfeifer, A., Ruth, P., Dostmann, W., Sausbier, M., Klatt, P., & Hofmann, F. (1999). Structure and function of cGMP-dependent protein kinases. *Rev Physiol Biochem Pharmacol*, Vol.135, pp. 105-149, PMID 9932482

Pihl, E., Hughes, E.S., McDermott, F.T., Milne, BJ., & Price, A.B. (1981). Disease-free survival and recurrence after resection of colorectal carcinoma. *J Surg Oncol*, Vol.16, No.4, pp. 333-341, PMID 7253653

Pinchuk, I.V., Mifflin, R.C., Saada, J.I., and Powell, D.W. (2010). Intestinal mesenchymal cells. *Curr Gastroenterol Rep*, Vol.12, No.5, (Oct 2010), pp. 310-318, PMID 20690004

Pinto, D., and Clevers, H. (2005). Wnt, stem cells and cancer in the intestine. *Biol Cell*, Vol.97, No.3, (Mar 2005), pp. 185-196. PMID 15715524

Pitari, G.M., Di Guglielmo, M.D., Park, J., Schulz, S., and Waldman, S.A. (2001). Guanylyl cyclase C agonists regulate progression through the cell cycle of human colon carcinoma cells. *Proc Natl Acad Sci U S A*. Vol.98, No.14, (July 2001), pp. 7846-7851, PMID 11438734

Pitari, G.M., Zingman, L.V., Hodgson, D.M., Alekseev, A.E., Kazerounian, S., Bienengraeber, M., Hajnoczky, G., Terzic, A., & Waldman, S.A. (2003). Bacterial enterotoxins are associated with resistance to colon cancer. *Proc Natl Acad Sci U S A*, Vol.100, No.5, (March 2003), pp. 2695-2699, PMID 12594332

Pitari, G.M., Baksh, R.I., Harris, D.M., Li, P., Kazerounian, S., and Waldman, S.A. (2005). Interruption of homologous desensitization in cyclic guanosine 3',5'-monophosphate signaling restores colon cancer cytostasis by bacterial enterotoxins. *Cancer Res*, Vol.65, No.23, (Dec 2005), pp. 11129-11135, PMID 16322263

Pitari, G.M., Li, P., Lin, J.E., Zuzga, D., Gibbons, A.V., Snook, A.E., Schulz, S., & Waldman, S.A. (2007). The paracrine hormone hypothesis of colorectal cancer. *Clin Pharmacol Ther*, Vol.82, No.4, (Oct 2007) pp. 441-447, PMID 17687268

Pitari, GM., Lin, J.E., Shah, F.J., Lubbe, W.J., Zuzga, D.S., Li, P., Schulz, S., and Waldman, S.A. (2008). Enterotoxin preconditioning restores calcium-sensing receptor-mediated cytostasis in colon cancer cells. *Carcinogenesis*, Vol.29, No.8, (Aug 2008), pp. 1601-1607, PMID 18566015

Polyak, K., & Weinberg, R.A. (2009). Transitions between epithelial and mesenchymal states: acquisition of malignant and stem cell traits. *Nat Rev Cancer*, Vol.9, No.4, (April 2009), pp. 265-273, PMID 19262571

Potten, C.S., & Loeffler, M. (1990). Stem cells: attributes, cycles, spirals, pitfalls and uncertainties. Lessons for and from the crypt. *Development*, Vol.110, No.4, (Dec 1990), pp. 1001-1020, PMID 2100251

Qian, X., Wang, T.N., Rothman, V.L., Nicosia, R.F., & Tuszynski, G.P. (1997). Thrombospondin-1 modulates angiogenesis in vitro by up-regulation of matrix metalloproteinase-9 in endothelial cells. *Exp Cell Res*, Vol.235, No.2, (Sep 1997), pp. 403-412, PMID 9299165

Ramos-DeSimone, N., Hahn-Dantona, E., Sipley, J., Nagase, H., French, D.L., & Quigley, J.P. (1999). Activation of matrix metalloproteinase-9 (MMP-9) via a converging plasmin/stromelysin-1 cascade enhances tumor cell invasion. *J Biol Chem*, Vol.274, No.19, (May 1999), pp. 13066-13076, PMID 10224058

Reya, T., and Clevers, H. (2005). Wnt signalling in stem cells and cancer. *Nature*, Vol.434, No.7035, (April 2005) pp. 843-850, PMID 15829953

Rhee, S.G. (2001). Regulation of phosphoinositide-specific phospholipase C. *Annu Rev Biochem*, Vol.70, pp. 281-312, PMID 11395409

Rozen, P., Fireman, Z., Fine, N., Wax, Y., & Ron, E. (1989). Oral calcium suppresses increased rectal epithelial proliferation of persons at risk of colorectal cancer. *Gut*, Vol.30, No.5, (May 1989), pp. 650-655, PMID 2731758

Sakatani, T., Kaneda, A., Iacobuzio-Donahue, C.A., Carter, M.G., de Boom Witzel, S., Okano, H., Ko, M.S., Ohlsson, R., Longo, D.L., & Feinberg, A.P. (2005). Loss of imprinting of Igf2 alters intestinal maturation and tumorigenesis in mice. *Science*, Vol.307, No.5717, (March 2005), pp. 1976-1978, PMID 15731405

Sanceau, J., Truchet, S., & Bauvois, B. (2003). Matrix metalloproteinase-9 silencing by RNA interference triggers the migratory-adhesive switch in Ewing's sarcoma cells. *J Biol Chem*, Vol.278, No.38, (Sep 2003), pp. 36537-36546, PMID 12847101

Schulz, S., Singh, S., Bellet, R.A., Singh, G., Tubb, D.J., Chin, H., & Garbers, D.L. (1989). The primary structure of a plasma membrane guanylate cyclase demonstrates diversity within this new receptor family. *Cell*, Vol.58, No.6, (Sep 1989), pp. 1155-1162, PMID 2570641

Schulz, S., Hyslop, T., Haaf, J., Bonaccorso, C., Nielsen, K., Witek, M.E., Birbe, R., Palazzo, J., Weinberg, D., & Waldman, S.A. (2006). A validated quantitative assay to detect occult micrometastases by reverse transcriptase-polymerase chain reaction of guanylyl cyclase C in patients with colorectal cancer. *Clin Cancer Res*, Vol.12, No.15, (Aug 2006), pp. 4545-4552, PMID 16899600

Schultz, R.M., Silberman, S., Persky, B., Bajkowski, A.S., & Carmichael, D.F. (1988). Inhibition by human recombinant tissue inhibitor of metalloproteinases of human amnion invasion and lung colonization by murine B16-F10 melanoma cells. *Cancer Res*, Vol.48, No.19, (Oct 1988), pp. 5539-5545, PMID 3416307

Shailubhai, K., Yu, H.H., Karunanandaa, K., Wang, J.Y., Eber, S.L., Wang, Y., Joo, N.S., Kim, H.D., Miedema, B.W., Abbas, S.Z., Boddupalli, S.S., Currie, M.G., & Forte, L.R. (2000). Uroguanylin treatment suppresses polyp formation in the Apc(Min/+) mouse and induces apoptosis in human colon adenocarcinoma cells via cyclic GMP. *Cancer Res*, Vol.60, No.18, (Sep 2000), pp. 5151-5157, PMID 11016642

Shapiro, S. (1992). Goals of screening. *Cancer*, Vol.70, No.5, (Sep 1992), pp. 1252-1258, PMID 1511372

Sheinin, Y., Kallay, E., Wrba, F., Kriwanek, S., Peterlik, M., & Cross, H.S. (2000). Immunocytochemical localization of the extracellular calcium-sensing receptor in normal and malignant human large intestinal mucosa. *J Histochem Cytochem*, Vol.48, No.5, (May 2000), pp. 595-602, PMID 10769043

Shipley, J.M., Doyle, G.A., Fliszar, C.J., Ye, Q.Z., Johnson, L.L., Shapiro, S.D., Welgus, H.G., & Senior, R.M. (1996). The structural basis for the elastolytic activity of the 92-kDa and 72-kDa gelatinases. Role of the fibronectin type II-like repeats. *J Biol Chem*, Vol.271, No.8, (Feb 1996), pp. 4335-4341, PMID 8626782

Siegel, R., Ward, E., Brawley, O., & Jemal, A. (2011). Cancer statistics, 2011: The impact of eliminating socioeconomic and racial disparities on premature cancer deaths. *CA Cancer J Clin*, Vol.61, No.4, (July-Aug 2011), pp. 212-236, PMID 21685461

Small, J.V., Anderson, K., & Rottner, K. (1996). Actin and the coordination of protrusion, attachment and retraction in cell crawling. *Biosci Rep*, Vol.16, No.5, (Oct 1996), pp. 351-368, PMID 8913526

Spruck, C.H., Won, K.A., & Reed, S.I. (1999). Deregulated cyclin E induces chromosome instability. *Nature*, Vol.401, No.6750, (Sep 1999) pp. 297-300, PMID 10499591

St-Pierre, Y., Van Themsche, C., & Esteve, P.O. (2003). Emerging features in the regulation of MMP-9 gene expression for the development of novel molecular targets and therapeutic strategies. *Curr Drug Targets Inflamm Allergy*, Vol.2, No.3 (Sep 2003), pp. 206-215, PMID 14561155

Stamenkovic, I. (2003). Extracellular matrix remodelling: the role of matrix metalloproteinases. *J Pathol*, Vol.200, No.4, (July 2003), pp. 448-464, PMID12845612

Steeg, P.S. (2006). Tumor metastasis: mechanistic insights and clinical challenges. *Nat Med*, Vol.12, No.8, (Aug 2006), pp. 895-904, PMID 16892035

Steinbrecher, K.A., Tuohy, T.M., Heppner Goss, K., Scott, M.C., Witte, D.P., Groden, J., & Cohen, MB. (2000). Expression of guanylin is downregulated in mouse and human intestinal adenomas. *Biochem Biophys Res Commun*, Vol.273, No.1, (Jun 2000), pp. (225-230), PMID 10873591

Steinbrecher, K.A., Wowk, S.A., Rudolph, J.A., Witte, D.P., & Cohen, M.B. (2002). Targeted inactivation of the mouse guanylin gene results in altered dynamics of colonic epithelial proliferation. *Am J Pathol*, Vol.161, No.6, (Dec 2002), pp. 2169-2178, PMID 12466132

Steinbrecher, K.A., & Cohen, M.B. (2011). Transmembrane guanylate cyclase in intestinal pathophysiology. *Curr Opin Gastroenterol*, Vol.27, No.2, (March 2011), pp. 139-145, PMID 21102322

Suzuki, K., Sun, R., Origuchi, M., Kanehira, M., Takahata, T., Itoh, J., Umezawa, A., Kijima, H., Fukuda, S.,& Saijo, Y. (2011). Mesenchymal Stromal Cells Promote Tumor Growth through the Enhancement of Neovascularization. *Mol Med*, Vol.17, No.7-8, pp. 579-587, PMID 21424106

Tang, Y., Katuri, V., Srinivasan, R., Fogt, F., Redman, R., Anand, G., Said, A., Fishbein, T., Zasloff, M., Reddy, E.P., Mishra, B., & Mishra, L. (2005). Transforming growth factor-beta suppresses nonmetastatic colon cancer through Smad4 and adaptor protein ELF at an early stage of tumorigenesis. *Cancer Res*, Vol.65, No.10, (May 2005), pp. 4228-4237, PMID 15899814

Thompson, W.J., Piazza, G.A., Li, H., Liu, L., Fetter, J., Zhu, B., Sperl, G., Ahnen, D., & Pamukcu, R. (2000). Exisulind induction of apoptosis involves guanosine 3',5'-cyclic monophosphate phosphodiesterase inhibition, protein kinase G activation, and attenuated beta-catenin. *Cancer Res*, Vol.60, No.13, (July 2000), pp. 3338-334, PMID 10910034

van Engeland, M., Derks, S., Smits, K.M., Meijer, G.A., & Herman, J.G. (2011). Colorectal cancer epigenetics: complex simplicity. *J Clin Oncol*, Vol.29, No.10, (April 2011), pp. 1382-1391, PMID 21220596

van Es, J.H., Jay, P., Gregorieff, A., van Gijn, M.E., Jonkheer, S., Hatzis, P., Thiele, A., van den Born, M., Begthel, H., Brabletz, T., Taketo, M.M., & Clevers, H.(2005). Wnt signalling induces maturation of Paneth cells in intestinal crypts. *Nat Cell Biol*, Vol.7, No.4, (April 2005), pp. 381-386, PMID 15778706

Waldman, S.A., Cagir, B., Rakinic, J., Fry, R.D., Goldstein, S.D., Isenberg, G., Barber, M., Biswas, S., Minimo, C., Palazzo, J., Park, PK., & Weinberg, D. (1998). Use of guanylyl cyclase C for detecting micrometastases in lymph nodes of patients with colon cancer. *Dis Colon Rectum*, Vol.41, No.3, (March 1998), pp. 310-315, PMID 9514425

Waldman, S.A., Hyslop, T., Schulz, S., Barkun, A., Nielsen, K., Haaf, J., Bonaccorso, C., Li, Y., & Weinberg, DS. (2009). Association of GUCY2C expression in lymph nodes with time to recurrence and disease-free survival in pN0 colorectal cancer. *JAMA*, Vol.301, No.7, (Feb 2009), pp. 745-752, PMID 19224751

Wang, H., Fu, W., Im, J.H., Zhou, Z., Santoro, S.A., Iyer, V., DiPersio, C.M., Yu, Q.C., Quaranta,V., Al-Mehdi, A., & Muschel, R.J. (2004). Tumor cell alpha3beta1 integrin and vascular laminin-5 mediate pulmonary arrest and metastasis. *J Cell Biol*, Vol.164, No.6, (March 2004), pp. 935-941, PMID 2172296

Warburg, O. (1956). On the origin of cancer cells. *Science*, Vol.123, No.3191, (Feb 1956), pp. 309-314, PMID 13298683

Weiss, L. (1990). Metastatic inefficiency. *Adv Cancer Res*, Vol.54, pp. (159-211), PMID 1688681

Whitaker, T.L., Witte, D.P., Scott, M.C., & Cohen, M.B. (1997). Uroguanylin and guanylin: distinct but overlapping patterns of messenger RNA expression in mouse intestine. *Gastroenterology*, Vol.113, No.3, (Sep), pp. 1000-1006, PMID 9287995

Whitfield, J.F. (1992). Calcium signals and cancer. *Crit Rev Oncog*, Vol.3, No.1-2, pp. 55-90, PMID 1550862

Whitfield, J.F., Bird, R.P., Chakravarthy, B.R., Isaacs, R.J., & Morley, P. (1995). Calcium-cell cycle regulator, differentiator, killer, chemopreventor, and maybe, tumor promoter. *J Cell Biochem Suppl*, Vol.22, pp. 74-91, PMID 8538213

Witek, M.E., Nielsen, K., Walters, R., Hyslop, T., Palazzo, J., Schulz, S., & Waldman, S.A. (2005). The putative tumor suppressor Cdx2 is overexpressed by human colorectal adenocarcinomas. *Clin Cancer Res*, Vol.11, (Dec 2005), pp. 8549-8556, PMID 16361536

Witz, I.P., & Levy-Nissenbaum, O. (2006). The tumor microenvironment in the post-PAGET era. *Cancer Lett*, Vol.242, No.1, (Oct 2006), pp. 1-10, PMID 16413116

Wolfe, H.R., Mendizabal, M., Lleong, E., Cuthbertson, A., Desai, V., Pullan, S., Fujii, D.K., Morrison, M., Pither, R. and Waldman, S.A. (2002). In vivo imaging of human colon cancer xenografts in immunodeficient mice using a guanylyl cyclase C--specific ligand. *J Nucl Med*, Vol.43, No.3, (March 2002), pp. 392-399, PMID 11884500

World Health Organization (WHO). (February 2011). Cancer, In: *WHO fact sheet N°297*, 29.07.2011, Available from: http://www.who.int/mediacentre/factsheets/fs297/

Yamaguchi, H., & Condeelis, J. (2007). Regulation of the actin cytoskeleton in cancer cell migration and invasion. *Biochim Biophys Acta*, Vol.1773, No.5, (May 2007), pp. 642-652, PMID 16926057

Yaroslavskiy, B.B., Zhang, Y., Kalla, S.E., Garcia Palacios,V., Sharrow, A.C., Li, Y., Zaidi, M., Wu, C., & Blair, HC. (2005). NO-dependent osteoclast motility: reliance on cGMP-dependent protein kinase I and VASP. *J Cell Sci*, Vol.118, No.Pt23, (Dec 2005), pp. 5479-5487, PMID 16291726

Yu, H.G., Tong, S.L., Ding, Y.M., Ding, J., Fang, X.M., Zhang, X.F., Liu, Z.J., Zhou, Y.H., Liu, Q.S., Luo, H.S., & Yu, J.P. (2006). Enhanced expression of cholecystokinin-2 receptor promotes the progression of colon cancer through activation of focal adhesion kinase. *Int J Cancer*, Vol.119, No.12, (Dec 2006), pp. 2724-2732, PMID 16998832

Yu, Q., & Stamenkovic, I. (1999). Localization of matrix metalloproteinase 9 to the cell surface provides a mechanism for CD44-mediated tumor invasion. *Genes Dev*, Vol.13, No.1, (Jan 1999), pp. 35-48, PMID 9887098

Yu, Q., & Stamenkovic I. (2000). Cell surface-localized matrix metalloproteinase-9 proteolytically activates TGF-beta and promotes tumor invasion and angiogenesis. *Genes Dev*, Vol.14, No.2, (Jan), pp. 163-176, PMID 10652271

Zhang, Q., Furukawa, K., Chen, H.H., Sakakibara,T., & Urano T. (2006). Metastatic potential of mouse Lewis lung cancer cells is regulated via ganglioside GM1 by modulating the matrix metalloprotease-9 localization in lipid rafts. *J Biol Chem*, Vol.281, No.26, (Jun 2006), pp. 18145-18155, PMID 16636068

Zucker, S., & Vacirca, J. (2004). Role of matrix metalloproteinases (MMPs) in colorectal cancer. *Cancer Metastasis Rev*, Vol.23, No.1-2, (Jan-Jun 2004), pp. 101-117, PMID 15000152

Zufall, F., Shepherd, GM., & Barnstable, CJ. (1997). Cyclic nucleotide gated channels as regulators of CNS development and plasticity. *Curr Opin Neurobiol*, Vol.7, No.3, (Jun 1997), pp. 404-412, PMID 9232810

Zuzga, D.S., Gibbons, A.V., Li, P., Lubbe, W.J., Chervoneva, I. & Pitari, G.M. (2008). Overexpression of matrix metalloproteinase 9 in tumor epithelial cells correlates with colorectal cancer metastasis. *Clin Transl Sci*, Vol.1, No.2, (Sep 2008), pp. 136-141, PMID 20443834

Zuzga, D.S., Pelta-Heller, J., Li, P., Bombonati, A., Waldman, S.A., & Pitari, GM. (2011). Phosphorylation of vasodilator-stimulated phosphoprotein Ser239 suppresses filopodia and invadopodia in colon cancer. *Int J Cancer*, (Epub ahead of printing), PMID 21702043

Permissions

The contributors of this book come from diverse backgrounds, making this book a truly international effort. This book will bring forth new frontiers with its revolutionizing research information and detailed analysis of the nascent developments around the world.

We would like to thank Dr Rajunor Ettarh, for lending his expertise to make the book truly unique. He has played a crucial role in the development of this book. Without his invaluable contribution this book wouldn't have been possible. He has made vital efforts to compile up to date information on the varied aspects of this subject to make this book a valuable addition to the collection of many professionals and students.

This book was conceptualized with the vision of imparting up-to-date information and advanced data in this field. To ensure the same, a matchless editorial board was set up. Every individual on the board went through rigorous rounds of assessment to prove their worth. After which they invested a large part of their time researching and compiling the most relevant data for our readers. Conferences and sessions were held from time to time between the editorial board and the contributing authors to present the data in the most comprehensible form. The editorial team has worked tirelessly to provide valuable and valid information to help people across the globe.

Every chapter published in this book has been scrutinized by our experts. Their significance has been extensively debated. The topics covered herein carry significant findings which will fuel the growth of the discipline. They may even be implemented as practical applications or may be referred to as a beginning point for another development. Chapters in this book were first published by InTech; hereby published with permission under the Creative Commons Attribution License or equivalent.

The editorial board has been involved in producing this book since its inception. They have spent rigorous hours researching and exploring the diverse topics which have resulted in the successful publishing of this book. They have passed on their knowledge of decades through this book. To expedite this challenging task, the publisher supported the team at every step. A small team of assistant editors was also appointed to further simplify the editing procedure and attain best results for the readers.

Our editorial team has been hand-picked from every corner of the world. Their multi-ethnicity adds dynamic inputs to the discussions which result in innovative outcomes. These outcomes are then further discussed with the researchers and contributors who give their valuable feedback and opinion regarding the same. The feedback is then collaborated with the researches and they are edited in a comprehensive manner to aid the understanding of the subject.

Apart from the editorial board, the designing team has also invested a significant amount of their time in understanding the subject and creating the most relevant covers. They scrutinized every image to scout for the most suitable representation of the subject and create an appropriate cover for the book.

The publishing team has been involved in this book since its early stages. They were actively engaged in every process, be it collecting the data, connecting with the contributors or procuring relevant information. The team has been an ardent support to the editorial, designing and production team. Their endless efforts to recruit the best for this project, has resulted in the accomplishment of this book. They are a veteran in the field of academics and their pool of knowledge is as vast as their experience in printing. Their expertise and guidance has proved useful at every step. Their uncompromising quality standards have made this book an exceptional effort. Their encouragement from time to time has been an inspiration for everyone.

The publisher and the editorial board hope that this book will prove to be a valuable piece of knowledge for researchers, students, practitioners and scholars across the globe.

List of Contributors

Boye Schnack Nielsen
Bioneer A/S, Kogle Allé, Hørsholm, Denmark

Tatyana Vlaykova and Denitsa Vlaykova
Dept. Chemistry and Biochemistry, Medical Faculty, Trakia University, Stara Zagora, Bulgaria

Maya Gulubova
Dept. General and Clinical Pathology, Medical Faculty, Trakia University, Stara Zagora, Bulgaria

Yovcho Yovchev
Dept. General Surgery, Medical Faculty, Trakia University, Stara Zagora, Bulgaria

Dimo Dimov
Dept. Internal Medicine, Medical Faculty, Trakia University, Stara Zagora, Bulgaria

Petjo Chilingirov
Oncology Center, Stara Zagora, Bulgaria

Denitsa Vlaykova
Regional Hospital, Burgass, Bulgaria

Nikolai Zhelev
University of Abertay Dundee, UK

Toshinari Minamoto, Masanori Kotake and Kazuyuki Kawakami
Division of Translational and Clinical Oncology, Cancer Research Institute, Japan

Mitsutoshi Nakada
Department of Neurosurgery, Graduate School of Medical Science, Kanazawa University, Kanazawa, Japan

Masanori Kotake
Department of Surgery, Ishikawa Prefectural Central Hospital, Kanazawa, Japan

Takeo Shimasaki and Yoshiharu Motoo
Department of Medical Oncology, Kanazawa Medical University, Uchinada, Ishikawa, Japan

Teodoro Palomares, Marta Caramés, Ignacio García-Alonso and Ana Alonso-Varona
University of the Basque Country, Spain

Stefania Pizzimenti, Cristina Toaldo, Piergiorgio Pettazzoni, Eric Ciamporcero, Mario Umberto Dianzani and Giuseppina Barrera
University of Turin, Italy

Hiroshi Y. Yamada
University of Oklahoma Health Sciences Center (OUHSC), USA

M.C. Langheinrich, V. Schellerer, K. Oeckl and R.S. Croner
Department of Surgery, University Hospital Erlangen, Germany

M. Stürzl and E. Naschberger
Division of Molecular and Experimental Surgery, Department of Surgery, University Hospital Erlangen, Germany

Barbara Szachowicz-Petelska, Izabela Dobrzyńska and Zbigniew A. Figaszewski
Institute of Chemistry, University in Bialystok, Poland

Stanisław Sulkowski
Department of General Pathomorphology, Medical University of Bialystok, Poland

Zbigniew A. Figaszewski
Faculty of Chemistry, University of Warsaw, Poland

Mehboob Ali and Giovanni M. Pitari
Division of Clinical Pharmacology, Thomas Jefferson University, Philadelphia, PA, USA